# Clinical Social Work

# Clinical Social Work
*A Narrative Approach*

## Gary W. Paquin

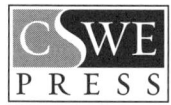

COUNCIL ON SOCIAL WORK EDUCATION
*Alexandria, Virginia*

Copyright © 2009, Council on Social Work Education, Inc.

Published in the United States by the Council on Social Work Education, Inc. All rights reserved. No part of this book may be reproduced or transmitted in any manner whatsoever without the prior written permission of the publisher.

Library of Congress Cataloging-in-Publication Data

Paquin, Gary W.
   Clinical social work : a narrative approach / Gary W. Paquin.
     p. cm.
   Includes bibliographical references and index.
   ISBN 978-0-87293-129-9 (alk. paper)
    1. Psychiatric social work. 2. Narrative therapy. I. Council on Social Work Education. II. Title.

 HV689.P37 2009
 362.2'0425—dc22

ISBN 978-0-87293-129-9


Printed in the United States of America on acid-free paper that meets the American National Standards Institute Z39-48 Standard.

Council on Social Work Education, Inc.
1725 Duke Street, Suite 500
Alexandria, VA 22314-3457
www.cswe.org

# Contents

| | | |
|---|---|---|
| Foreword | | vii |
| Introduction | | ix |
| Chapter 1: | Introduction to Narrative as an Approach to Social Work | 1 |
| Chapter 2: | Power, Narrative, and Social Work | 35 |
| Chapter 3: | Social Work Ethics, Postmodern Ethics, and Where the Twain Shall Meet | 59 |
| Chapter 4: | Problem Definition as a Tool of Power: Externalization | 87 |
| Chapter 5: | The Effect of the Problem on the Person | 123 |
| Chapter 6: | The Effect of the Person on the Problem | 141 |
| Chapter 7: | Richer Alternative Stories Along With Problem Stories | 157 |
| Chapter 8: | Written Work to and for Clients | 173 |
| Chapter 9: | Teams: Audiences, Reflecting, and Ending With Pomp and Appreciation | 203 |
| Chapter 10: | Narrative and Conflict: Advocacy and Mediation | 235 |
| Chapter 11: | Narrative Approaches in the Area of Children and Families | 257 |
| Chapter 12: | Narrative Approaches in Health and Gerontology | 297 |
| Chapter 13: | Narrative Approaches to Mental Health and Substance Abuse | 319 |
| Epilogue | | 339 |
| References | | 341 |
| About the Author | | 365 |
| Index | | 367 |

# Foreword

Social work practitioners, educators, and students have long needed a book that integrates narrative practice into social work, and this is it. Gary Paquin gives us a volume deeply rooted in social work values and traditions and focused on the use of narrative practice where social workers work, backed up by thorough knowledge of social work practice literature as well as mastery of the narrative and postmodern literature.

The volume begins with an excellent introduction to narrative theory. It moves on to spell out the practice in a clear and lively way and, finally, demonstrates the use of narrative work in specific fields of practice and with particular populations.

Throughout the discussion, the author continually turns to practice examples and segments of interviews to illustrate the points being made, and the client is always at the center. The perspective is also truly psychosocial, in that practice is contextualized and the larger issues of oppression, injustice, power, and destructive dominant discourses are always part of the picture. The author makes clear the worker's responsibility to deconstruct those contextual issues and to advocate for the client. This, of course, means that the work is very sensitive to issues of diversity. Michael White and his followers have taken "psychosocial" to a new level of sophistication, and the author builds this into his presentation. The theory is, in some respects, quite complex, but the author makes it truly available to the reader.

It is a wonderful text, complete with many classroom exercises and other learning aids, and those teaching social work practice will find it an enormously rich resource for themselves and their students. Students will like the fact that the book is full of how-tos. Gary Paquin demonstrates how to shape the interview and, most important of all, how to ask good questions, which is at the heart of narrative work.

I welcome this wonderful volume. It makes an important and needed contribution to the profession and to social work education.

Ann Hartman

# Introduction

Does social work need another text on yet another approach to working with people? This introduction discusses some of the challenges facing professional social work, as well as how an approach that listens to suffering as more than evidence of symptoms and that approaches people as separate from their problems is particularly important now.

Social work is under attack and continues to struggle for its identity in a sea of helping professions. It has been accused of losing its mission to the poor and disadvantaged (Specht, 1990), becoming instead enchanted with popular therapies for the "walking wounded" of the middle class. Yet the practice of social work increasingly is governed by a diagnostic system used for financial reimbursement that it has had little input in developing (Kutchins & Kirk, 1997) and by policies that may run counter to the profession's expressed values.

In the early 1900s Abraham Flexner declared social work unable to claim itself a profession because it could not point to a unique and exclusive knowledge base (Flexner, 1915), and the criticism remains fresh despite decades of attempts to rectify the situation. Social work has claimed the person-and-environment relationship as its domain, yet that domain has been encroached upon by marriage and family therapists, community and ecological psychologists, ecology-based counselors, clinical sociologists, and wellness-focused psychiatric nurses.

Areas of special professional expertise, such as child welfare, are being declassified by state agencies, with formal professional social work education and skills declared unnecessary. Some functions performed by social workers are being privatized, typically to the detriment of providers' income and employment benefits. Privatization intensifies the demand on direct-practice social workers to do more with less, to be more efficient.

Health professionals of all kinds struggle to provide efficient and effective services under the pressure of fiscal restraint. This situation has led to the 15-minute physician visit, as-brief-as-possible treatment models, and a continued emphasis on clients being seen as diagnostic categories upon which a treatment plan is executed for the remediation of the problem. This pressure to mimic medical procedures has led to the development of problem-specific, research-based best practice models. Examples of these models are cognitive behavioral strategies, which are derived from psychology, and wraparound services for children and adolescents (Reid, 2002). Sound business principles—maximum productivity, hierarchical control of professionals with accountability resting on the providers, minimum waste of resources, and reduced government support with a focus on the market—are seen as the best way to confront today's health care and social service crises.

In this practice environment, narrative treatment represents a new and increasingly popular approach to helping people. It focuses on people over problems. It, like the solution-focused approach (Walter & Peller, 1992), was developed primarily by social workers. By exploring the power of self-narratives, stories, and discourses (societal stories), people can be helped to tap into their skills and understandings to find ways to cope with the often monumental problems in their lives. What results is a strengths-based form of social work that honors clients' views of both their problems and their lives. This approach is a far cry from research-derived models that apply techniques to the "real" problem, as defined by the social worker.

Letting people tell their stories and helping them to expand and enrich those stories can result in powerful changes in people's lives. Arthur Kleinman (1988), author of *The Illness Narratives*, goes into graphic detail about his experience with a young patient while he was a medical student that led to his understanding of the importance of narratives in healing:

> The first patient was a pathetic seven-year-old who had been badly burned over most of her body. She had to undergo a daily ordeal of a whirlpool bath during which the burnt flesh was tweezered away from her raw open wounds. This experience was horribly painful to her. She screamed and moaned and begged the medical team, whose efforts she stubbornly fought off, not to hurt her anymore. My job as a neophyte clinical student was to hold her uninjured hand, as much to reassure and calm her as to enable the surgical resident to quickly pull away the dead, infected tissue in the pool of swirling water, which rapidly turned pinkish, then bloody red. Clumsily, with a beginner's uncertainty of how to proceed, I tried to distract this little patient from her traumatic daily confrontation with terrible pain. I tried talking to her about her home, her family, her school—almost anything that might draw her vigilant attention away from her suffering. I could barely tolerate the daily horror: her screams, the dead tissue floating

in the blood-stained water, the peeling flesh, the oozing wounds, the battles over cleaning and bandaging. Then one day, I made contact. At wit's end, angered at my own ignorance and impotence, uncertain what to do besides clutching the small hand, and in despair over her unrelenting anguish, I found myself asking her to tell me how she tolerated it, what the feeling was like of being so badly burned and having to experience the awful surgical ritual, day after day after day. She stopped, quite surprised, and looked at me from a face so disfigured it was difficult to read her expression; then, in terms direct and simple, she told me. While she spoke, she grasped my hand harder and neither screamed nor fought off the surgeon or the nurse. Each day from then on, her trust established, she tried to give me a feeling of what she was experiencing. By the time my training took me off this rehabilitation unit, the little burn patient seemed noticeably better able to tolerate debridement. But whatever effect I had on her, her effect on me was far greater. (pp. xi–xii)

Sharing the story of her suffering and her efforts to get through the pain helped the little girl to endure the ordeal. What this passage does not say is that many professionals do not ask their clients to share what they are experiencing because they are afraid of what they will hear and they do not know if they will have the courage to truly listen. Listening to stories is no small task, and the effects can be mutual on both the storyteller and the listener.

This book begins with an overview of the strengths-based approach to working with people. I describe the unique contributions of postmodern theory (that there are many truths, not just one truth about situations). In particular, I discuss social constructionism (meanings and truths are constructed through language in social interaction), which provides the philosophical foundation for using the narrative metaphor to guide clinical social work practice. I then present a coherent, teachable model of narrative social work.

Clients are seen as the experts on their problems. But when the client is in the role of expert, what is the role of the worker and how is it affected by context-specific material on both values and diversity? I describe how a narrative approach profoundly shifts the worker role from expert to facilitator and collaborator. I also show how narrative work emphasizes the ways oppression operates in the definition and maintenance of problems. I discuss how information is gathered through skillfully listening to and questioning the cultural, class, and racial meanings of actions. Values are examined at both micro and macro levels.

A narrative approach produces a different set of questions to fundamental assumptions. For instance, how does the social worker's thinking and behavior make his or her values known to clients? How do social workers recognize and minimize the power disparity between themselves and their clients, and why would they want to? How do larger political forces make problems more or less amenable to change? Can organizing with others who struggle against such problems assist in placing the problem in context?

Narrative theory has opened up new definitions of self and new methods for helping people. I present some of these methods here to show the array of options for working with people that this approach offers. In addition, I discuss techniques for using this approach with children, adolescents, adults, and families, as well as in settings where health, mental health, substance abuse, and child- or family-centered services are offered.

Although providing a model, I am aware that this is a model only in the broadest sense. Given the demands on, and initial anxiety of, social work students to get "techniques," it should be noted that these techniques will not be useful without accepting some of the philosophy underlying the narrative model. Postmodernism, and narrative in particular, questions many firmly held assumptions. Without an appreciation of the forces that help shape how we think about problems, the idea that a different self-narrative can transform people probably seems far-fetched.

To truly embrace a narrative approach, we need to acknowledge that our experience of reality is fluid and based on language, that social messages are important, and that we have no one true self that we must seek out and understand before we can change. Without these understandings, the relationship that develops between worker and client will be a false one, with the social work student still maintaining the "expert on the problem" mentality. As with any form of social work practice, if the work is inauthentic, the relationship is less likely to be helpful and the intervention more likely doomed to failure. As O'Hanlon (1994) notes,

> If externalization is approached purely as a technique, it will probably not produce profound effects. If you don't believe to the bottom of your soul, that people are not their problems and that their difficulties are social and personal constructions, then you won't be seeing these transformations. When Epston or White [developers of this approach] are in action, you can tell that they are absolutely convinced that people are not their problems. Their voices, their postures, their whole beings radiate possibility and hope. (p. 28)

*Clinical Social Work* presents a basic model of narrative therapy, but as McKenzie and Monk (1997) note, models have their dangers. It becomes too easy for beginners to follow the model's map instead of following the client, and, as a result, get themselves back into the "expert position," pulling the client through the model. Using the model in that way can lead to a lack of emotional connection in the relationship and a minimization of feelings. The model is portrayed for teaching purposes because it provides a coherent way to make sense of the narrative approach; however, it is important to remember that this model is but one story among many.

Students often find it difficult to grasp postmodern philosophy, which is the theoretical basis for the narrative approach. I attempt to reduce the confusion arising from terms such as *discourse, knowledges, power, privileges, constituting reality, landscapes of the mind*, and *performances of meaning*. I include a great many examples of questions, not because the particular questions are transformative in themselves, but because they nicely demonstrate the narrative viewpoint.

In a narrative approach, the questions asked during a treatment session are likely to be different from those used in other approaches. Many, if not most, of the questions presented in this book are not my own, but those of master therapists. Madigan (2003) mentioned at a workshop that when he started out learning the narrative approach, visiting its developers in Australia and New Zealand, he developed a "question notebook." He found this very helpful in seeing how the approach was actually played out in therapy. I offer many questions so that you, too, can begin a question notebook.

For ease of reading, I use the word *client* to describe those who consult us, either on their own or through coercion. However, the term implies that such people are in need of being taken care of by an expert who will work to solve their problems, and, as such, goes against an important narrative assumption: that the story of the person seeking consultation is more important than the listener's version of it (Cowger, 1998). Alternative terms or phrases would be awkward, so *client* is used throughout, although the reader is cautioned to remember that the person on one side of the conversation is little different from the person on the other side.

I also use the word *treatment* in keeping with social work's traditional terms. Narrative therapists may object to the use of this word because treatment implies that the client has a problem and that the social worker negotiates with the client for a treatment of that problem. Although a narrative approach takes a somewhat different stance, I have kept the word *treatment* because most social workers will be working in modernist agencies and must adapt to those agencies' paperwork requirements. Objecting to the word *treatment* is a losing battle in most agency settings given the conditions for receiving financial reimbursement. If all third-party payers require paperwork that follows a medical model, then protesting that model will be fruitless without a major change in the health care system.

What this text does not have are separate sections on assessment, diagnosis and medication, and treatment planning. A narrative perspective does not emphasize these steps, though undoubtedly agencies will require paperwork that identifies these skills. Assessment in narrative practice generally involves naming and mapping the impact of the problem, as well as articulating the beginnings of an alternative story that could lead to a preferred outcome.

Diagnosis is important as the basis for using tools such as medication. A narrative approach sees a biological explanation of behavior as one story among the many other stories available. It recognizes the value of medication as a tool to help people get control over aspects of the problem that have taken control away from them. The point is not to take away the option of medication or deny its usefulness, but to emphasize that medication is of use only when the client takes it regularly and also receives assistance with developing his or her own strategies for standing up to the problem when breakthrough symptoms occur.

A narrative approach attempts to contextualize problems in their sociocultural milieus. Treatment planning, which assumes that the social worker and client will each carry out certain tasks to facilitate the client's reaching an agreed-upon goal, is not as important in a situation in which the client is seen as an expert on his or her problems. There are times, however, when the worker can intervene in systems to better equalize the playing field, and this is especially important when the client has very little power and the other party in a conflict has a great deal. Chapter 10, which discusses narrative mediation and advocacy, is included for this purpose.

An approach that focuses on the communication of subjective experience requires experience to learn it. Each chapter of this volume has exercises that can be performed in class. Discussion of the experience of the exercises will demonstrate that you can assume this different posture and can use more of who you are as a person in your work with clients. You will also learn that clients have much to teach us.

CHAPTER 1

# Introduction to Narrative as an Approach to Social Work

Narrative treatment is part of a new movement that is having an impact on direct social work practice by challenging its traditional frameworks and assumptions (Biever & Franklin, 1998; Kelley, 1995; Laird, 1995; Pozatek, 1994; Reid, 2002). It represents a model of working with people that is transportable to many different populations and problems. Postmodern philosophy, specifically social constructionism (Foucault, 1988), narrative psychology (Gergen & McNamee, 2000), and anthropology (Myerhoff, 1982, 1986), make up its theoretical foundation. Consistent with this theoretical orientation, narrative treatment emphasizes the constitutive power of *stories, narratives,* and *discourses* (White & Epston, 1990, chap. 1). Its de-emphasis of social worker expertise and its elevation of client knowledge and skills fit well with multicultural and feminist concerns about imperialistic and patriarchal approaches to social work treatment (Kelley, 1995, 2002). These characteristics also make it compatible with a strengths-based approach to social work, although its definition of strengths (client knowledge, understandings, and skills) is more fluid than is typically considered in social work.

## Clinical Social Work

This is a book about clinical social work, a narrowing of the broader profession of social work. Clinical social work focuses on providing therapeutic assistance to individuals, families, and groups through the application of social work practice knowledge and skills. It is often associated with working in the area of mental health. In its 1984 statement, the National Association of Social Workers (NASW) defined the goals of clinical social work as the "enhancement and maintenance of psychosocial functioning" based on social work ethics and recognized in its definition the necessity of "client-centered advocacy" (as cited in Dorfman, 1996, p. 2). Social work has attempted to focus on the person-environment interaction, but most other helping professions have seen this as an area of interest and have claimed expertise here also.

Most states in the United States have special licenses for clinical social work, which is considered an advanced form of social work practice. Yet the fact that each state has its own definition adds to the confusion over what clinical social work is. The statute describing the privileges of receiving the advanced license in Ohio, for example, mentions the practice of something called sociotherapy.

States that license clinical social workers typically require a passing score on the Association of Social Work Boards' written examination in addition to specified hours of supervision and practice experience. The clinical examination purports to test for the minimum knowledge needed to be a clinical social worker and is based on the results of extensive surveys of clinical social workers to find out what they do and need to know to do it. The clinical examination differs from the advanced generalist examination in a number of areas. The clinical examination emphasizes human development theories; clinical practice theories; use of the American Psychiatric Association's (2000) *Diagnostic and Statistical Manual of Mental Disorders*, known by the acronym DSM; and clinical practice techniques and issues. Compared to the advanced generalist test, the clinical examination has fewer questions on research and service delivery (Association of Social Work Boards, 2006).

As this discussion suggests, a practice theory for clinical social work must encompass several key points: First, it must be based on social work values and ethics. Second, it must examine people's ability to function in their environment and the environment's ability to offer them a fair opportunity for success. Third, it must address not only what happens between the client and the worker but also what happens between the client and the environment, using advocacy when necessary. A strengths-based approach to social work meets these criteria.

## Strengths-Based Social Work

Alongside social work frameworks such as problem solving (Compton, Galaway, & Cournoyer, 2005; Perlman, 1957), systems (Pincus & Minahan, 1973), and the life model (Germain & Gitterman, 1996), is the strengths model (Rapp, 1998; Saleebey, 2002a, 2002b), which has steadily gained adherents. Strengths-based social work has been provided to clients with severe and persistent mental illness (Rapp, 1998), individuals with substance abuse problems (van Wormer & Davis, 2003), the elderly (Fast & Chapin, 2002), youth (Benard, 2002), and those involved in the child welfare system (Dunst, Trivette, & Deal, 1994). <u>Strengths-based social work means recognizing and using the resources available to clients so they can accomplish their goals.</u>

Assuming a strengths-based approach is challenging in the face of funding requirements, recording requirements, and a theory/practice focus on deficits and problems. Psychopathology, rather than resilience, is taught in most clinical social work courses. Much of social work education is devoted to training students to find the causes of and solutions to clients' problems. Strengths are rarely emphasized.

Strengths themselves are vague because they are context specific. For example, the ability to physically defend one's self may be an important "strength" in the military but less so in a seminary or convent. However, strengths usually are seen as including capacities, resources, and assets (Saleebey, 2002b). Madsen (2007) quotes an unnamed workshop participant who succinctly summed up the matter: "Competence is quiet, it tends to be overlooked in the noise and clatter of problems" (p. 32).

## The Benefits of a Strengths-Based Approach

A strengths-based approach, which assumes the client, not the worker, has the ability to handle the client's problem, offers social workers a number of benefits. Saleebey (2002a) identifies several limitations of a problem-based approach. First, although there may be some value in naming problems as problems, problems once named can become owned by the person struggling against them. The person then comes to be defined as the problem. Moreover, the label can become the person, and the individual is then treated as that label. subjugation

For example, years ago when I was an attendant in a hospital while working my way through school, I was assigned to sit with a man who had gotten drunk, passed out in a snowbank, and gotten badly frostbitten feet as a result. He was in a good deal of discomfort due to the condition of his feet as well as to being on a cooling bed to lower the fever from his infection. The nurses were less than sympathetic to his plight, referring to him as a "drunk." The next week when I returned, one of his feet had been removed and he was in great pain. I helped when they removed his dressing, exposing what looked like a foot sawn neatly in half. The man thought he still might be able to work at his blue-collar job even with his amputation, and he told me that what was keeping him going was the knowledge that they were somehow going to save his other blackened foot. As I was getting ready to leave my shift the next morning, the medical resident came in and told the man that he was not to eat any breakfast because they were going to "take the other foot off" that day. He then left without another word. The man was in shock, and I spent some time trying to calm him. I doubt that he would have been treated so uncaringly, with so little attention to his trauma, if he had not been seen as a drunk. <u>From the label came a view of who this man was, and his treatment was less sensitive as a result.</u>

Second, deficit labels bring with them a sense of pessimism. Many labels lead people to believe that they are restricted to rather narrow lives. Imagine if you were led to believe that your mind was defective to the point where you thought of yourself as disabled. Whereas some may see the possibility of receiving Supplemental Security Income (SSI) as a haven, think also about what restrictions being classified as disabled can put on a person's dreams and aspirations. If you were in such a person's shoes, what might being disabled mean to you and to those around you? Might they expect less of you as a person? If so, how might this affect how you would see yourself? Or, if you have been labeled this way already, what have you had to confront to get to where you are that those who are "able" have not had to cope with? How did the ability/disability label affect your struggle? For many, such labels can become the rationale for hopelessness and constrained actions.

Third, a natural extension of a problem-focused approach is the production of case records in which certain data are strung together to reach an assessment of a person. These often serve to create distance between the client and the worker. The case notes found in these records typically treat the client in the third person, not as an actual party in the interaction that has occurred. The writing style is supposed to be factual, yet of course it is the personal view of the worker. Sometimes workers refer to themselves, but when they do it also is often in the third person, as "this worker" or "the worker." At a community meeting with a state task force on mental health, a consumer discussed the way it was assumed that consumers were trying to cheat and lie to their workers. This consumer testified about how angry she became when young workers with clean clothes and a car who only knew her from her case file would blithely say, without any sense of the ordeal involved, that she needed to get herself to a Laundromat. As she stated, "Taking a bus with laundry and detergent to a Laundromat when you don't feel particularly well, as most of us don't, is really hard." And when getting to the clinic takes two bus rides, missed appointments should be expected. It is perhaps a wonder that clients can get there at all.

Fourth, problem-based assessments encourage individual rather than ecological understanding. It is difficult when focused on the problem to see the context in which the problem is occurring and is being defined. This focus on the individual is particularly apparent when psychiatric diagnoses are required. Configurations of troubles make up symptoms, which, in turn, make up disorders, and medication is typically prescribed for these disorders despite the environmental supports for the symptoms. It is not uncommon for assessment to miss such factors as the obligations clients have to others, the impact of grinding poverty on their worldview, and the inability they have to muster resources through legitimate means. The strengths-based approach was developed to both respond to these issues and bring social work back to its roots, away from a medicoscientific paradigm and toward a more humanistic one (Cohen, 1999).

## Specifics of a Strengths-Based Approach to Social Work

The strengths-based approach is seen less as a model than as a perspective—a focus on client strengths. Saleebey (2002a) lays out several principles of this perspective, which can be summarized as follows: First, every individual, family, and neighborhood has strengths and resources. Second, difficulties bring wisdom and knowledge as well as injury and pain. Third, people's hopes and dreams should always be taken seriously, and social workers should collaborate with clients as the clients strive to reach their goals. Finally, understanding the context of behavior is central to recognizing strengths, and caring, over technique, remains an important component in working with people.

This form of helping is more akin to rehabilitation. Where treatment strives to alleviate symptoms, rehabilitation strives to restore functioning (Cohen, 1999). For example, medication and psychosocial interventions may be the appropriate methods for handling problems clients have with "voices." However, medication often does not entirely clear up the voices but simply reduces their intensity and volume. Sometimes, voices break through the medication when the person is under considerable stress. To function, people who hear voices must be able to get along in spite of them. They need to develop their own strategies for standing up to the voices so that the voices do not force them to lose what they want in life.

Benard (2002) has perhaps provided the closest thing to a strengths-based model by laying out the following steps:

> Listen to their story
>
> Acknowledge the pain

> Look for strengths
>
> Ask questions about survival, support, positive times, interests, dreams, goals, and pride
>
> Point out strengths
>
> Link strengths to client's goals and dreams
>
> Link client to resources to achieve goals and dreams
>
> Find opportunities for client to be teacher/paraprofessional (p. 217)

This last point about clients sharing what they have learned with others is discussed in some detail in chapter 9.

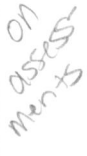

A strengths perspective focuses as much, if not more, on the abilities the person brings to the clinical session as it does on his or her deficiencies. Given the emphasis on problems that most assessment frameworks have, the shift to strengths is a major change (Cowger & Snively, 2002; Kristhardt, 2002). Despite the difference between problems and strengths, it is not uncommon to hear workers who come from a problem-based perspective describing their work as strengths-based because they incorporate client strengths in some of their interventions.

Strengths-based social workers must start with the problems presented and give problems their due recognition. Clients do not come to social workers to have their strengths confirmed; they come, or are sent, because of their problems, and shifting too fast would lead clients to feel they are not being heard.

Historically, problem-focused workers have been involved in capacity building (McMillen, Morris, & Sherraden, 2004). However, considerable differences become evident when the traditional problem-solving model, particularly when diagnosis is included in it, is placed alongside Benard's (2002) model. Engagement and assessment involve listening to the client's story and acknowledging the pain. Contracting involves developing client goals and dreams; intervention involves looking for, probing for, and pointing out strengths, and linking them to the client's goals. Ending and evaluation are not discussed extensively by Benard, except that the knowledge and skills the client has found might be extended to assisting others. The client role is different in this model, because it is mainly the client's expert knowledge of his or her life that is seen as most relevant, rather than the expert knowledge of the worker. It is also the worker's determined focus on client strengths that distinguishes this model from problem-based approaches.

The strengths perspective also considers the power of narrative as an important source of strength for individuals and communities (Saleebey, 1994).

Through the practice of social work, a transformation of meaning occurs. The meanings given to client behavior by the worker through the worker's theories meet the client's experience as described in the client's stories, and both unfold within the context of the myths and themes inherent in the culture (Saleebey). Freudian theory, though it has lost popularity in the mental health professions, continues to have a strong influence on popular culture. It is not uncommon for people to enter treatment expecting their childhood experiences to be the primary area of interest. It is in the cultural stories that theories are developed and the important themes of people's lives are shaped. As a result, the idea of development and origins often leads clients to emphasize stories related to their early life as being the foundation of who they really are. But as this example illustrates, both theory and stories are influenced by culture. There are stories in the culture that indicate who we should be, and what we, social workers, should do.

Narratives can lead to contradictory expectations. In class, social work students have often identified being compassionate and competent as the ideal for their careers. Stories of what these two words mean can occupy many hours, particularly when they are seen as contradictory. Saleebey (1994, p. 355) provides an example of a student returning an "I love you" to a young man dying of AIDS, an entirely compassionate and authentic expression of feeling, but one that some might see as indicating poor boundaries and an inappropriate blurring of the social work role.

Narratives of who a person is and what is expected of him or her can often be contradictory, and this itself can leave a person confused if he or she expects one story to fit all. Postmodern theories of "who we are" would lead us to expect this, particularly in times of cultural change, because their definitions of "self" tend to be flexible. Given that this is such a novel approach, a theoretical and philosophical foundation for the narrative perspective is explored.

## Theory Behind Narrative Work: Postmodernism

Postmodernism emerged in many fields as a philosophical reaction to the empiricist, positivist view that all reality can be known. Much of modern truth is described as having been developed through observation using the scientific method to examine the "essential" parts of a phenomenon. Postmodern thought sees reality as constituted by language, through which we construct our experiences of the world in interaction with others (Freedman & Combs, 1996). Postmodernists are aware that language is only a symbol or representation of experience, not the experience itself, and that the meaning given to the experience through language determines the reality experienced by the person. Stories become reality.

For example, in describing the conservative revolution in the United States during the Reagan administration, Thomas "Tip" O'Neill (1987), the former Democratic leader of the House of Representatives, writes that "the most depressing thing of all was the hatred of the poor that developed all across America. . . . People don't develop new attitudes out of thin air. These grasping and uncaring views had to come from somewhere, and I blame the president for allowing this kind of selfishness to become respectable" (pp. 346–347). He describes how the Reagan White House would tell the story of a "black welfare woman in Chicago who lives lavishly and supposedly collects something like a hundred and three welfare checks under different names" (p. 347). O'Neill reports that the head of the Department of Health, Education, and Welfare (now the Department of Health and Human Services) noted in three separate letters that the story could not be confirmed, but this did not stop the story from being continually cited.

The myth became the rallying point for those opposed to welfare; it became real by repetition. Even welfare recipients, when interviewed, distinguished themselves from those "other" recipients. The statistics showing that most families on Aid to Families with Dependent Children were White, had about the same number of children, on average, as the rest of the population, and received benefits for limited time periods were irrelevant (Abramovitz, 1996). The war on poverty had turned into a war on the poor. The poor were the problem, not poverty, and welfare was the cause. The power of an emotional narrative to define reality for the majority must never be dismissed.

Worldviews can be short stories or bigger cultural stories. Gonzalez (1998) summarizes the ideas of social psychologist Kenneth Gergen, who said there have been three different Western worldviews during the past few centuries: premodern, modernist, and postmodern. Premodern thought placed a strong emphasis on faith and loyalty. It focused on people's character, soul, and breeding. Meaning resided in the person, internal feelings were of central value, and individual effort defined success. Premodern thought has been characterized as displaying romanticism because it so emphasized the function of the soul and the deep interior of the individual.

Modernist thought, which sees outside reality as completely knowable, follows a pattern that started with the Enlightenment and accelerated with the Industrial Revolution. It focuses on progress through objectivity and rationality. It emphasizes knowledge acquired through systematic observation and reasoning based on positivism (all useful knowledge comes through science) and empiricism (all useful knowledge comes through observation and experiment). This view is buttressed by technology.

According to modernist thinking, external reality is studied to produce objective knowledge that will apply universally. Objective truth can be made visible, and reality can be measured. People can be categorized and their traits precisely assessed. Life and people are treated within a mechanistic framework, in that people are seen as having qualities that can be measured with skill and accuracy. With repeated observations and (sometimes) study, the knowledge obtained is portrayed as truth, giving it certainty. Those who hold the truth (researchers and professionals) are given expert status, and this knowledge confers on those who possess it certain power over those who do not (Parton & O'Byrne, 2000). The expert can find out (and define) who a person really is.

Modernist thought also leads to partializing problems to solve them. A nice illustration of this is offered by Pierre Bourdieu, an anthropologist, who described a West African woman as saying, "In the old days . . . folk didn't know what illness was. They went to bed and they died. It's only nowadays that we've learned words like liver, lung, stomach, and I don't know what!" (as cited in Frank, 1995, pp. 4–5).

The West African woman's comments about modernist talk—of organs, symptoms, and syndromes—demonstrate where the patient vanishes and the language of the medical profession becomes dominant. Bennett and colleagues' (2005) discussion of a science advisory from the American Heart Association is a case in point:

> The primary property of this class of drugs is the inhibition of cyclooxygenase (COX). COX enzymes have 2 major classes. COX-1 is broadly considered to be expressed constitutively (constantly) in most tissues, whereas COX-2 is induced in inflammation. Both COX-1 and -2 enzymes use arachidonic acid to generate the same product, prostaglandin H2 (PGH2). A number of enzymes further modify this product to generate bioactive lipids (prostanoids), including prostacyclin, thromboxane A2, and prostaglandins D2, E2, and F2, which influence immune, cardiovascular, GI, renovascular, pulmonary, central nervous system, and reproductive function. The COX-2 inhibitors vary in their selectivity for the COX-2 versus the COX-1 enzyme (for medications currently or formerly on the market in the US, rofecoxib > valdecoxib > parecoxib > celecoxib). Other COX-2 inhibitors are under development and may be introduced onto the US market in the

future. The differences in the biological effects of COX inhibitors are a consequence of the degree of selectivity for COX-2 versus COX-1 and tissue-specific variations in the distribution of COX and related enzymes that convert prostaglandin H2 into specific prostanoids. For example, several prostanoids, including prostaglandin E2 and prostacyclin, are both hyperalgesic (i.e., elicit an increased sense of pain) and gastro-protective. Thus, nonselective COX inhibition with agents such as aspirin, ibuprofen, indomethacin, and naproxen, which inhibit both COX-1 and COX-2 enzymes, provides effective pain relief for inflammatory conditions but carries with it a risk for erosive gastritis and GI bleeding. Selective COX-2 inhibitors (valdecoxib, rofecoxib, celecoxib, and others yet in development) were developed to minimize GI toxicity because of the relative paucity of COX-2 expression in the GI tract and the relative abundance of COX-2 expression in inflamed and painful tissues. (pp. 1713–1714)

It is easy to skim this piece and notice that only processes and symptoms are discussed, not the people who are the subject of the warning, and feel that whereas in the old days we had only aspirin, we now have unpronounceable enzymes and who knows what else. The modernist approach accepts completely this type of knowledge as truth and applauds it as a mark of progress. Yet progress can also heighten anxiety.

From a modernist point of view, the case record is the official story and, therefore, contains the truth of the illness or trouble (Frank, 1995). But there also are other truths.

The questioning of these grand narratives of progress and the recognition of the conditionality of most truth have led to the postmodern turn in thinking seen in many fields. Postmodernism takes note of, and reflects, the transformations occurring because of the increased pace of change; growing attention to difference and plurality, not just similarity; greater awareness of relativities; and heightened recognition of the socially constructed nature of reality (Parton & O'Byrne, 2000). Truth is seen as more local, more focused on the specific case at hand than on cases in general. A singular conception of knowledge is supplanted by *knowledges*, the multiplicity of simultaneously existing truths (White & Epston, 1990, p. 20).

The views of White, middle-class, able-bodied males have been embedded in modernist truths about people and society, though these truths are presented as universal and neutral. Movements of those who are oppressed and disenfranchised, such as gay men and lesbians, older adults, and the poor, have attempted to look at the implications of knowledge being socially constructed and understand how their stories have been silenced. Members of the dominant culture may see these considerations as being "politically correct," a code term for factitious and trivial. However, when women, minorities, or others are not identified as contributing to the common cause, even though they have been purposefully excluded from the "great narrative," they are diminished and their stories will not live on when those of others of equal accomplishment do. This diminishment leads to distinctions of difference and to "less than" comparisons between the dominant and nondominant groups.

The postmodernist perspective gives voice to the experience of the sufferer and those who suffer with the one who is suffering. Sufferers recognize that more is involved in their trouble than what official records tell. The postmodern turn occurs when people reclaim the capacity to tell their story in their own voice. Frank (1995) characterizes illness as an experience that incorporates one's body, self, and expected destination in life. A postmodernist perspective gives primary attention to the person's experience of the illness or trouble, not simply to the compilation of symptoms, though both are important stories.

Postmodern ideas are making considerable contributions to social work knowledge (Biever & Franklin, 1998). Postmodernism sees the world through many different lenses and finds that there is not one central conception of reality. People's subjective experience of reality is what counts. Their ability to conceptualize many different beliefs about human functioning—from biological and genetic to behavioral and cognitive—supports this viewpoint. Clearly, these different worldviews sit side by side.

Postmodernism is a product of our postindustrial service/information economy. People are saturated with contact with new ideas through globalization as well as advancements in transportation and media technology (Gergen, 1999). Far greater flexibility of self is required to survive in this environment. This is a difficult transition given our desire for a consistent self from which we can feel centered. In the field of psychology and in the helping professions, postmodernism has developed into two distinct approaches: constructivism and social constructionism. These approaches are discussed next.

## Constructivism

Constructivism is a view that places the subjective experience of the world above the objective experience of it. It forms the basis for cognitive therapy by indicating that thinking can change how people see the world, which, in turn, can change their emotions and behaviors. The emphasis is on the cognitive structure more so than on the societal factors that produce that structure. According to Ecker and Hulley (2000), constructivism is based on a number of principles. Some that are valuable to consider are as follows:

- Internal representations of the world are all we have of our reality and these representations are actively developed by the individual, not simply copies of the "objective" world.
- How a person perceives, anticipates, and responds to "reality" is determined by his or her mental constructs.
- Problems and symptoms seen in treatment are products of these internal constructs.
- These constructs can be dissolved or discarded, but people are not usually conscious of these processes.
- The mind is self-organizing in that there is a structural ordering, with deeper processes influencing the more surface ones.

Constructivism, therefore, tends to focus on cognitive structures such as organizing principles and schemas about the self (Franklin, 1998).

This point of view does have biological credibility given the research of Lettvin, Maturana, McCulloch, and Pitts (1959), who found in their study of frogs that the world frogs perceive is very different from the world people perceive. In contrast to human beings' double visual system, frogs possess a single visual system, and their eyes and brains pick up only four functions. However, those four functions are vital to frogs' survival, allowing them to detect the movement of insects on which they feed. Yet if what we experience of the world is vastly different from what other species experience, what makes our reality superior to those of other species? We experience only a small slice of reality, and our cognitive structures further constrain the amount of information we receive and process.

Constructivist therapists take their lead from George Kelly (1955), a psychologist who developed personal construct theory and therapy in the 1950s. Constructivist approaches tend to focus on the characteristics of the narrative itself under the assumption that a well-organized self-narrative enables people to have a more cohesive sense of self and allows them to exercise their coping skills more usefully. Corrections to these structures are possible (see Fisher, 1991; Goncalves, 1995; Guidano, 1991; Mahoney, 2003; Markus & Nurius, 1986). One branch of family therapy, which was developed by the Mental Research Institute and is sometimes termed the *communications approach*, has used these insights (Hoffman, 1981; Watzlawick, 1976).

## Social Constructionism

Social constructionism is a postmodern viewpoint that sees the experience of reality as determined by the cultural instructions and meanings people acquire in the world. Social constructionism is interested in "the processes by which human communities generate meaning" (Gergen & McNamee, 2000, p. 334) as well as how these meanings, including the values, traditions, and interests embedded in them, come to be expressed through culture, custom, and language. Thus, for example, "when one credits people with the capacity for 'independent thought,' one acts to sustain a tradition of democracy; when one attributes to them a spiritual dimension, one favors the sustenance of religion" (p. 334). Culture provides the glasses we use to see the world.

Social constructionism, from which narrative treatment ideas arise, de-emphasizes the labeling of constructs in individuals (e.g., character, personality, disorder) and looks instead at their social origins. Culture can constrain people's reality through definitions and scripted stories. Language is important in this approach, and "because the very terms in which we construe ourselves are cultural artifacts, our selves are deeply penetrated by the vocabularies of our place and time, expressing dominant modes of discourse as much as any unique personality" (Neimeyer, 2000, p. 209). Some social constructionists would say that the entire personality is made up of the unique characteristics of time, place, and culture. Not surprisingly, those who hold a social constructionist orientation focus on language, narratives, and sociocultural/historical processes (Franklin, 1998).

The approach to working within a narrative metaphor that I describe in this book is associated with the work of social workers Michael White and David Epston (1990) and psychologists Jerome Bruner (1986) and Kenneth Gergen (1999). Although there are a number of postmodern-based approaches to assisting people in coping with their problems (e.g., cognitive constructivist, solution-focused, and dialogic or conversational), this text focuses on the narrative approach.

A narrative approach to working with people, which depends on a social constructionist view of the world, sees most problems that people confront as being defined by society. The socially constructed meanings of problems can reduce the number of possible options available to a person. However, what can be socially constructed can be socially deconstructed, which can offer new, more useful definitions of problems. These new definitions, in turn, can provide new and more helpful strategies for coping.

Constructs such as race, gender, social class, sexual orientation, age, and different abilities are socially constructed. Examining these constructs and the impacts they have on individuals from a narrative perspective can provide people with the flexibility to make changes in their behavior. The postmodern clinician must always be alert to dominant discourses, to whose interests they serve and whose they oppress, and to how they influence what clients bring in as their understanding of their situations (Laird, 1995). Problems must be seen in their cultural context to separate them from the person of the client.

## A Narrative Approach to Clinical Social Work

A narrative approach to working with those who consult us corresponds well with the demands of clinical social work. The social constructionist view it is based upon is compatible with person-in-environment and ecosystem perspectives, because the person is never seen either as a victim of the environment or as a fully independent actor (Witkin, 1991), although power differentials are often overlooked in these latter two perspectives. According to Madigan and Epston (1995), a narrative approach

1. Privileges the person's lived experience.
2. Encourages a perception that change is always possible and occurring through linking lived experience across the temporal dimension.
3. Encourages multiple perspectives and acts to deconstruct claims of "expert knowledge."
4. Encourages the carnival of possible futures through the reconstruction and rerembering of alternative stories.
5. Invites a reflexive posture and demands that therapists be accountable for their therapeutic stance.
6. Acknowledges that stories are coproduced and endeavors to make the clients the privileged authors of their own experiences.
7. Believes that persons are multistoried. (p. 261)

In traditional treatment, the information given to the worker by the client is generally fit into the theory the worker espouses. Part of what treatment does is teach people the "truth" about their feelings, actions, and thoughts. A problem behavior might be in response to a biological malfunction, a traumatic event in the past, a reinforcing consequence, anxiety in a family system, or deprivation in the social environment, to name a few rationales. The behavior is seen as the result of a cause that is not the behavior itself. Therefore, traditional therapeutic interviewing will involve asking questions and gathering data to pinpoint where the cause might lie.

A narrative approach gives preference to the client's story rather than to the worker's theory. Listening to the story as a story is different from listening to the story as the key to the client's suffering. Some clients are lost in their pain, and through communicating a concern for their wounds, which are little different from our own, people can come to feel less lost in their stories (Frank, 1995). This type of interviewing is called *curious questioning* (McKenzie & Monk, 1997, pp. 87–89), because the worker's questions are generated by his or her genuine interest in the client's story.

A narrative approach sees change as always occurring. Single stories cannot include the entirety of a person's life, but problem stories can overshadow the rest. A person struggling with depression who gets up in the morning and takes a shower (because he or she is supposed to be doing that anyway) does not appreciate what a stand against depression such behavior is. Problems are rarely 100% intensity 100% of the time. Instances when people have taken stands against a problem by doing behaviors or thinking thoughts they might not be expected to if the problem had a complete hold on them may be noted as changes but often go without full recognition.

A narrative approach encourages multiple perspectives and actions to deconstruct claims of expert knowledge. Most people who have problems in the individualistic culture of the United States have been told the "truth" about themselves by others who know what the problem is. These others may be professionals, authorities, loved ones, or the media. The presumption of these authoritative others that they know the person better than the person knows himself or herself often results in a shorthand label, such as delinquent, bedwetter, abuse victim, phobic, bipolar, or something less esoteric, such as fool, drunk, loser, or bitch. Internalizing these problem labels places people in the position of either accepting the label and any help they can get to "fix" the label, or fighting the label.

In a narrative approach workers and clients together look at the assumptions behind the labels to see what part clients agree with and what part they disagree with. I might agree that the problems that get my life mixed up match what the DSM (American Psychiatric Association, 2000, pp. 382–401) calls bipolar mood disorder, but I might not accept that I am defective although I find that medication helps control my moods. I might even strive to find ways to produce the productivity and pleasure I feel in the early stages of my manic episodes through meditation, affirmation, and/or journaling.

A narrative approach encourages a multiplicity of possible futures through the recollection and reconstruction of *alternative stories* (White & Epston, 1990, p. 41), which are those that suggest a person's ability to influence the problem and that point to a preferred outcome. Mikhail Bakhtin, a Russian literary theorist and philosopher, talks about a *carnival* of possible futures, by which he means the situation or mind-set of openness and incompletion from which come new possibilities and viewpoints (as cited in Irving & Young, 2002, p. 25). Because no one story can contain the entirety of a person's lived experience, there are always other stories, some of which have been overshadowed for different reasons. Those overshadowed stories can point to futures very different from the future suggested by the person's current *dominant story* (White & Epston, p. 11), and through the process of developing an alternative story, the person can *re-author* his or her life (Brown & Augusta-Scott, 2007, pp. xxxiii–xxxiv).

For example, I may see myself as a coward for backing down from a fight when I was an adolescent. I do not see my ability to work with inmates in prison or to skydive as indications of courage; they just are. If I am struggling with certain problems because I am not acting more assertively, I might confirm my view of myself as a coward, not as a person who can access bravery when I need to. Yet some people in my life have praised my ability to do difficult and demanding things. Accessing what allows me to work behind bars or to jump out of an airplane might become a story that will help me ask for a raise or ask my neighbor to lower the volume on his stereo. With assistance, people can often reclaim these other stories and see how they are foreshadowed by other events and comments.

A narrative approach invites a reflexive posture and demands that therapists be accountable for their therapeutic stance. With clients' stories having center stage, workers will frequently ask if what they are doing is helpful, to increase their accountability. As a result, workers and clients together reflect on the treatment process, where it is going, and what options are available at the moment. Course corrections thus can be made along the way.

A narrative approach acknowledges that stories arise from people's social interactions, which occur within a specific cultural context. Epston (1999, p. 137) coined the term *co-research* to describe the collaboration between the worker and the client to bring to the fore often forgotten client knowledge and skills that can be harnessed in opposition to the problem. Consistent with this stance, narrative treatment endeavors to make clients the privileged authors of their own experiences. By the questions workers ask, the conversation can take a variety of turns. Focusing on success rather than failure can lead the conversation in an optimistic direction.

A narrative social worker believes that people are multistoried. People are more than their labels, or even how they see themselves. When in the room with a hostile couple during marriage therapy, for instance, it is important for the social worker to remember that this is not the only story about the relationship. If the hostility and bitterness often displayed in couple treatment were the only story, the worker would quickly feel overwhelmed and have little hope of success. There are other stories that are now overshadowed by the hostility. How does the couple interact with friends, get the trash taken out, pay the bills, or do the laundry?

There are always other stories waiting to be recognized. Author Anne Lamott (1994, pp. 47–48) quotes from a short story by Andre Dubus on this point:

> I love short stories because I believe they are the way we live. They are what our friends tell us, in their pain and joy, their passion and rage, their yearning and their cry against injustice. We can sit all night with our friend while he talks about the end of his marriage, and what we finally get is a collection of stories about passion, tenderness, misunderstanding, sorrow, money; those hours and days and moments when he was absolutely married, whether he and his wife were screaming at each other, or sulking about the house, or making love. While his marriage was dying, he was also working, spending evenings with friends, rearing children; but those are other stories. Which is why, days after hearing a painful story by a friend, we see him and say: How are you? We know that by now he may have another story to tell, or he may be in the middle of one, and we hope it is joyful.

Although narrative therapy does not follow a specific model, an approximate one can be explored. It would look something like this: The social worker first wants to find out what the problem is and how it affects the person's entire life as well as the lives of those around the person. The worker then asks about those times when the person was able to stand up to the problem and influence its effect on his or her life. Next, alternative stories are explored. An *audience* (White, 1995, p. 26; see also Lobovits, Maisel, & Freeman, 1995), or group of appreciative others, for this new story of self is identified and recruited to reinforce the alternative story as an important one in the person's life.

Abels and Abels (2001), experienced social work educators, discuss five reasons why narrative is an appropriate approach for social work. First, narrative reflects the historic mission and purpose of the social work profession. Second, it provides unique practice principles and a socially contextualized perspective that arise directly from the philosophy on which it is based. Third, narrative deals with the person's situation in the context of his or her social environment. Fourth, it emphasizes collaborative mutuality between the worker and the person consulting the worker. Fifth, it minimizes self-blame and offers ways for people to move in desired directions.

A narrative metaphor takes the strengths seen in individuals', families', and communities' stories and develops them to assist people in reaching the outcomes they prefer for their lives. In what follows, I explore the broad foundation behind the approach beginning with the concept of narrative.

## Narrative and Stories

This book describes a narrative approach to clinical social work. As the word implies, *narrative* relates to stories, to a sequence of events strung together across time and connected by a theme that gives meaning to events. In attempting to make sense of life, people arrange their experiences into sequences over time. This helps them to develop a coherent view of themselves and the world in which they live (White & Epston, 1990).

Let us look at a simple story:

> I am walking down the street and a large snake crosses the sidewalk in front of me. I have just come from a lecture on reptiles at my local community college and my initial reaction is shock because large snakes do not usually cross the sidewalks of my town and snakes can be dangerous. I know that they can be dangerous because I have seen signs at the zoo saying that they can be, and I have seen people killed by them on television. However, because of the lecture, I am fascinated by and curious about the snake. As a result, instead of running away or trying to kill the snake, as I might usually do, I follow the snake and watch how it moves and notice its colors until it finally moves down into a deep hole. All the time I watch, I am wondering if this is a smart thing to do because I am concerned that snakes are dangerous, even though the lecturer said that few snakes actually are.

Not a terribly exciting story perhaps, but a story nonetheless. Or is it so uninteresting?

When I first saw the snake and all the stories of snakes from my past came to mind, how did I keep from becoming overly anxious? What in the lecture intrigued me so much that I rejected the anxiety and fear and watched instead? How close did I get to the snake and what was I feeling at the time? What were the snake's colors and how did it move? What fascinated me most about the snake? How did I feel when it went down the hole? What did I do or think next? Did I tell anyone about my encounter? Who? What does it say about our relationship that I told that person about this? What was his or her reaction? How did I respond to the reaction?

[margin note: Q to ask clts abt their stories]

Through these and other questions my little story can be expanded well beyond the mundane; it can be examined in greater detail and its impact on me developed. If you are terrified of snakes you might be interested in how I was able to watch calmly, and my experience might give you ideas about how you might confront your own disgust or fear of snakes, if this is something you are convinced you need to change. Virtually any story can be expanded and explored so that the ordinary becomes exotic, special. My snake story can be seen by me as indicating my heroics or my foolishness, or it may simply not even register in my memory after a day or two. Narrative therapy takes events that are assumedly unimportant (the quiet competence) and develops a different story of people's lives, one that runs parallel to those other troubled stories they have but that promises a different future.

My simple story also provides a good opportunity to distinguish stories from beliefs. Beliefs, and the cognitions that support them, are the focus of cognitive therapies. As noted by Griffith and Griffith (1994), a story is the organization through language of an immediate experience, whereas a belief is an abstraction, an interpretation of that experience. In my story, what I did with the snake is the story; what it means are beliefs.

A collaborative stance, as used in narrative treatment, recognizes the client as the expert on the story. The worker, though no longer claiming expertise on the story per se, can see himself or herself as the expert on the beliefs surrounding it and find that instead of taking a reflective position he or she becomes more challenging and assumes more authority when addressing beliefs. This can change the dynamics of the worker-client relationship, as may happen in cognitive therapy, in which beliefs are assessed as rational/irrational or true/false.

Listening to stories and not questioning their interpretation can lead to more and richer stories from which can develop a more helpful story that addresses a person's ability to find sources of strength. The client owns the story; the narrative practitioner helps to expand it.

Writing or repeating stories can have a beneficial effect on people's health. A study by Pennebaker (1993) provides evidence suggesting that the repetitive construction of a narrative of a traumatic event that includes words portraying strong negative emotions (i.e., anger, sadness, fear, depression) can in and of itself have a helpful effect on both mental and physical health. In this investigation, those who appeared to cope best with their trauma wrote about their negative emotions and created stories that over time showed increased self-awareness and narrative coherence (Pennebaker). The ability to construct a cohesive narrative of the events in a person's life serves an important mental health function.

We all try to understand the meaning of the events in our lives. Stories are the natural way for developing this understanding. Stories can also be limiting. If I tell you my snake story, you might find it vaguely interesting, but, of course, it would not be the whole experience—all the sensory information I received, all the history I have, all the encounter's impact on me. The questions I ask at the end of the story give a small indication of how a story can be expanded simply by bringing to awareness different dimensions of it. Even if I told you of my prior history with snakes, that would not provide you with all my experiences, both direct ones and what I have learned through books, other media, and conversations. Any story represents only a thin slice of the whole pie of a person's lived experience. This is an important concept: It is all the rest of individuals' lived experiences—those slices of the pie not represented by the story—that creates the space for social workers to help those who consult them. Not all events or experiences in life are storied; in fact, most are not.

Some experiences are given meaning and treated as important. Narrative workers call the process of making experiences important and giving them meaning to *perform meaning* (Combs & Freedman, 1994, p. 74). For example, if in the snake story the snake had a flat, triangular head, I might not register that information, even though I saw the snake's head, and it simply would not be part of the story. However, if during the lecture on reptiles I learned that poisonous snakes have triangular heads, then I would perform meaning on the experience of seeing the snake and perceive the snake's head as highly important information. Similarly, if I were in Freudian psychoanalysis at the time, I might consider my fascination with the snake through the lens of sexual symbolism; my interest would take a very different turn and I would perform meaning on the incident in a very different way. Later in this book I discuss how the philosophy of social constructionism enables social workers to develop unique tools for helping people perform meaning on their stories in the presence of others, which can turn previously unconsidered events into reality for clients.

Let us take a look at another story:

> I am sent to see you, a social worker, because I am a "tough kid" who has gotten in trouble with the law. I have a history of fights at school. You ask me what happened and how it is I get into these situations. I tell you I do not know; the fighting just seems to come naturally because people are always pushing me and testing me. I give you the reasons why I need to be a tough kid. I go away from our meeting knowing that another expert figures I am a tough kid and I am further confirmed in this tough kid identity. What you cannot know from our discussion on fighting is that I really care about my girlfriend and my grandmother and that there was a teacher a couple of years back who thought I was special and I really liked her. You cannot know that I do a lot of the housekeeping in my home. Nor can you know that I am good at taking care of my mother and that several friends think I am a very loyal guy because I have taken raps for them on a couple of occasions. Actually, I do not really think about these things much because they do not fit the tough kid way I see myself. My exploits as a tough kid create a very limiting story for me, one that does not fill in all the gaps of my identity.

In this story, it is the feelings and behaviors that relate to the tough kid image that receive attention and shape how I will confront life. It is a very narrow story. It is also a bit unrealistic because people have many stories going on in their lives and are usually somewhat aware of them. Having one story may be a way to provide an example, but people are more complex than that. People are multistoried, though one or two stories can become primary or dominant for a person and lead the individual to not see all the others.

## Stories and Who We Are

Through the plots of our stories, we develop meaning for our experiences. These stories in effect create our lives and our reality. If I am deeply engaged in gang life, being in a gang is not a problem for me, or a situation I am involved in, or even a way to meet my needs; it is simply my life and who I am. Postmodernists talk about stories constituting, or shaping, people's lives and identities. White and Epston (1990) note that Edward Bruner, an anthropologist, said, "It is in the performance of an expression that we re-experience, re-live, re-create, re-tell, re-construct, and re-fashion our culture" (p. 12). Most important, Bruner stated, "The performance does not release a pre-existing meaning that lies dormant in the text.... Rather the performance itself is constitutive" (as cited in White & Epston, p. 12). It is the retelling and reworking of a story based on new information or events that create a new reality to the situation.

For the snake story, one of the questions asked relates to how I pushed back my anxiety and fear in that circumstance. Now, I may never on my own have come to the conclusion that in following the snake I had overcome my anxiety and fear of it, but then the more I think about it, the more I do see it that way. The more questions asked about the whole experience, the more I think about it. I also am asked to name the strategy that I used, rather than suggest what someone else could have done. I am required to think of my *agency* (White & Epston, 1990, p. 82) in the story: what I said or did on my own behalf and how I did it.

Another example of how stories can be changed over time is how a divorced woman looks at her prior marriage as a failure and a farce, with little appreciation of the love experienced during the relationship. The woman may look at that relationship and be amazed she did not earlier see all the falseness in her ex-husband. Periods of affection and caring are reinterpreted as sneakiness and calculation: "He was faking it." With repeated tellings of this story, either to herself or to supportive people who agree with her, the story becomes real, despite her prior experience of the marriage. The reinterpretation has developed a new truth, which redefines not only the prior marital relationship, but also the woman's identity, how she will see others, and perhaps even her view of the world.

How people interpret their life defines how they will see themselves as living it. How they see themselves as living their life will affect where they will put their energy. And through their interactions with others, they will continually create their self. This view of the self as being defined and changed through social interaction has been termed *constitutionalism*, which White (1993b) succinctly, if obtusely, summarizes as follows:

> Constitutionalism brings with it the proposition that, upon entering into life in the social world, persons become engaged in particular modes of life and thought—or, according to Foucault, particular practices of power and knowledges about life that have achieved or been granted a truth status. According to this perspective, these practices and knowledges are not radically invented—the individual person does not simply "dream them up." These practices and knowledges

have been negotiated over time within contexts of communities of persons and institutions that comprise culture. The social formation of communities and institutions compose relations of forces that, in engaging in various practices of power, determine which ideas, of all those possible, are acceptable—they determine what is to count as legitimate knowledge. (p. 124)

This is an important point to consider because it suggests that the stories we created to explain many of life's psychological and interpersonal problems not only may have contributed to the development of those problems, but also may have made those problems worse. These stories are restricted by the discourses, or wider cultural stories, that make some stories, rather than others, more available to us. A discourse includes our taken-for-granted assumptions (e.g., marriage is for life; everyone must work; people are not for eating); our unexamined daily habits (e.g., husband talks over wife in an argument; father gets enraged by son's disobedience and mother protects son); and the economic, political, and cultural institutions in which these assumptions and actions exist (Madsen, 2007). It often sets the standards for how people are seen by others, how they are expected to be, and whether they are viewed as measuring up. Problems develop when people internalize stories and discourses that do not allow them to access the full range of their lived experiences and that therefore limit their ability to access other choices (Adams-Westcott & Isenbart, 1995).

## Narrative Conception of Self

The self is a story. As Drewery and Winslade (1997) note, "Thus, we make sense of our lives in the context of our social history, shaping stories about the groups we belong to and about how we came to be who, how, and where we are. Such stories constitute something of our identity; they are the background context that gives the possibility of coherence to our lives" (p. 34). Identity comes through participating in interaction with others and through cultural messages.

Gergen (1999) proposes that the self be conceptualized as "relational." Some definitions of self are privileged based on a society's power relations; others are not. The difference between being a patriotic freedom fighter and a terrorist/rebel is a good example. The definition depends on who is doing the defining. Where many in the American colonies saw people fighting the British as patriots fighting for their country, those in Britain saw treasonous rebels. If the vast majority of colonists held the latter view, then colonists who fought the British would have been labeled "rebels." The discourse is typically written by the victors of power struggles, and where terrorism and freedom fighting become mixed is when the former terrorists are the victors, as was the case in Algeria and Israel.

In a social constructionist perspective, the self is not a single entity but is composed of multiple voices from the past and the present that interact and are amended with continual social contact. In the postmodern era, people have so many different roles and requirements that it is difficult to "be yourself" in all of them (Gergen, 1999). Just as there is not one great truth in social constructionism, there is not one great "self" who is the "true" person.

Traditionally, Western civilization has considered the self to be the inner core of the person from which he or she functions. As an example, the relationship among ego, superego, and id forms the core of personhood from which functioning is determined, according to Freudian theory. This semi-closed system is self-centered, with environmental input being something with which one of the parts copes. The unified self is seen as becoming more clearly formed through a process of development. Adolescents' task is not so much about learning how to fit into society as it is about "finding yourself."

If you have ever watched a James Bond movie, then you have seen someone being the same person in every new situation that arises, being, in essence, a singular, unified self. No matter what novel situation James Bond gets himself into, he always acts like James Bond, a continuity that is perhaps feasible because he has a working knowledge of every skill known to humankind. But is this your life experience?

When thinking about how true to oneself a person can be, it is also worth considering where and how we learned what our true self is. An important aspect of narrative work is the understanding that people have strong preferences about how they like to see themselves, how they like to act, and how they like others to see them. This composite makes up a person's preferred view of self, or his or her *preferred description* (McKenzie & Monk, 1997, p. 87). "People are at their best when they act, think of themselves, and imagine that others regard them in ways that confirm who they wish to be" (Eron & Lund, 1999, p. 293). The "wish to be" is psychologically important because it implies more plasticity in the self than has been accorded by other approaches.

The "true self" is itself a social construction through which the culture prescribes different stories. Usually we pick one of these types of stories and see it as meeting our own unique desires. People acquire preferred values and commitments from their culture, and these values and commitments create what feels like a unified, solid self. In fact, people's behavior does not always honor these values and commitments, and what is emphasized can affect their sense of cohesion.

A way to think of this is to imagine if all your failures were raised up to you for correction as the most important aspect of your life by those who care for you. How would your life be different? Now imagine if all your successes were raised up instead. How would you see yourself? Would you think of yourself differently? In both cases, you would have the same experiences in your life except some would be more strongly accented to you than others. As a result of what is spotlighted, you might have a very different perspective on your life and the world. Social constructionism considers the center of the person to be actually outside the person in the collectivity with others (Andersen, 1995).

The degree to which people can look back at their lives and see a consistent narrative leads to a feeling of continuity in their sense of self. An event is integrated into someone's perceptions through the identification of those properties that match the person's sense of personal continuity (Arciero & Guidano, 2000). Those events that fit the dominant story of self get priority. Therefore, acquiring a new sense of self requires taking an alternative story based on a present event or two and following it back in the person's life, or *historicizing* (White & Epston, 1990, p. 117) the new, preferred self-description. Historicizing requires looking for additional past events that are precedents for or predictive of the current event as a way to develop a consistent new self-narrative. These prior events indicate that the person has longstanding relationships with certain skills, knowledge, and attitudes.

Problems are located in the cultural discourse, and people develop stories of their experiences in ways well prescribed by the culture. These stories create versions of a person, some of which fit the individual's dominant story, some of which do not. When some of these versions do not fit either the person's dominant story or the culture's definition of normal, then they can be seen as problems (Neal, Zimmerman, & Dickerson, 1999).

The dominant culture sees problems as located in the individual, offering people little alternative but to see themselves or others with whom they are in conflict as defective. If the links between these cultural truths and the individual's experience of problems are not challenged, then the person's "negative experiences of identity" are reinforced (Neal et al., 1999, p. 365). Questions to clients about how the problem has led them to see themselves provide a way to initiate exploration of this dimension. Does the problem try to convince the person of positive or negative things about himself or herself (White, 1995)? Seeing the story of one's identity as only one of several possible stories gives people choices they may not have had otherwise.

In summary, as Franklin (1998) notes:

- It is impossible for us to interpret our experience in a vacuum. A frame of intelligibility, usually of a cultural nature, is necessary for interpreting any lived experience.
- Such frames provide a context for our experience and make the attribution of meaning possible.
- The meanings we derive in the process of interpretation have real effects on the shape of our lives and on the steps we take in life. Thus, such meanings are not neutral in their effects on our lives.
- The personal story or self-narrative provides the principle frame of reality for our lived experience.
- The personal story or self-narrative is not radically invented inside our heads. Rather, it is something negotiated and distributed within various communities of persons and the institutions of our culture.
- The personal story, or self-narrative, structures our experience. It determines what aspects of our stock of lived experience are selected for expression.
- The personal story or self-narrative determines the shape of the expression or particular aspects of our lived experience.
- The stories we have about our lives actually shape or constitute our lives.
- Our lives are multi-storied. No single story of life can be free of ambiguity and contradiction. No single personal story or self-narrative can handle all of the contingencies of life. (pp. 67–68)

Working with people from a narrative perspective allows social workers to listen to clients' actual stories, without having to try continually to deduce stories' hidden meanings. Actually listening to people's stories reduces workers' evaluative statements about clients being "less than." By reducing the expert, superior position of the social worker and encouraging a *not-knowing* stance (Freedman & Combs, 1996, pp. 44–45) (i.e., a position of openness, curiosity, and willingness to listen to and learn from clients), conflicts and differences in the worker-client relationship can be diminished and made available for examination. *Deconstruction* (White, 1993c, p. 34), in which everyday definitions and taken-for-granted assumptions are subjected to examination, opens up issues of diversity in a direct manner and looks at the discourses that might be affecting the treatment relationship.

## Criticisms of a Narrative Approach

A number of criticisms have been raised about using the narrative approach in clinical social work practice. First, if all stories are valuable, then it would seem that values are relative, too. So where are the profession's obligations in this model? From a social constructionist point of view, all stories may have a value, but some stories can lead to oppression and even terror through the exercise of power. Stories that say men should control the lives of women or that minorities are never as good as majority group members lead to oppression and pain. Questioning the assumptions behind societal truths encourages people to look at where these ideas come from and whether they make them the kind of people they would prefer to be. By recognizing the importance of difference and subjugated voices, social work values are upheld.

Second, social workers have social control obligations that require them to assess for and report or intervene in such situations as family abuse, suicidal ideation, or homicidal intentions. How can we take a curious, not-knowing stance with such obligations when we believe the client is initially lying? Do postmodernists believe in lying? Lying is a problem in a narrative approach because there are some social work roles that require investigative functions. When a person has a history of troubling behavior, the person's reputation, and any behavior that might give the appearance of furthering that reputation, can be questioned and treated appropriately. If a client has attempted suicide, that client has therefore acquired a suicidal reputation. Behavior that seems to extend that negative reputation can be questioned. If the client isolates himself or herself and reports taking medication while actually stockpiling it, the person's suicidal reputation will be extended regardless of his or her intent. Does the client prefer a suicidal reputation? What needs to happen for this reputation to be removed? The appearance becomes the cause of concern, rather than the specific intent, and this shift in focus reduces the level of conflict. Lying is not ignored; it is instead addressed from a different perspective.

Third, as social workers we see clients who are faced with multiple material resource problems such as lack of housing, food, and income. This is not a discourse problem; this is real. Although narrative approaches attempt to diminish workers' expert role and focus on clients' expertise, workers have unique expertise in bureaucracy and locating resources, the same way a psychiatrist might have expertise in medication. A worker providing a client with resources and referrals is not taking away the client's expertise but is making further tools available to the person so that he or she can develop a preferred outcome (i.e., a result the client wishes to achieve). When required, workers can provide mediation and advocacy services to clients, if both see it as appropriate. Even where material needs are not at issue, both worker and client can work together to advocate for an alternative story to be heard by the appropriate authorities.

Finally, a frequent criticism is that a narrative metaphor does not lend itself to a researchable model. Part of the difficulty in researching the impact of narrative treatment is that the followers of this approach distrust the modernist scientific enterprise. A research approach that objectifies and quantifies clients and their problems runs counter to a social constructionist view of subjective reality as primary. That said, research studies have been done on narrative work. Some of these investigations have used qualitative research techniques, which fit better into the narrative framework.

## Exercises

### Exercise 1: Questioning About Stories That "Create" Social Workers

An important part of a student's social work education involves developing a professional identity as a social worker, and the task is for social work educators and field instructors to work with students to construct this story (Winslade, Monk, & Drewery, 1997). This often is a complicated task in MSW programs because many students enter with extensive social work experience and see themselves as social workers already. It is not uncommon to see faculty and students struggle over this socialization process, with students feeling faculty are out of touch and coercive and faculty questioning the commitment of students to the profession, interpreting their pursuit of the degree as simply a way to get a pay raise.

Winslade and colleagues (1997), in discussing counselor education, describe the advantages of looking at students' and faculty members' professional development as an unfolding story of their accomplishments. Development of a professional identity as a social worker involves the formulation of a self-description consistent with the performance of the values and skills of social work (see McKenzie & Monk, 1997 in relation to counselor education).

Introduction to Narrative as an Approach to Social Work         29

The following exercise, which is based on an activity developed by McKenzie and Monk (1997), is designed to help you think about your professional identity. Have students break into pairs and interview each other for about 30 minutes. McKenzie and Monk (pp. 86–87) tell their students to "consider sharing with your partner your own history and life experiences that will be useful to you in the development of your preferred description" as a social worker.

In the language of narrative treatment, someone's preferred description is how that person would like to see himself or herself and have others see him or her. If your viewpoint is that people have many different identities and that those identities are malleable in social contexts, then focusing on what your preferred description is can act as an anchoring point. Your preferred description can also be deconstructed to see what discourses are leading you in that direction and if others would better suit you. McKenzie and Monk (1997) suggest several questions as guides for the interviewers, who should take a genuine, curious stance toward the interview, keeping in mind that what is important is not what the conversation means to them (i.e., searching for data for hypotheses) but, rather, what it means to the interviewee:

1. What experiences have you had in your life . . . that have assisted you in moving toward your preferred description of yourself as a counselor [or social worker]?
2. How have you been curious about your work with your clients and yourself, and what came from that?
3. How have people been responding to you differently as you move toward or embrace your preferred description?
4. How do you account for these changes?
5. Are these changes similar to any you have experienced on other occasions in your life, or are they absolutely new? (p. 87)

Here are examples of the first two questions:

**1. What experiences have you had in your life that have assisted you in moving toward your preferred description as a social worker? Can you think of specific incidents or events? May we discuss these in some detail?**

*People have told me that I'm the kind of person who can listen and make others feel better. I remember a time when a friend was going through a difficult time with her boyfriend and she talked to me for about 3 hours, crying all the time. I was 17, and she and I had been friends for 3 years, ever since we met in middle school. She said that she couldn't talk to anyone else and didn't know what she would have done if it hadn't been for me. She was pretty upset. It made me feel good that she trusted me like that and said I was helpful. See, her boyfriend, whom she had dated for about a year, was going out behind her back. When she found out, he decided to drop her. He was the creep, yet she got mistreated. It wasn't fair. Oh, we met in her bedroom; I remember calling home and letting my parents know where I was and that I was coming home late. She kept saying that she really cared about him and that she really tried, and that she really felt cheated and betrayed by his behavior. She wondered why she didn't see this about him before and got angry at herself for getting used. I guess I got angry seeing her so upset and wondered why they couldn't work it out. I tried to stay neutral and she appreciated me not dumping on her boyfriend or on her. I felt exhausted by the end of that talk, but it seemed to be what she really needed.*

*I remember another, earlier occasion. I was in church and heard the minister talk about the struggles of poor people in the congregation as well as in the country in general. I was maybe 6 years old at the time—it's hard to remember. I recall how upset I was by this and I wanted to do something. I was too young at the time, but later when I was 12, I volunteered and took hot lunches to older people who needed them. I enjoyed helping them out, and I think I got more from them than they got from those hot lunches. I remember how an older woman told me she had been a social worker at the Boston Psychopathic Hospital. I had never heard of it. She said that she was one of the first social workers there and that she thought I was the kind of person who would like social work. She thought that I was a good listener and that I enjoyed helping people who needed help. I can still see her today as I talk about her, though I am sure she is long gone. Her apartment, in the Back Bay area of Boston, was a little musty and old looking. I remember hearing the clock ticking when things were quiet. She was such an interesting person that those moments of stillness weren't very often. She would talk about the kinds of things she did, like checking out people's homes to make sure they could come home and talking to people who were leaving the hospital about what they wanted to have happen with their lives. There was no psychotropic medication then, so I can't imagine how difficult it was.*

2. **How have you been curious about your work with your clients and yourself? What came from that curiosity?**

*I wonder sometimes if I still come across as a person who is concerned about helping or if I am more detached from people. I have been wondering if social work school hasn't stolen my soul. It is just too easy to see people as big problems and write up a treatment plan clients barely understand, and I find myself doing it just to meet the agency's paperwork requirement. I sometimes wonder what happened to the old me who so badly wanted to go to social work school to help people. Some of the stuff we learn is interesting, but things at my placement rarely seem to work out the way they do in the books. That part confuses me and makes me wonder if I can ever really do this work right.*

Reflection on these sorts of incidents can result in bringing to life many stories that reorient students to their goals of developing themselves as social work professionals and completing a professional education program.

## Exercise 2: Practicing Curious Questioning

This is an interviewing exercise, based on the work of McKenzie and Monk (1997), in which students have the opportunity to practice curious questioning with each other about a nonsensitive topic. Divide the class into pairs. One student will be the interviewer, the other the storyteller.

Instruct the interviewers to interview the storytellers on their morning rituals. These can include getting out of bed, showering, getting breakfast, and interacting with others in the home during this period of time. Explain that the interviewers are to get more detail than might normally be provided. Possible questions include: When do you get up? Do you use an alarm clock? What kind: alarm or radio? Which side of the bed is it on? How did that come about? What kind of soap do you use? What color is it? What does it smell like? How is it you chose that sort of soap? What do you think that says about you?

Inform the interviewers that they are to be respectful and genuinely curious about the storytellers' story of their morning routine. Explain that the trick is to avoid interrogating the storyteller and trying to find hidden implications in the individual's actions. The purpose is to help the storyteller discover new information about himself or herself or about an activity by discussing it in detail.

Ask students to switch roles. After this second interviewing process, allow students at least 10 minutes to process what it was like interviewing and being interviewed and, in particular, to note if at any time the interview felt like an interrogation and how this came about.

Here is an example:

**Interviewer:** I would like to interview you about your morning routine. I will try to go into as much detail as possible. You can refuse to answer any question I ask without explanation. I am interested in doing this to practice curious questioning. I am told that you may also get a different viewpoint on things as a result. Would you be interested in letting me interview you?

**Storyteller:** *Yes, that's okay.*

**Interviewer:** What time did you get up this morning?

**Storyteller:** *I guess about 5:45.*

**Interviewer:** Did you use anything to help you get up?

**Storyteller:** *Yes, my alarm clock.*

**Interviewer:** Could you describe your alarm clock to me?

**Storyteller:** *Well, it's gray and it has an alarm and a radio.*

**Interviewer:** Do you wake to the alarm or the radio?

**Storyteller:** *The alarm, which actually wakes up my boyfriend and he tells me to get up.*

**Interviewer:** Is the clock on his or your side of the bed?

**Storyteller:** *His. He gets up easier.*

**Interviewer:** When the alarm went off this morning and your boyfriend told you to get up . . . By the way, how did he tell you to get up?

**Storyteller:** *Oh, well, very sweetly. Actually he just told me the alarm went off and it was time to get up. . . . He didn't yell; he understood I needed to get up extra early to work on my policy paper before work.*

**Interviewer:** Did you get right up when you heard this?

**Storyteller:** *No, it took me about 3 or so minutes.*

**Interviewer:** Were you thinking about anything before you got up?

**Storyteller:** *Yes, I was thinking about how I wish I didn't have to do this paper and how I would like to stay in bed.*

**Interviewer:** Anything else?

**Storyteller:** *Yes, that I needed to get it done and the sooner I got up the better, so I got up.*

**Interviewer:** Did you find yourself noticing anything in the room while you were lying in bed?

**Storyteller:** *No.*

## Exercise 3: Recognizing Strengths

This exercise is ongoing and involves each student in the class. During the class sessions, in role-plays, and in discussions, students tend to show their abilities and interests. These often go unnoticed. For the rest of the course, when you notice that a fellow student gives some indication of his or her abilities, knowledge, skills, or experience that predicts a good future in social work, make a note in the margin of your class notes of the person's name and the event that led you to that conclusion. Try to notice an event for every member of the class, especially if your class is a smaller one. Toward the end of the course, these could be compiled and people in the class could receive these comments anonymously. This exercise requires you to build up your ability to notice strengths; you will also begin to see how the strengths you notice affect your attitude toward others.

CHAPTER 2

# Power, Narrative, and Social Work

Social work is a values-based profession. Although our practice as clinical social workers involves working with individuals, families, or small groups, we cannot ignore the economic, social-structural, and cultural environments. Issues of power, oppression, and discrimination are always considerations in what we do. It is only right, therefore, to ask: Does a narrative approach address these issues? Does it help to advance our profession's commitment to social justice?

Narrative work, in fact, deals directly with these concerns. In this chapter, I describe how a narrative approach offers a particularly effective way to address issues of power, difference, and disadvantage. I begin by discussing the empowerment perspective in social work and how a narrative approach complements that perspective. I then examine how societal discourses are constructed; how they can reinforce the power of particular groups; and how they can act to separate people, defining some as "less than" or "other" and some as "better than" or "dominant." I also look at power in therapeutic relationships and how narrative therapy attempts to shift power between workers and clients as well as how clients' and workers' narratives can have an impact on each other. I conclude the chapter with a discussion of the use of the DSM-IV-TR in clinical practice.

## Empowerment

There is growing interest in social work in the uses of power in both professional relationships and clients' relationships in the outside world. Social work has had a long history of engaging in what are called empowering practices (Lee, 2001; Simon, 1994; Solomon, 1976). The word *empowerment* is confusing because it indicates that someone is given power of some sort. In fact, it often involves giving people the space to discover their own power.

On the micro level the term is used to signify a personal sense of empowerment, or feeling more in control of one's life, whereas a more macro view of empowerment involves people receiving rights and resources from the environment that give them greater personal control of their lives and a sense of being counted. Feeling empowered and having greater power to control one's position in the environment, though related, are not identical (Zimmerman, 1990). Macro level empowerment arises from considerations of social justice and a commitment to alleviate poverty, oppression, and discrimination (Lee, 2001). Thus, I can be empowered when a great love relationship and a reduced sense of hopelessness result in my feeling in control of my world, but I can still be oppressed by a poverty-wage job and discrimination.

An empowerment perspective emphasizes a collaborative worker-client relationship that engages capacities, not incapacities, and focuses on the person and the environment. Empowerment arises from the person and the community, not the worker (Lee, 2001). Clients are treated as people with rights, responsibilities, and claims on their society, an important point for members of groups who have a history of being oppressed (Simon, 1994). Gutierrez, Parsons, and Cox (1998) add that empowerment practice also entails educating clients about their rights and ways to defend them.

Lee (2001) lays out a set of assumptions upon which, she argues, an empowerment practice can be built:

1. All oppression is destructive of life and should be challenged by social workers and clients.
2. The social worker should maintain holistic vision in situations of oppression.
3. People empower themselves: social workers should assist.
4. People who share common ground need each other to attain empowerment.
5. Social workers should establish a mutual and reciprocal relationship with clients.
6. Social workers should encourage the client to say her own words.
7. The worker should maintain a focus on the person as victor and not victim.
8. Social workers should maintain a social change focus. (p. 60)

Much of empowerment practice is built upon the work of Brazilian educator/scholar Paulo Freire (as cited in Lee, 2001). According to Lee, Freire recommended that people look at the cultural and class biases in themselves and in the environment around them by posing critical questions about their social reality. How is it, for instance, that women are abused so frequently in this country? What effect does that have on all people in this society? The same sorts of questions can be asked about racial or gender differences in economic levels or about age differences in employment patterns. Freire saw this process of consciousness-raising producing a critical awareness of people's positioning in the society; this critical awareness can, in turn, lead to praxis, a process of reflecting, acting, and reflecting once again in light of the awareness gained through action (as cited in Lee).

Like deconstruction, Freire's critical perspective involves questioning the dominant reality. Such questioning can give rise to collective action, as exemplified by the problem-specific *leagues* (Madigan & Epston, 1995, p. 261) that have arisen from narrative work. These leagues, which embody self-help organizing, are willing to use social action to stand up to the problem-enhancing messages of the culture. The activities of leagues are discussed in chapter 9.

An example of empowerment practice designed to assist a child who is having difficulty with school might involve helping the parents become able to stand up to and be assertive with the school. This work might require initially educating the parents on their rights and coaching them so that over time they are able to make their presence known on their own. Intervention might also involve offering information about advocacy groups that could support and assist them.

As will be seen, a narrative approach to social work shares many of the same assumptions as the empowerment perspective: the need for collaborative, strengths-based relationships; the clarification of rights through deconstruction; and the recognition that individuals, particularly those who are members of minority or outsider groups, are not given equal access to resources. A narrative approach assumes that a community, more so than an individual, can stand up to and protest injustice, though individuals, in their own way, protest all the time and are frequently seen as deviant as a result.

## Social Construction and Power

Social constructionism generally, and narrative therapy in particular, look at how power is used in treatment relationships to replicate the problem, depriving a client of power, albeit on a different scale. In thinking about these sorts of issues, narrative workers have turned to the work of Michel Foucault, a French philosopher/historian. It is important to consider power matters at this point because they represent a key aspect of narrative practice that may be overlooked. Not paying attention to power in relationships can lead to forcing people into a narrative approach through a lack of patience, and workers once again wind up telling clients what the clients' problems are. Those reading this text have had extensive schooling where they have acquired the skill of showing people how smart they are and it is easy to fall into that mode when, as workers, they feel anxious with a client. Making space in conversations for clients to identify their own preferences and strategies is not easy.

## Culture and Power

Narrative treatment is certainly not the first approach to examine the cultural dimensions of what appear to be people's individual problems. Feminist psychologists and treatment providers have long studied the impact of culture to foster a broader understanding and heightened consciousness of how political factors affect women. Feminist writers note the difference between distress and pathology, arguing that some distress may actually represent a form of resistance to oppressive social norms (Brown, 2000). Historically, individuals who are not part of the mainstream, dominant culture (White, middle-class, heterosexual, young, able-bodied, Christian, male) are seen as less rational, physically closer to nature, weaker, and less mentally fit (Hacker, 1976). In a patriarchal society these attributes are seen as negatives and typically are assigned to women. Diagnoses are developed to describe an excess of femininity (hysteria, dependent personality) but not masculinity (Brown). For these reasons feminist theorists are reluctant to assign pathology to individuals in whom the distress is the result of oppression (sexism, racism, institutionalized violence, discrimination, inaction to social problems by the government, unequal distribution of resources, etc.; Brown, 2000).

Power is an important aspect of people's problems. When something is defined as a problem, society can exercise its power and have an impact on the problem by making judgments about it. All cultures "order" their members so as to enforce an internal commitment to the culture's standards of normality and reduce the need for coercion. People learn what is right and good, and when we look at other cultures we often sit in wonder. Some years ago, in the United States, a Japanese woman walked into the sea with her infant in response to the shame of her American husband leaving her. What made perfect sense to her and what traditional Japanese culture might have seen as acceptable, if not expected, behavior was viewed as shocking and aberrant in her new country. Yet our culture's taken-for-granted discourses on such issues as individualism, consumerism, self-interest, freedom, and competition might seem aberrant to those from other cultures.

We rarely consider the values embedded in our culture's discourses because they are "the way things are supposed to be." They, like White, male, middle-class privilege, are the air, or some might say, the smog, we breathe (Tatum, 1997) and are not noticeable. Although the ordering that occurs in a culture keeps it running smoothly, it also establishes an evaluative structure that has a negative impact on people. These evaluative criteria are least favorable to the very people (labeled as poor, minority, vulnerable) social workers are likely to help.

Foucault was interested in how the way we normally do things and enact "the obvious" in our lives leads to restricting our thoughts, actions, and feelings. He looked at how institutions exercised social control through promulgating worldviews and habits that have turned people into "things." He was particularly interested in how truth leads to the acquisition of power in relationships between people. Foucault did not see truth as something plucked out of nature, but as socially constructed, as what is made to be true. It is always easier to see the fallacies in past truths, such as slavery, the importance of breeding within one's class, or the inability of women to cast rational votes, than in current truths.

Foucault also was interested in how societal truths lead to divisions between people and affect the development of the self. He examined these issues by looking at current institutions (those responsible for punishing crime, relieving mental illness, and treating the sick) and their practices and tracing them historically to show the shifts in truth and the societal impacts of such shifts (Foucault, 1965/1973, 1973/1975, 1977/1979). He noted how truth has been used over the centuries to separate, and in some cases eliminate, those individuals different from what the society says is normal. Given the impact truth can have on people's lives, those with special knowledge of it can have great power over those lacking such knowledge. According to Freedman and Combs (1996, p. 38), Foucault saw the relationship between knowledge and power as so strong and so fundamental that he argued "power is knowledge and knowledge is power."

Foucault's ideas have particular relevance to social work, which some have characterized as a "normalizing" profession, helping people to accommodate to their environments (Epstein, 1999, p. 9). Few would doubt that most of our efforts as social workers go toward assisting clients to fit into the society rather than working to make the society more just (Specht, 1990). Most social work practice theories are focused on how individuals adapt to environmental demands and do not look at the roles of power, conflict, oppression, and violence, which play such a large part in the life of many groups in the United States (Saleebey, 1993). Foucault's analysis highlights the need for practice theories and methods that explicitly take into account power and its impact on the lives of our clients.

## Separating Practices

People are separated from each other through a process that begins with normalization. Normalization categorizes people and distinguishes those who are "normal" from those who are "abnormal" according to medical, psychological, or other standards.

In a modernist world, the categories of normality are founded on the best science available at the time, and society sees them as true because they are based on science. Scientific truth trumps the subjective experience of the people who are categorized. The categories then leave open the possibility of developing dividing practices that turn the subjective experience of people into the object of scientific knowledge. Because the dividing practices are based on what is true, most people go along with their subjugation without comment, believing it is the right thing to do. However, wherever there is power there is resistance, and individual acts of resistance can lead to further pathologizing and disciplining practices.

For example, if you are struggling with emotions that you have been told look like depression, then you might go to a mental health clinic. As part of the mental health intake process, you likely will be asked if you use alcohol or illegal drugs, if you have ever been physically or sexually abused, or if you have ever been traumatized. Disclosure is expected of you because you are seeking help and are being considered as a client. If you refuse to give this information, stating you do not see its relevance to giving you relief, you may be told that this can be important information for helping depressed people and that its collection is required by the state agency that makes policies for the mental health clinic. The worker may note on the intake form that you are "guarded," which is seen as an indication of suspiciousness or paranoia. This means there is potential for a more serious diagnosis should your resistance continue. You then will be given a DSM diagnosis or two (categorized) and will likely be asked to see a medical practitioner who will evaluate you for medication. If you refuse the medication prescribed (a protest against the dominant discourse) and continue to have depressive symptoms, and you indicate that you have feelings of helplessness and hopelessness ("wish it would just end") and perhaps mention that as a hunter you have guns in the house, then you might be convinced to sign yourself into a hospital for a bit. This seems logical to protect you, though you do not want either the humiliation or stigma of going into a psych unit. If you refuse to do so and say there is no need, and you also refuse to get rid of your prized guns or give them to someone else (another protest), you might find yourself under the threat of being committed to a hospital against your will for at least 72 hours. If you continue to refuse, police will be called to take you to the hospital. Your emotional state will have led you into a fairly dire situation because you failed to become more passive and not protest the practices of those who were attempting to help you. Although this is perhaps a glib anecdote, in busy clinics it is not outside the possible, especially when workers are held liable for their clients' actions.

The culture exercises control of its members through the use of knowledge that constitutes the truth, which is treated as more real than an individual's subjective experience. Here is another example: In an involuntary commitment hearing, the social worker states that the patient, a young man, suffers from paranoid delusions and is a danger to himself, given his symptoms. The patient, who may feel that his every desire has been ignored and that control of his life has been taken from him, states that his loss is so bad that people on television are talking to him and telling him to do things like kill himself or others. He says he does not really wish to do this and talks about struggling against these voices that stay in his head after he shuts off the television. The worker is trying to protect this person and those around him from the physical danger these voices could produce. Is the patient's experience respected in this situation? Does reducing his experience of fears and compulsions to symptoms and signs respect his viewpoint, which does not fit the viewpoint of the dominant culture? Was his cooperation sought for the hospitalization? What would happen if the patient's viewpoint was respected and the difficult situation he is in was recognized? What impact might these changes have on the situation?

Social workers often feel a sense of helplessness when they consider their own power, and it may seem like clients hold all the power. We all know that community mental health clients have a poor rate of keeping appointments. At the same time, a medicalized mental health system requires social workers to see clients for a certain percentage of the time they are at work, if they are to keep their positions. Office-based strategies have mixed results in working with oppressed populations, and it can feel like clients merely cycle through treatment, sometimes repeatedly, at their own discretion. Worker frustration can be exacerbated by the incomprehensibility of the disability pension system and the experience of the law as a barrier to hospitalizing people who are not really making it yet who fall outside the statute's criteria for involuntary hospitalization. But despite these reasons for feeling powerless, workers do have power and their words are seen as more reliable and accurate than the words of their clients.

The case file captures the lives of people and fixes them in time. It can produce a totalizing view of the person, from the perspective of the person's mental illness, medical illness, poverty, or criminal behavior (Madigan, 1998b). Readers of the file will likely see and treat the person as he or she is described in the file—as a member of a stigmatized category, not a whole person. The power of the file is best seen in the decision of most legal jurisdictions to eliminate from circulation, or expunge, the files of juveniles involved in criminal activities. The life-influencing nature of the file, or criminal record, is recognized and our society wishes to give youth a second chance.

## How Oppression and Discrimination Are Based in Stories of the Other

Several authors have seen narrative as an important method for understanding diversity between workers and clients (Abels & Abels, 2001; Kelley, 1995). Truly listening to and validating a person's narrative can have a powerful effect on both the worker and the client. Narrative practitioners see cultural discourses as important contributors to the problems that individuals experience. The effects of some discourses can be seen in certain attitudes and habits that people take on, in the damage caused by the exercise of power, and in the effects of oppression. If sexuality were not seen as so important in this culture and women were not expected to meet a certain ideal form, would anorexia still be such a widespread problem today for young women in the United States?

Clinical social workers who are working with poor, minority clients are more likely to recognize psychiatric problems than the impacts of cultural, socioeconomic, and gender-based discourses. Yet problems such as depression and anxiety can also be seen as arising from situations in which a person experiences marginalization, feels not good enough, does not meet the societal standard, or does not have access to adequate resources (Neal et al., 1999).

Drug company–sponsored continuing education workshops rarely focus on the sociological aspect of symptoms. As Waldgrave (1990) notes, we collude with the forces of oppression when we treat depression solely as the personal illness of an individual who is unemployed because of structural changes or discrimination.

Relationship problems also can be seen as a result of societal discourses. What a person owes another in a relationship is based on the culture's stories about relationships and about how power should be distributed in them. What are you entitled to in your relationships? Relationship conflicts can reflect the "*effects* of the contradictory cultural prescriptions people use to make sense of themselves and to guide them in their relationships" (Neal et al., 1999, p. 361, emphasis in original). In cross-gender relationships, men's tendency to discount women's views because of supposed lack of rationality is an example of how this mechanism can work. This discounting encourages women to distrust their own experience to get along in relationships (Neal et al.); it leads to a continuation of male dominance and female submissiveness. Upsetting this balance has led to negative reactions toward women who stood up and had the courage to endure in their belief in themselves.

Cultural discourses can even split people's selves, with one part judging the other part. Foucault (1988, p. 16) notes how "technologies of the self" (such as social work treatment) are designed to promote changing people's selves to be more in line with cultural standards. These cultural prescriptions operate as forms of power over people, telling them they are never good enough, through either others' reactions or their own narratives.

Cultural discourses about race also can be seen as leading to often harmful separating practices. Race is not a biological concept but a cultural one. Definitions of race rest upon cultural characterizations of bloodlines, which often serve as the legal basis for race and which can vary from country to country. Even from a modernist's point of view, race is not a biological concept, because there is as much or more genetic diversity within races as there is between races. The meaning of race is based on the myths, themes, and rituals of the culture, reinforced by historical and current stories and by media portrayals. These narratives live on in current relationships and can lead to external oppression (denial of rights and resources to the minority group members) and diminished internal resources (questioning one's personal adequacy in a world that defines you as different in a negative way), as well as rage directed at members of the dominant culture.

These same stories influence dominant-culture social workers, who are brought up on them and have not had to question the assumptions behind them. In most situations, workers are more privileged than clients, often because of class and socioeconomic status and sometimes because of race or gender. Privilege blinds social workers to these differences, which feel natural and as things should be. We enact racist thoughts without even realizing we have done so, because they are within the very histories and discourses that shape our identity (Akamatsu, 2002). The ease with which we can replicate the mandates of societal discourses in the therapeutic relationship should come as no surprise.

"Remembering not to forget" (White, 1997, p. 140) is remembering there is a privilege of power that the worker has and that affects everything occurring in the treatment interaction. The dominant discourse leads social workers to forget or ignore their privilege because they are there to "treat a disease" or to "develop resources for people" or whatever the task is. When workers deconstruct the treatment as well as the client's presenting problem and name the sources of oppression and inequity, a new perspective becomes available on both the treatment situation and the person's problems in the world. The more visible these power relations are made, the easier it is to stand beside clients in their attempts to protest them.

The importance of making privilege and difference visible is perhaps clearest in those situations in which the worker and client are of different races or genders. Pointing out the obvious to clients—stating that you, the worker, may not "get it" and requesting that they let you know when that happens (assuming they see it and feel they can trust you)—sets the stage for bringing up issues of difference. Coming back to this issue every few sessions can eventually open up the topic for discussion. Lobovits et al. (1995) report that Archie Smith Jr., a cultural consultant who has worked with them, observed:

> If an African American client chooses to value a white therapist's nondominant ways of behaving, he/she must then live simultaneously in two worlds. . . . According to Smith, the African American client "may exhibit a double consciousness towards a non-subjugating therapist which is a mixture of genuine gratitude on the one hand and suspicion . . . on the other." Both sides of this consciousness need to be developed and expressed. . . . If the therapist fails to allow for the expression of this suspicion, he/she ignores the reality of racism and may imply that the client can and should expect nondominant behavior from the other whites in positions of power outside the context of therapy. (p. 238)

For example, I worked with a man who was a devout Black Muslim. I brought up our racial difference in the first session. It was treated both politely and jokingly. The client asked me about the lack of African American males on staff at the agency, and, despite all my training, I got a bit defensive. When I calmed down, I wondered about racial oppression when he mentioned some of the problems he faced. Several months later, he discussed the humiliation of coming to see me about a problem he thought he should have been able to fix without my help. This opened up the opportunity to reexamine the issue of race, which is rarely done with in treatment, although we often treat it as an obstacle to be gotten around. As with many stories, "closure" is in the mind of the storyteller, but the story continues for the characters in it. This gentleman and I came around to issues of racism several times in our work together.

Race and gender are emotional issues in this culture. Although they are obvious, clients may not want to bring them up, particularly if they have come to like and trust the social worker, for fear of damaging the relationship or embarrassing the worker. During a workshop at the Ackerman Institute, family therapist Ken Hardy (2004) remarked that "race is so important that we can't talk about it."

Social workers need to seriously ask themselves how comfortable they are with these issues. It is not uncommon for people to act like they are receptive to feedback yet become defensive when the inherent patriarchal and racist attitudes endemic in this society are pointed out in them. Tamasese and Waldgrave (1993, p. 75) say that the initial reaction of dominant-culture workers is to feel attacked and to display one of several responses: "paralysis," where workers' feelings of culpability and shame prevent them from taking any action; "individualising," where workers separate themselves from the histories that helped place them in their lives and claim to be exempt from the collective effect of (and responsibility for) oppression; or "patronising," where workers claim to understand and be able to represent the experiences of a discriminated-against group better than the actual members of that group. Again, truly listening to a client without defensiveness is challenging, and committing to specific changes in one's relationship with a client gives away the social worker's power and control. Workers are not supposed to have problems, and seeing these problems in oneself can be particularly threatening.

Most dominant-culture social workers have been exposed to and educated into these negative stories, and the ability to reach beyond them requires no small amount of honest questioning and self-examination. The stories that minority clients bring to the relationship about dominant-culture professionals are likely to affect and reinforce each party's opinion of the other. Authenticating the complaints of those who have experienced discrimination and oppression is not an easy task, as Tamasese and Waldgrave (1993) note:

> We are not interested in "politically correct guilt" or "white and male flagellation." Our concern springs from the pain of our [minority and female] colleagues, who feel we have failed them. We trust their pain and their ability to discern the significant obstacles, and they trust us to take them seriously and act honourably. The process is a vulnerable one for both sides. (p. 36)

Even though most White social workers and most male social workers would avow antiracist and antisexist practices, the difficulty is that they seldom experience what people who have been marginalized experience (Tamasese & Waldgrave, 1993). Whites often do not even see themselves as having a race, as the title of Janet E. Helms's (1992) book *A Race Is a Nice Thing to Have: A Guide to Being a White Person or Understanding the White Persons in Your Life* suggests. The impact of this ignorance can be profound. Peggy Davis, an African American law professor, coined the term *micro-aggression* to describe the daily oppressive experiences of minorities caused by majority-culture people who would deny their actions were racially biased, even though they were based on stereotypes (as cited in Silver, 2002, p. 227).

Racial stereotypes are a major discourse in our culture; as a result, they are not experienced as a story per se but as the way the world is ordered, as the truth. Most dominant-culture members are not even aware of these stereotypes influencing their behavior, although, in fact, tacitly they do (Lawrence, 1987). Micro-aggressions are subtle, often automatic, nonverbal put-downs of Blacks by Whites; they are incessant and cumulative assaults on Black self-esteem from an attitude of presumed superiority. They can be seen in the way minority-member comments might be subtly written off, not given full credence, or treated as needing further confirmation. All this is conveyed in the look on the listener's face, by the turning of the head or eyes.

A group of narrative therapists in New Zealand has developed what it calls "just therapy" (Tamasese & Waldgrave, 1993). These therapists assume that the best judges of injustice are members of those groups that have been treated unjustly. As a result, White therapists often have Maori consultants to assist them in seeing areas of injustice that come up not only in the treatment of Maori families but in the organization itself.

Such collaborations between members of dominant and nondominant groups can make important contributions to reducing the blindness and the perpetuation of unjust practices caused by privilege. However, members of oppressed groups should not be placed in the position of always having to explain themselves to dominant-group members, a situation that is not uncommon in social work classes when issues of diversity arise and minority students are put on the spot to represent their racial or ethnic group.

## The Micropolitics of Social Work Practice: The Therapeutic Relationship in a Narrative Approach

Narrative treatment attempts to address questions of culture, power, and social influence initially through finding ways to address the imbalance of power in the treatment relationship, and then by looking at the sociopolitical dilemmas clients face. Narrative work requires social workers to be sensitive to the power politics of gender inequities, heterosexual dominance, race discrimination, cultural differences, and class inequalities, both within relationships and in the construction of problems. With this knowledge, practitioners can work on ways to help clients identify, embrace, and honor their resistance to their oppression. By focusing on clients as experts in their own lives and being open to alternative knowledge from them, narrative practice seeks to subvert the expert power of the worker and the institution. Finally, a narrative approach requires social workers to confront the moral and ethical responsibilities resulting from their actions; workers can do this, in part, by making their work accountable to clients (Franklin, 1998).

Positivist research indicates that the treatment relationship is important for helping people change (Orlinsky, Ronnestad, & Willutzki, 2004). However, the therapeutic relationship is typically explained in a one-way direction. What do you, as the worker, need to do to effect change in the person coming to see you? Depending on the worker's theory, he or she initiates a relationship through joining with a family (Minuchin, 1974) or engaging with individuals (Compton et al., 2005). Minuchin talks about developing a personal connection with each member of the family as well as with the family as a whole. Compton et al. identify social workers' initial tasks as inviting participation, understanding the presenting problems, comprehending what the person(s) wants, and clarifying expectations/developing a preliminary contract for working together. Psychodynamic writers, who recognize that the treatment relationship can be affected by clients as well as by workers, discuss the importance of being aware of transference reactions of the client to the worker, which are said to be based on the client's early caretaker experiences, and countertransference reactions of the worker to the client, where it is the worker's early experiences that influence the interactions.

The dynamics of the contemporary world of practice frame the treatment relationship. Typically, the client goes or is sent to see the worker because he or she is troubled or needs to be "fixed." The worker is an allegedly untroubled and unbroken person with expertise in helping people who are in need of fixing. When the client comes in for treatment, the conversation is usually lopsided, with the worker asking questions and the client giving answers, or at least being expected to. The worker is an expert with expert knowledge and the client is the subject of that knowledge.

The narrative approach also considers the relationship between worker and client to be important, though the understanding of that relationship differs from the conceptualizations of traditional treatment models. Although narrative practitioners acknowledge that the relationship between worker and client can never be truly equal, they do not see themselves as experts. Instead, they talk about trying to become an "appreciative ally" (Madsen, 2007, p. 22). This relationship stance comprises connection, respectful curiosity, openness, and hopefulness. Connection means taking the time to get to know someone before intervening. Respectful curiosity means thinking about what it might be like to be the person and to experience his or her life under the circumstances. Openness requires workers to be receptive to the good and the bad of people and to take them for who they are. Finally, hopefulness means focusing on what could be instead of what is not. A belief in the resourcefulness of people, families, and communities takes precedence over the idea of brokenness or deficiency. Madsen, in discussing the importance of practitioners' attitude in clinical work, talks about the empowering ability of workers who make themselves accountable to the clients by working *with* clients instead of *on* clients.

## The Impact of Client Narratives on Workers and the Worker's Impact in Response

The impact on social workers of the work they do has been given very little examination because the treatment relationship has been viewed as one-sided. A two-way approach to looking at the therapeutic relationship, as encouraged by narrative therapy's diminution of power relations, emphasizes the life-changing nature of this work on the social worker (White, 1997). What is it in clients' telling of their stories that enriches the lives of social workers? How can social workers use this experience to help them work with others? How can social workers let clients know what they have contributed both to the worker and to others? The actions arising in response to these questions have been termed *taking-it-back practices* (White, p. 132).

Moving from a one-sided to a two-way view of the therapeutic relationship affords workers a number of new options. White (1997) discusses an array of opportunities that become available through a two-way approach to the treatment relationship, including "inclusion"; "new associations"; "re-engagements"; "re-membered lives"; "re-voicing therapy"; "solution knowledges"; "skills of therapeutic practice"; and "purposes and intentions, values and commitments" (pp. 132–142).

Inclusion means realizing the privilege social workers have in being included so powerfully in other people's lives. It is easy to get so involved in completing paperwork and worrying about failed appointments that workers forget how difficult it is to open up to a stranger about one's life. When the difficulty and vulnerability required of clients is recognized by workers, they can embrace the significance of this in their own lives (I am a person who is privileged with the sensitive information of people's lives) and appreciate the trust that is being extended to them. Workers might then be more understanding of clients' reluctance and fears about attending sessions, more sensitive to their guardedness, and more aware of keeping clients' confidences. They might also appreciate what is being asked of clients when a large diagnostic or intake form has to be filled out in the initial session. If social workers indicate to clients that the requirement of so much personal information is a burden that must be jointly met, the initial interview can more readily be separated from the treatment relationship.

New associations come about when social workers help clients attribute alternative meanings to their actions and find new, previously unrecognized meanings in areas of their lives. For example, a client might cry during a session when talking about a painful sequence of events. The social worker may wonder out loud if those tears are tears of pain or tears for oneself that indicate the person is now taking care of himself or herself. Through this process, the particular meanings and events in a worker's own life can be experienced and expanded. The worker in this example may begin to consider whether recent tears he or she has shed over losses or pain might also be an indication of self-care and whether this is a sign of his or her own progress.

Re-engagement occurs as the little events and acts that contradict the problem-saturated stories of people's lives are given greater significance. By working with clients to draw out these small instances and to explore their potential as points of entry into alternative stories, social workers may begin to consider previously overlooked aspects of their own lives. As a result, workers can look at the history of their own lives in a nonblaming fashion and identify moments that can provide them with a more useful self-definition. For example, as clients discover and string together events that indicate they can stand up for themselves and draw boundaries—perhaps letting go of a disrespectful boyfriend or girlfriend, refusing to work late when their child needed them, or standing firm with their child on certain rules—workers may begin to reconsider what they have done in their own lives and may come to see themselves differently.

Re-membered lives are recovered as social workers help clients look at those people in the clients' lives who have or who would support an alternative, positive view of themselves. As a result of these therapeutic encounters, workers may find themselves reviewing their own histories and having conversations with people they might not otherwise have contacted. For instance, as a client talks about the impact a teacher had and how the teacher believed the client was better than the messages given by his or her family, the client may consider trying to seek out the former teacher to let that person know what he or she meant to the client. The worker, too, may find himself or herself considering which teachers were important and what messages they gave. The worker also may consider whether to seek out these individuals. If it turns out that both the worker and the client are successful in locating and talking with these former teachers, the worker could let the client know how his or her courage influenced the worker to seek out the teacher and the importance of that reconnection. The client is thus respected for a mutual contribution.

Re-voicing occurs when social workers find themselves recalling the image of clients they previously worked with and using what they learned from those individuals in their work with other clients and in confronting concerns in their own lives. Social workers in hospice settings often talk about what they learn about life and death through their work with terminally ill clients, and the courage that such work generates. It is interesting that this work, which tends to be less formal and not as treatment oriented, is a place where stories have always been important and where workers have given voice to their privilege of being with people at this time in their lives and to the benefits they accrue from the clients' courage.

Solution knowledges are obtained when workers recognize the creativity people use to manage the issues before them and to develop solutions, some of which work and some of which do not. Solution knowledges are coproduced through the worker-client interaction. Accumulating this information over time can give social workers an array of examples of how people can and do cope, a valuable resource that can be provided to other clients and can be used by the practitioners themselves when they face dilemmas in their own lives. For example, a single mother faced with loneliness entering her life may have found that "goofing around" with her teenaged daughter helped her avoid the more intense self-criticism and sadness that loneliness brings. As the social worker helps the client put together this story of protest against loneliness, the worker may consider how his or her own child has helped in such situations and how, perhaps, he or she might spend a bit more time with the child that night. The social worker may also consider exploring with future clients who experience loneliness or sadness whether positive time spent with their children has served the same function for them.

When social workers ask for feedback from clients about what seems to be working and what seems to be most useful, they receive information that can be used to help them improve their skills. When workers get into the habit of asking clients at the end of each session whether the conversation was useful and what makes the client say it was or was not, they can use this feedback to focus their skills. This benefit accrues not just to the workers themselves, but to their other clients, too. For instance, a worker could say, "Before we set our next appointment, could you tell me whether the talk we had today felt useful or not to you?" If the client responds that the talk was useful, the worker could then ask, "What do you think made it useful to you? Anything specific I said or we discussed? What might be more helpful to you now?" Similar questions can be posed if the client states the session was not useful. Obviously, conversational approaches that receive good feedback may be used more often than those that receive negative feedback.

Finally, when social workers ask people to see their problems outside themselves and think about how these problems have influenced them to do, think, or say things against their better judgment, they are recognizing the moral aspect of people's lives and asking them to think about their purposes and intentions as well as the values and commitments they hold dear. Engaging with clients as they assess what is important to them may lead social workers to undertake a reevaluation in their own lives. For example, a couple may complain that fighting and arguing are not how they want to run their lives and that their behavior in their conflict is not who they want to be. But when conflict enters their relationship, they lose their better judgment. As a result of the discussion, the worker may start thinking about how he or she gets locked into emotional conflict with his or her partner and may come to understand how this behavior is not "who they really are" and does not reflect "who they want to be."

When social workers ask clients to specify what their better judgment is and what principles stand behind it, the clients are defining what they value and what obligations and duties they stand by. In the process, both the clients and the workers have the opportunity to consider what their values are in establishing the basis for their better judgments. People can begin to explain what they stand for in life. In the previous example of the couple who engage in fighting and arguing, the discussion might become one in which the clients talk about what seems to be behind the need to win and discover that having a say, being heard, and maintaining control over their lives have become important values. If engaged in their narrative, workers, as well as clients, can become more aware of the moral effect of their actions in the world.

■ ■ ■

A few years ago when I was leaving a social service agency, clients were pleased to find out that I would not forget them and their work by including them in this book. We discussed what I would use of their experience, and that process let them know that the story did not end with my leaving. Knowing that you, the client, are a person and not a case is important in developing relationships; knowing that we, the social workers, can learn from our clients is important in developing ourselves professionally and personally.

## The DSM and Professional Language as Tools of Power

The DSM-IV-TR (American Psychiatric Association, 2000) is a useful instrument for prescribing medications and collecting medical insurance reimbursements. It can also be valuable for some clients to know that what they are experiencing has a name and that they are not alone in having the problem. Some clients consider DSM-IV-TR diagnoses to be the names of diseases that attack them and not a statement of their personhood (Wetchler, 1999), though the views of mental illness expressed in popular psychology tend to push in the other direction (Focht & Beardslee, 1996). Diagnosis can offer hope to people, who then think a treatment may be available, and the classification and the naming of symptoms as a disorder can provide relief to family members who may have been blaming themselves for another member's feelings, thoughts, and behaviors. (Mothers seem to have to endure a disproportionate amount of the blame here.)

The difficulty occurs when the diagnosis locates cultural disorders and problems in the body of the client. Such descriptions do not take into account what is occurring outside the body but instead locate difficulties in the body as a disease, making medical interventions the treatment of choice. Diagnosis can become a problem, in particular, when the person is seen as the object of the process, with little to no active role in his or her own life. This process of objectification (Drewery, Winslade, & Monk, 2000) can be especially troublesome when the client entirely accepts it. For example, a woman comes to an intake stating that she has an intermittent explosive disorder and she brings her partner, who is often the subject of the explosions, because she "can't remember what triggers it, but the partner will know." In this way, the client abdicates any personal responsibility for her actions and eliminates from consideration the possibility that she might have control over them.

Compare this to a woman who comes in saying that she is depressed but knows that drugs alone are not the answer and would like to figure out ways to fight her depression if she can. In the first instance, the client has no sense of agency, no belief that she can take an active role in her own life; as a result, she has very few options other than taking a pill. In the second, the client sees herself as taking an active role in managing her depression and wants help to determine how she can best do this, realizing that medication may have a part to play in her efforts.

Biochemical explanations can be a great help in developing tools to control symptoms but can also be used to cover up issues of oppression, as the mother's little helpers did in the 1950s and 1960s for depressed married women. Drewery et al. note,

> We believe that it is possible to show that it is more politically advantageous and more personally healthy to be positioned as an agentic subject—as a speaker in, and therefore a producer of, the conversation that produces one's life—than as an object of a conversation about oneself. . . . Objectifying people, reifying mental concepts, transforming the person into a subject, and inviting to take up more or less passive positions are all actions that are achieved though linguistic forms. (pp. 252–253)

They argue that a DSM diagnosis may work in ways "that erase the sufferers, totalizing their existence as the diagnosis" (Drewery et al., p. 257) if workers and clients accept that invitation.

Even as a scientific instrument, the DSM can be attacked for being low on reliability and validity and for having categories subject to political processes (Kutchins & Kirk, 1997). For example, based on a vote of the members of the American Psychiatric Association, the diagnostic category of homosexuality as a mental disorder was redefined in the DSM-III to apply only to those who were not satisfied with their sexual orientation; in the DSM-IV, homosexuality was eliminated altogether as a mental disorder (Coleman, 1984). "The concepts of normality and abnormality, even those offered in the DSM-IV, are inventions more than discoveries" (Raskin & Lewandowski, 2000, p. 16).

Constructionists are contemptuous of systems like the DSM that claim scientific objectivity at the expense of the subjectivity of the person experiencing the problem. However, because social workers wish to be employed in the mental health system, they live with this method of categorization and find ways to address its difficulties. Like any other facet of the treatment process, diagnosis can be a tool; it is not an end in itself.

## Exercises

### Exercise 1: Deconstructing Common Beliefs in Social Work

Have students break into groups of about six students each. Ask each group to nominate a reporter who will take notes on the discussion that ensues as each group answers the following questions:

1. Social work takes a *person-in-situation* or *person-in-environment* view of client problems. What does this mean? Where does this perspective come from? What are the assumptions behind it?

2. Social work takes a firm stand on issues of *social justice*. What is social justice? Where does this concept come from? What are the assumptions behind it?

3. Social work takes a strong stance on *self-determination*. What does this mean? What are the exceptions? Where does this concept come from? What are the assumptions behind it?

An example of what might result from such a discussion follows:

1. **Social work takes a firm stand on *confidentiality*. What does this mean? What are the exceptions? Where does this concept come from?**

   *Confidentiality means keeping what you learn in a conversation secret. Or, does it mean not telling people who might use the information against the person who told it? Any injury received by your disclosure could lead to both malpractice and ethical charges against you. The information is only as confidential as the client wishes it to be. Clients can tell anyone what they told you or what you said. You are not supposed to do the same.*

*There are many exceptions to client confidentiality because many different interests are concerned about obtaining information. Client information is circulated in agencies through supervision and case presentation. Clients are not usually invited, so maybe what is said in supervision about the confidential information is more confidential than the information itself. Information put in records can be seen by quality assurance personnel and auditors for insurance companies, Medicaid, and Medicare. Legally, you are supposed to report to the proper authorities any information specific to danger to others or to the client as well as any reasonable suspicions of abuse. Reporting crimes is confusing: If your state does not protect you and your ethical code says you should not make such reports, you are in a bind. If the client gives written consent, you are supposed to share information. If you are subpoenaed, you need to look at the state law to see if you have a legal privilege to protect the information.*

*The ideas behind confidentiality are twofold. One idea is that if people cannot trust that their information will not be used against them, they have less incentive to provide it. If the social worker's practice theory requires him or her to obtain sensitive information to provide help, then such information must be acquired if the treatment is to be halfway successful. Keeping communications confidential is important because society sees being able to seek treatment for problems as important. Losing access to some information is a cost society is willing to pay if it means that more people receive help through treatment. A second idea behind confidentiality has to do with professionalism and power. Developing confidential relationships is an important aspect of most professions, and social work needed to claim this ability if it was to be seen as a profession. With the duty of confidentiality, you show yourself as a professional who has some power because what is said to you is important. If you are set up professionally to protect secrets, then clients might expect to tell their secrets to you.*

*Confidentiality accords supreme value to the integrity of the individual. Having your own secrets protected is an important individual right of privacy. However, with confidentiality you strip away the client from his or her loved ones by not being allowed to talk to them without permission, usually written, from the client. It is an ethic that focuses on separateness and that at times can discourage community.*

After the groups have discussed the questions, have them rejoin the class as a whole and ask the reporter for each small group to report, question by question. Pull together the different group comments on the board. Then ask if anyone sees patterns and if some basic assumptions, such as individualism, the idea of human rights, a capitalist economic system, or democracy, have had an impact on these concepts. Students also could be asked: How does social work's need to professionalize affect the interpretation of these concepts? Can you conceive of a different kind of social work that might reach a different interpretation?

## Exercise 2: Discussing an Experience of One's Own Marginalization

This exercise, developed by Freedman and Combs (2003) and with their permission presented in its entirety, represents an attempt to get beyond a "who's right" view of oppression, which shuts down communication and understanding. Because it asks students to reflect on their own experiences with difference, oppression, and marginalization, it can leave them feeling vulnerable. Thus, sensitivity and care on the part of the instructor and students are needed.

General instructions for facilitators:

> Set the frame for these questions by telling your group you will ask some questions to invite each of them to share some stories of times, places, or contexts in which he or she has experienced marginalization in a de-legitimizing or disempowering way.
>
> *Say that different group members will have come from backgrounds that offered each of them different degrees of privilege, and therefore each person's experience will be quantitatively and qualitatively different. Nonetheless, we are asking for stories of some sort of hurtful marginalization, and we believe that everyone has experiences of this sort in one way or another.*
>
> Take these questions one at a time, giving each person in the group a chance to share his or her answer before moving to the next question. (Our intention is to facilitate an *interweaving* of people's individual stories, *not* for each person to experience the complete process in turn.)
>
> Ask group members to wait until the last part of the session for interaction and commenting on each other's stories. We are interested in people having an experience of their stories unfolding. Our experience is that this is more likely to happen if participants go

through the entire structured experience before stepping out of it to reflect on it. Assure people that they will have a chance to respond to each other at the end.

Keep one eye on the clock. Try to save a half hour at the end for an interactive group experience.

Questions for participants:

1. You have probably already reflected at some time or other on how the culture (if not at home, then at school, in the neighborhood, religious institutions, the media, etc.) modeled norms, standards, ideals, values, hierarchies, and the like for you. The stories you saw being lived out within the influence of these norms showed you who was a legitimate member of society; they told you whether you qualified for positions of power and influence in the world. What *specific incident* can you recall in which you got the message that you didn't "measure up" or belong (by virtue of race, class, gender, or membership in some group)?

    Facilitator—encourage the story of a *particular incident*, rather than a generalization. If the person insists he or she never experienced marginalization, or says he or she was never bothered by such experiences when they did occur, encourage them to pass for the moment and to keep searching as they listen to other people's stories.

2. What was the meaning of this incident to you? What generalizations did incidents like this one invite you to make?

    Facilitators might want to ask: Anything about who "counts" and who doesn't? About who has a voice and who doesn't? About what the possibilities were for your future? What paths were open to you and what ones were closed? What did the incident teach you about power and privilege?

3. What have been some of the effects of this marginalization on your life and your relationships?

4. Even though this marginalization occurred, what is an example of a time you were able to act outside of its limits? (To experience voice, agency, choice, freedom to act according to your own values, etc.)

    Facilitator—encourage the story of a particular incident.

5. How were you able to transcend the stories and the models offered by the marginalizing stories, practices, and ways of being? What does it mean that you were able to act as you did in this new incident? What person or people stood by you through this or went before you letting you know this was possible? What does it show you give value to? What did you learn in the process that might help clients transcend similar models?

6. What possibilities might it open for your future if this way of being becomes even more available to you? How would relationships between people that you work with in therapy be different if this way of being was part of the dominant societal norms and values?

   Facilitator—now offer an opportunity for people to respond to anything they have heard from each other. Then, if there is time, ask them to comment on the process.

CHAPTER 3

# Social Work Ethics, Postmodern Ethics, and Where the Twain Shall Meet

This chapter concentrates on the role of values in the social work profession and looks at the function of ethical codes and the National Association of Social Workers Code of Ethics (NASW, 1999) in particular. I discuss the core social work values that are seen as flowing from the profession's mission and the ethical principles identified as being consistent with those values. Following that, I talk about the purposes and shortcomings of ethical codes. I then look at how a narrative approach to social work meets the profession's value test. I frame my discussion of how ethics are approached from a narrative perspective by focusing on the fundamental moral obligations of social workers who take on caring roles and how sharing stories leads to certain duties. Finally, I discuss several ethical dilemmas.

## Social Work Values and the Profession

Social work is a profession not only of skills and knowledge but, perhaps more important, of values. Though values are most obvious when social workers engage in political action to promote social justice, they are continuously involved in direct practice, too. Social work practice theories are never neutral or value free (Laird, 1995). All practice theories have assumptions about what is important and desirable, what means are legitimate to meet ends, and what rights professional expertise confers on workers to allow them to ignore client requests or desires "for their own good." How the social work profession wishes to see itself, and be seen by others, is well encapsulated in the preamble of the NASW *Code of Ethics* (1999, Preamble section, para. 1–2), which states:

> The primary mission of the social work profession is to enhance human well-being and help meet the basic human needs of all people,

with particular attention to the needs and empowerment of people who are vulnerable, oppressed, and living in poverty. ...Social workers promote social justice and social change with and on behalf of clients.... Social workers are sensitive to cultural and ethnic diversity and strive to end discrimination, oppression, poverty, and other forms of social injustice.... Social workers seek to enhance the capacity of people to address their own needs.

The NASW *Code of Ethics* (1999) starts with a mission statement, goes on to describe six core social work values that distinguish the profession, then presents broad ethical principles associated with the core values, and finally defines specific ethical standards of conduct that apply to different types of professional relationships. The standards tend to structure conduct in the template of a traditional psychodynamic treatment relationship. Great care is given to protecting the inviolability of the treatment relationship with clients, while recognizing that some of those clients may be organizations or communities.

Codes of ethics serve a number of purposes. They protect clients by stating what behavior should be expected of professionals. They provide education and guidance to professionals on how to handle ethical issues. They enhance the profession's status, because such standards are part of the criteria for a "position" to become a profession. Similarly, they create a professional identity by stating the profession's core purpose and the values to which members are to aspire. They allow for self-policing of the profession by providing professionals the ability to sanction those of their own who have violated the ethical code (Banks, 2003).

Ethical decision making in social work tends to be a top-down affair. As mentioned, ethical codes are based on ethical principles and, as such, they make the decisions behind certain actions justifiable. The values in the codes are developed by professionals and have little client input. Unlike legal precedents, which are modified by case facts, codes of ethics, being derived from principles, are meant to be proactive, not reactive. The necessary vagueness that results may be beneficial because it requires workers to use ethical judgment (Murphy, 1997). There are two traditions of ethical analysis that social workers can draw on when making these decisions: applying broad ethical principles that help to define whether an action is inherently right (or good) or inherently wrong (or bad, deontological), or determining the rightness (or goodness) or wrongness (or badness) of an action based on assessing what will be the consequences for all involved (teleological; Reamer, 1999).

Codes of ethics are also used to regulate worker behavior. Most states that license social workers have ethical codes in their statutes or regulations, and these function in addition to the code promulgated by NASW. Sometimes these two codes, the state and the professional, do not match up, particularly where a state's code of ethics is meant to cover a variety of helping professions, such as counseling and marriage and family therapy as well as social work.

If a state's code of ethics is violated, the social worker risks losing his or her license to practice. This action can greatly restrict a person's employment opportunities in the field. Most states have Web sites that allow people to check the status of individual professional licenses; states often inform other licensed social workers of sanctions against specific workers through newsletters. If the professional standard is violated, the social worker risks losing his or her professional standing by removal from the voluntary professional association (e.g., NASW or the Clinical Social Work Association) and by sanctions that are made public in the professional newspaper. Most states have agreements with the state professional committee so that violations of professional ethics are made known to each board.

All states require reporting the abuse or neglect of children, the elderly, and the developmentally disabled. Most authorities recommend, and some state statutes require, reporting to designated authorities and warning third parties when clients have made serious threats to other people's physical well-being or real property. Some states do not give social workers immunity from reporting felonies, and they usually have the same responsibility as ordinary citizens to report to the police. In some states, social workers are required to report domestic violence against adults to the police or to the adult protective service agency. Information about these statutes can be spotty, requiring social workers to either contact the state professional association or delve into the statutes themselves. (In talking with two traditional agencies in one state that had a spouse-abuse reporting requirement, neither appeared aware of the law, which had been enacted more than 10 years earlier and was covered in professional education.) These statutes are reinforced by professional codes of ethics that have a statutory exception to the confidentiality of client communications, stating that the law will take precedence over the ethical code.

## Social Work Ethical Principles

The core social work values, as described in the NASW *Code of Ethics* (1999, Preamble, para. 3), are "service, social justice, dignity and worth of the person, importance of human relationships, integrity, and competence." All forms of social work practice must be weighed on the scales of these values. These core social work values may seem generic, but compare them to the values underlying medical bioethics, which is based on autonomy (self-determination), nonmalfeasance (do no harm), beneficence (act for the benefit of others), and justice (treat people fairly; Beauchamp & Childress, 2001). Social work values are not as generic as they at first may appear.

The six core social work values (service, social justice, etc.) are further delineated through ethical principles. A major problem facing the profession is that these ideals are becoming ever more difficult to maintain in the current practice environment. To fulfill one's duty of service, the principle suggests that the social worker "help people in need and address social problems" (NASW, 1999, Ethical Principles section, first principle). Ideally, service should weigh more heavily for social workers than self-interest. One function of a professional social worker is to gain people's trust, which is fostered by the belief that the worker has the client's best interests at heart. Consider the betrayal that clients would experience if they were to learn that hospital social workers were discharging them only to those services in which a group of doctors at the hospital owned shares, despite cost and need considerations.

Realistically, social workers find themselves in multiple ethical dilemmas that place their livelihood and self-interest in conflict with their ability to serve others. Some workers struggle with their personal desire to keep "easy" clients and discharge "difficult" ones. In fact, the organizational systems of many agencies promote this situation. Agencies that provide clinical services operate on the medical model with a requirement of diagnosis before treatment, and agency finances are dependent on treatment being billed based on services provided. If a client does not show up for a session or cancels late, it is unlikely that the worker can fill that time. In third-party payer situations (private insurance or Medicaid), it will be difficult to collect for the missed hour unless the client agrees to pay directly.

Social workers, whose profession proclaims a commitment to working with the poor and who are typically less expensive helpers than psychiatrists or psychologists, are likely to see clients with limited financial resources. Even if the client could be billed, social work clients are unlikely to be able to compensate the agency for the time they used. Most agencies require workers to deliver a minimum number of hours of direct client contact per month to justify their position (service units), which leaves workers with the problem of filling up any time lost with another billable client hour. Some studies (see Garfield, 1994, for a review) have shown that a significant proportion of clients do not show up after the first or second outpatient session; as a result, workers must book almost every hour to be sure they have the billable units required by the end of the month or year. This situation creates barriers to social workers who wish to use an unrushed, patient approach to working with hard-to-reach clients, because the workers are penalized by this system when clients miss appointments.

The value of social justice is important to social workers, and the profession commits practitioners to challenge social injustice. Yet, social workers often find themselves as "instruments of the state" and placed in situations in which they are expected to continue oppressive policies. For example, social workers in one state are not exempted from reporting felonies, whereas a variety of other professionals, including psychiatrists and psychologists, are. Despite its intent, this policy functions to provide heightened policing of vulnerable, lower income populations, who are not likely to receive the extended services of higher-waged helping professionals, and to make social workers the "police."

As a new worker in a mental health clinic, I was asked to do suicide assessments for inmates in the nearby county jail. The inmates I saw were already on suicide watch, which meant they were each in a small cell with a thin mat, no toilet seat, and under surveillance 24 hours a day by video camera. In addition, they were forced to wear a paper gown that inevitably was torn off or in tatters by the time I got to interview them. Essentially, I was interviewing naked men under very stressful conditions to decide whether they were still suicidal. In hindsight, it is somewhat embarrassing to say that I was introduced to this situation as "the way things had to be to protect the inmate," and I accepted the status quo and conducted my interviews. Fortunately, the local legal aid society was more astute and eventually the practice was abandoned because of a federal court order. Social workers do have opportunities to address social injustice, and inculcating the value of social justice can help them see the injustices occurring in everyday life.

When truly using a person-in-situation perspective, social workers often do notice the way in which the situation patterns the problem behavior, despite the focus on the individual. If a social worker's treatment model, such as cognitive therapy or solution-focused treatment, does not incorporate a political dimension to the work being done, then the primary focus will be strictly on individual change without a sense of the broader context. The current models of social work, and those encouraged in most brief treatment approaches, do not examine the political issues of power in the relationship of worker and client or in that of the client to the rest of society. When workers ignore the voices of their clients, they risk reinforcing clients' oppression.

Social workers respect the inherent dignity and worth of the person, and, in many ways, this is the most essential of social work values. The client's right to self-determination is derived from this value. The extent to which we objectify clients is the extent to which we may abuse our power over them "for their own good." Arguably, any model that focuses solely on diagnoses, labels, or narrow treatment goals diminishes the inherent worth of the individual. If people are simply passive problem carriers who are to follow the suggestions of the social worker, where does the person's agency (i.e., ability to take an active role in one's own life) and human dignity come into play? An understanding of diversity and the many ways people experience the world is important for a full appreciation of the dignity and worth of the individual. Every person brings to the therapeutic encounter his or her own unique story of successes, hardships, and failures.

Social workers should recognize the central importance of human relationships. Practice models based on systems and ecological perspectives tend to highlight the central importance of human relationships and areas such as social support. From a person-in-situation perspective, the human environment is critical in determining the health and happiness of individuals. Some models of treatment give a great deal of importance to the client's relationship to the worker, over which some semblance of control can be obtained, but do not see the client's environment as the source of coping and change. As a nod to acknowledging the importance of the environment, clients in managed-care settings are often discharged to self-help groups to maintain whatever progress has been achieved. Although self-help groups can be helpful, think of what gains might accrue to clients if social workers took on the more difficult, but potentially more effective, work of engaging clients' specific environmental resources.

Social workers must demonstrate integrity and behave in a trustworthy fashion. Can social workers always tell the truth? Should they? Integrity and trustworthiness would seem to be important prerequisites to securing the trust of clients. Counseling educator Derald Wing Sue (2005) points out that a minority client might ask a worker if he or she has ever laughed at racial jokes. The client assumes a worker in this culture has, and the question is not whether the worker is a racist, but whether he or she will be honest with the client. Or, when social workers use pejorative labels for clients in lunchroom gossip or even in supervision sessions, have they betrayed the trust of the relationship when they next meet with clients and act as if those thoughts do not exist? Workers often give the rationale for such behavior as "keeping them sane," but does such talk in any way change the dynamics of the treatment relationship? Does it put more distance between the worker and the client? Does it misuse clients' trust in social workers?

Social workers often have social control functions required by statute that override any trust relationship with a client. Reporting suspicions of abuse or the worker's belief in the potential for violence to others acts against the trustworthiness of the relationship. With the Health Insurance Portability and Accountability Act, social workers, as health care providers, are now required to provide clients with extensive information about the actual confidentiality of communications within the treatment relationship, although this often is treated in a perfunctory manner through repetition. Despite legal responsibilities, social workers are often torn over whether to report a suspicion of abuse or neglect to an overworked and often mismanaged child welfare system. Workers (and students) wonder if they are being untrustworthy when they make reports about clients. Have they misused the client's trust to get the client into trouble? Being transparent in work with clients means letting them know what the social worker is doing or will have to do. Working collaboratively with clients helps to reduce the number of situations in which the worker believes he or she is acting in an untrustworthy manner.

Social workers practice within their areas of competence and develop and enhance their professional expertise. Workers should not assume knowledge they do not possess, particularly when using evidence-based practices. Given the economics of treatment today, brief treatment modalities that have empirical support are highly valued. These models, particularly those derived from cognitive/behavioral theory, make assumptions about what the cause of the problem is and, based on the underlying theory, what specific techniques should be applied to alleviate the problem. When a social worker assumes specific knowledge of the cause of a problem, then he or she also assumes specific knowledge about intervening in it or referring the client to another professional who can.

A social worker exhibits his or her competence by making a suitable referral for specialized care based upon reasonable information. The responsibility to make a referral is clear when the underlying problem may be physical. For example, when a client comes in complaining about severe headaches, it is important to refer the client to a competent physician for an examination of possible physical causes before delving into emotional or social causes. Time wasted can be highly detrimental to the client, not only in terms of resources, but also in terms of the potential risk of further deterioration. In one instance, a woman expressed mood swings, sadness, and headaches. She was treated for depression without a full medical examination. One day at work, her headache became particularly intense and she went to a hospital emergency room. A CAT scan showed a very large brain tumor, whose symptoms included depression and headache. The client had always considered the problem to be different from a psychological one, but her therapist had convinced her otherwise. The professional value of competence encourages social workers to increase their expert knowledge, but possession of expert professional knowledge should not lead workers to ignore clients' unique expertise and first-person knowledge of their particular problem.

Unfortunately, competence often focuses on the need to acquire more information about how people function and what different, often simplistic, models are available for working with them. However, most social workers work in areas of great complexity, requiring flexibility in order to "do what needs to be done." Social workers assist people with intricate problems that occur in varying contexts and involve numerous people who have differing interests (Parton, 2003). Experienced social workers routinely confront uncertainty and must be open to change aspects of the work that are poorly addressed in simple treatment paradigms.

Competence is also an issue in a competitive market of clinicians who attempt to develop niches for themselves in their advertising. For example, being a trauma specialist can be a marketable subspecialty, and clients rightfully assume that some type of rigorous training is involved for those who specialize in this area. Yet licensing cannot keep up with all possible subspecialties, and accreditation is often under the jurisdiction of those who provide the training. Clients, thus, are left on their own without some ethical obligation on the part of social workers to work only in areas in which they are trained or are in training for.

## Social Work Values and a Narrative Approach

Is a narrative approach to social work consistent with social work values? Does it satisfy the profession's value test? Let us examine each of the core values described in the NASW *Code of Ethics* (1999).

### Service

Narrative treatment offers a strengths-based approach that goes beyond addressing just the difficulties of clients to recognizing and building on their prior successes. The focus of narrative work is on the client's stories—both the problem story and new, more beneficial stories that can exist alongside the problem story. The techniques used encourage an extension of the worker-client relationship by writing letters (Freedman & Combs, 1996; White & Epston, 1990), inviting friends and family to sessions (Lobovits et al., 1995), developing audiences for new stories (Lobovits et al.), and holding parties or celebrations for clients (Epston, White, & "Ben," 1995; Freeman, Epston, & Lobovits, 1997). Use of a *reflecting team*, where colleagues who have observed a session switch places with the worker and client, who then observe these colleagues discussing their observations about the session (White, 1995, pp. 172–198; see also Freedman & Combs, 1996), can help to expand the client's stories, bring new understandings to the worker and client, and offer a form of supervision and feedback to the worker. The amount of time a worker allots also may extend beyond the traditional 50-minute hour to meet the needs of clients. These actions are time-consuming and can be demanding on workers who see service as an important commitment.

## Social Justice

A narrative approach, through its focus on oppression, power, and the impact of dominant discourses, presents a unique opportunity for developing organizations or communities around values and problems. Clients can exercise their knowledge and skills in these new forums for their own and others' benefit. With its sensitivity to values and culture, narrative work involves a commitment to advocating against oppression and to recognizing the blindness that comes with privilege. The establishment of problem-based leagues to protect, support, and advocate against problems; the recognized power of stories to heal; and a commitment to not retraumatize those already victimized are all ways in which a narrative approach can advance social work's commitment to social justice. Sometimes, the promotion of social justice takes symbolic form. For instance, in the case of a major narrative conference being held on ground that was colonized by Western powers, the representatives of the indigenous peoples are often recognized and paid rent by the conference organizers for the use of what had been their land.

## Inherent Dignity and Worth of a Person

Stories provide the medium through which people's character and integrity are made apparent. By listening carefully to the story of how the problem has affected the client and by focusing on the brief moments that show resistance to the influence of the problem, the worker is able to underline the client's worth and dignity, often when the client feels most bereft of such qualities. For example, when people die, no matter what their economic status, it is their stories that live on after them if those stories are witnessed and expressed. A narrative approach helps clients construct their stories to maintain their preferred outcomes. It also helps clients develop an audience for their stories to ensure they are witnessed. In addition, because the person is seen as separate from the problem, his or her ability to resist the problem is recognized and valued.

## Centrality of Human Relationships

From a narrative perspective, it is through a person's relationship with others that some stories come to be dominant and others marginalized. The community is the audience to clients' changes and is crucial to maintaining them. Discourses are developed and enacted in the community, so community and the human relationships that comprise it are important in creating and supporting change. In addition, narrative social workers are sensitive to the power dynamics inherent in the worker-client relationship and seek out clients' abilities rather than demonstrate their own expertise of the problem.

## Integrity

Transparency is used as a way to keep as much power as possible in clients' hands so as to not further their oppression by the problem. Transparency is evident in making notes available to clients, writing letters to describe and expand upon session events, using reflecting teams that assist rather than evaluate clients, and understanding that the words used to describe a person have an impact on one's relationship with that person.

## Competence

The narrative perspective approaches expertise differently, and narrative social workers' competence is exhibited when they coconstruct new stories with clients and help them stand up to their problems. Competence is seen in narrative workers' skillful attempts to externalize problems, find alternative stories, use questions to flesh out stories, and understand that there can be many stories to each problem. This latter point is especially important because it encourages narrative workers to recognize the boundaries of their expertise and to refer clients when appropriate to other professionals. Successful narrative social workers display competence by recognizing and extending the competence of their clients.

■ ■ ■

As this discussion suggests, social work is a values-based profession and its theories and methods should be congruent with the profession's mission and core values. Therefore, a social work practice approach should strive "to enhance human well-being and help meet the basic human needs of all people, with particular attention to the needs and empowerment of people who are disadvantaged, oppressed, and living in poverty" (NASW, 1999, Preamble section, para. 1). It should promote social justice and social change with and on behalf of clients and be sensitive to cultural and ethnic diversity. It should foster empowerment by enhancing the capacity of people to address their own needs. Furthermore, it should focus on service to the client and recognize the dignity and worth of the person, the importance of human relationships, integrity, and competence. A values-based approach to clinical social work practice would try to integrate all these elements into its makeup; a narrative approach explicitly attempts to do so and, thus, meets the profession's value test.

## The Trouble With Codes of Ethics

Ethical reasoning differs from simply applying a particular section of a code of ethics to a particular situation. Ethical reasoning focuses on what is good and moral rather than on what is correct. In this way, ethical principles can sometimes even preempt laws and regulations formed by consensus or policy. Governments can make bad laws, some discriminatory to vulnerable populations. Moral judgment may supersede legal arguments, as seen in cases of civil disobedience in which social workers (and others) have been willing to pay the penalty rather than concede their moral judgment to the law.

For example, some social workers who assist undocumented immigrants find themselves in such a bind. If the U.S. government has good relations with a repressive government, for economic or ideological reasons, individuals who are asylum seekers from that country may be denied refugee status. If you are seeing a client who is not legally in the United States, who in other circumstances could seek asylum, and whom you reasonably believe would be returned to persecution in his or her homeland, would you fulfill your legal duty and report the person to the government? In earlier times, would you have returned a runaway slave? Would you have complied with Jim Crow segregation laws in your agency? Would these actions constitute ethical professional behavior?

Though we say that social workers follow the laws we so scrupulously teach in MSW programs, many, in fact, do not disclose their suspicions of abuse despite statutory requirements. Reporting is at least partially conditioned on workers' experiences with the local child welfare system and the general state of that system, though reporting laws do not make these considerations. If a social worker had previously reported a similar case and it was not followed up, the worker might be less likely to report again.

Even when willing to report, social workers often struggle with deciding when suspicion rises to the level of "reasonable suspicion" for reporting purposes. Though the drafters of principles and statutes would like to provide clear-cut guidelines for practice, people's lives are always more complex and one set of rules is never adequate to meet all situations. Short of seeing wounds and hearing about direct abuse, what constitutes reasonable suspicion to report child abuse? The answer is always case specific and many workers would disagree about when the criteria are met. It should come as no surprise that some practitioners decide to wait to report "until they know more," despite the law's requirement to the contrary, or use utilitarian analyses (i.e., what will be the consequences?) to determine their response, despite potential for liability for injury or possible criminal and professional misconduct charges. And if the local child welfare system is overwhelmed (unfortunately, an all too common occurrence under current fiscal constraints), the social worker's benchmark for reasonable suspicion might move a bit higher. Perhaps these are not justifiable excuses for not reporting under the law, but it would be naive to believe this analysis does not occur.

Despite disclaimers in the NASW *Code of Ethics* that state it is just one tool in ethical decision making, a 21-page ethical code constitutes a rule book. Some sections of the code, such as Ethical Standard 1.03 Informed Consent (NASW, 1999), which discusses the information clients should be given before receiving services, go into such detail that they can only be thought of as constituting specific rules.

A traditional ethical analysis that makes use of an ethical code essentially follows the same form of argument as a legal analysis. In an ethical analysis, the situation giving rise to the ethical dilemma is placed in a context that allows the features of the dilemma to be identified. The professional isolates the essential pieces of information relevant to the ethical code and focuses only on those. Similarly, in a legal analysis, lawyers listen to clients' stories and ask questions that pull together the elements of either a civil cause of action and possible exceptions or a crime and possible defenses. The events as laid out in the clients' stories must be lined up into professional categories for the lawyer to do his or her work.

Ethical dilemmas presented to social work students in course work are described according to the standards or values of the profession. However, various ethical standards can be used to justify opposite positions in ethical dilemmas. Reamer (1999), therefore, proposes a ranking of values and duties, which results in a set of six principles. These six principles, Reamer argues, can be used to guide ethical decision making, and the social worker should be able to determine which of these six principles is most important in a given scenario and act in accordance with that principle.

Ethical analysis based on predetermined standards has been called "principlism" (McCarthy, 2003, Principlism section). NASW (1999) recommends not using its code in this manner. NASW says the code is not intended to be a set of rules to prescribe how social workers should act in all situations, although it does recognize that professional ethical decision making should be consistent with the spirit as well as the letter of the code. Spirit, however, is a difficult concept to define.

Codes of ethics, and the belief that such codes can "take care" of ethical issues, are problematic in several ways. First, the principles in codes can seem unrelated to the ethical and moral issues workers experience on a daily basis. It is not uncommon for field liaisons from schools of social work to go on agency visits, ask students and field supervisors how they have resolved ethical issues in practice, and receive somewhat shocked looks because the students and field supervisors are unable to see any ethical issues in their practice. Is it an ethical issue how you decide which services to provide to a client? Where does your responsibility begin and end toward clients? What happens if a client does not return for a session? If the person is under the influence of a problem, be it emotional, such as depression, or social, such as lack of transportation, does the worker have a greater obligation or does the agency's ironclad rule apply in all cases? Are extended phone conversations with clients who do not come in seen as enabling in all circumstances, or can they be seen as beneficial in some situations to strengthen the relationship? When does loyalty to a client give way to other interests? These are often rarely discussed yet vital questions for students and social workers to consider. Deconstructing the assumptions behind these practices is important if workers are not to be mere functionaries but professionals using their ethical judgment.

Second, although codes of ethics give social workers some basic format for understanding their ethical obligations, they also serve to protect workers against liability in court litigation. Codes of ethics indicate what an ethical standard of care is in the profession, an important element in determining negligence in professional malpractice cases. The standard of care is the behavior owed to a client by a reasonable professional. For social workers, NASW's code acts to circumscribe what can be reasonably expected of practitioners. Codes of ethics, therefore, can be seen as attempts to restrict the obligations of workers.

Although generally reluctant to assign professionals ethical duties beyond their codes, courts have on occasion developed a standard of care beyond the professional code, such as in the case of *Tarasoff v. Regents of the University of California* (1976). In the Tarasoff case, the California Supreme Court found mental health professionals had a duty to breach confidentiality and inform both the police and endangered third parties of serious threats to them from clients. This constitutes an ethical obligation beyond what had been imagined in the professional codes. Thus, the legal system sometimes can extend professionals' obligations to others further than the professional group wishes to go, though in general it enforces ethical standards in client-initiated malpractice actions.

Third, codes of ethics assume that there are clear-cut and well-known principles that can be applied to most situations. Is a client's attendance at meetings confidential? Are the rules around confidentiality always good? What are "compelling professional reasons" for disclosing confidential communications without client consent? What are the rights of a parent to the records of a minor child? When clients consent to insurance companies auditing their records, does that constitute informed consent given it is a requirement for reimbursement? Should clients always know when their records would be discussed in supervision or in case conferences? These questions, and a myriad of other similar ones, suggest how complex these practice situations can be and how difficult it would be to articulate clear-cut principles that are generally applicable.

As typically presented in classes, ethical dilemmas are stories that are often of little help to students because they are essentialist, a vast simplification of the situation. The way ethics stories are usually framed diminishes the multiple viewpoints of different actors in the situation (Nelson, 2002), minimizes the actual results of the decision, and denies the emotional pull of responsibility on people. The voice presented in most ethical dilemma problems is the professional's, not that of the client or others who will be affected by the decision (Poirier, 2002). As a result, the history and context of the client is usually absent, the reasons and character of the people involved are either taken as given or ignored, and the future consequences of an action are often not considered except with regard to legal liability. In short, individual circumstances are minimized and the case is examined according to generalized rules that appear objective. This provides students an illusion of certainty in a chaotic world, though they are soon frustrated by the problems this illusion creates.

Because the professional's decision is relevant to an action that is to be made either in the present or near future, the ethics story given is one with a definable ending: the decision made. As can be imagined, the life of the client, or at least that of his or her community, will continue after the authors of the ethics story put down their pens. Life stories continue long after the contact with the social worker.

## Narrative Ethics

Principlism (i.e., applying predetermined standards in ethical analyses) is only one way of reaching an ethical decision. Narrative ethics, according to Rita Charon (1994), a physician, go beyond the application of universally applicable principles and adjudicatory rules to looking at individual circumstances in a particular situation involving a specific person who exists in a specific context and has a unique history.

A narrative approach to ethics assumes each moral situation is unique and has unique meaning to the individuals involved. For example, a social worker working with a client who is elderly would need to listen carefully when making an ethical decision about placement in assisted living and not assume that all older adults feel they need to stay at home or that they have the same reason if they wish to do so. Ethical decision making can be understood only in terms of its fit with the life stories of clients. Decision making in narrative practice does not occur through unifying moral beliefs, but through open discussion that can challenge accepted views and norms (McCarthy, 2003). Professional values are not written in stone; they are the result of societal discourses and their use is influenced by the social worker's life story.

Taking an expansive view of a client's situation helps the social worker recognize the coherence of the person's narrative, identify who is telling and hearing the person's story, determine the misinterpretations and ambiguities surrounding the story, and better appreciate the meaning of an event in the individual's life (Charon, 1994). Opening up to a worldview that treats people with dignity is different, Griffith and Griffith (1994) argue, than upholding this principle because it is an ethical injunction. The need for an ethical injunction implies a "flawed reality" (p. 92) where such behavior would not exist naturally. "Selecting the reality, rather than enforcing the action, is the more therapeutic path to follow" (p. 92). Selecting a position of hope and respect for people as a new reality, rather than because hope and respect are professional injunctions ("what must be done"), helps the social worker fall more in line with the needs of the client.

Philosophers and ethicists have examined the duty owed to others in relationships. Do we as social workers only provide techniques that constitute services and clients are simply consumers of those services? Or, do we also engage in a human relationship that has its own moral obligations beyond those of buyer and seller? Philosopher Immanuel Kant's categorical imperative, reflecting the premise that good and bad are constant and clearly distinguishable, suggests that people should be treated as an end in themselves, and not as a means to an end (as cited in Kimmel, 1988).

The people who come to see us are people in trouble either with themselves or with others. Trouble is a narrative idea and there is always a story behind it. Clients are people with a plight and that plight must be recognized through their own experience of it (Bruner, 2002). They are people with a plight for whom the social worker has assumed some responsibility. It is through witnessing the story of people's plights, which social workers are in a unique position to do, that we develop a responsibility to them. Despite the enabling implications, we develop a responsibility *for* people. Service derives from this deep moral responsibility.

## An Ethics of Caring

Women, who make up the majority of social work professionals, tend to take into account the relationship between people and the significance of that relationship in making moral decisions. Feminist ethics recognizes that caring is an important factor in any decision (Tong & Williams, 2003). Knowing that a mother's caring for her child would overcome the need to "win" a dead child, the biblical Solomon asked that the child be cut in half and then awarded the child to the woman who was willing to back out of the contest rather than see the child harmed. Her relationship and loyalty to her child were more important than winning a contest against a woman who was seeking to steal the child from her. An ethic based on caring requires a richer description than just the principles involved.

Perhaps there is a more basic moral ethics that is involved in listening to clients' stories, and that is the need to be *for* clients and not merely *with* them. In physician Arthur Kleinman's book *The Illness Narratives* (1988), he talks about a client who describes her many fears, including her fear of death after an amputation because of diabetes. She asks him, "Can you give me the courage I need?" (p. 39). This very human cry for help cannot be addressed through drugs or techniques. A possible response might be: "I wish I could but perhaps together we can find you courage to tap into."

*Externalization* (White & Epston, 1990, p. 16), in which the problem is seen as separate from and outside of the client, allows the worker to be outraged at what the problem is doing to the client rather than at the client's inability to behave in a way that will reduce the problem. The question is not so much "How can we stop your fear or how irrational is it?" but "What is that damn fear doing to take away your hope?" Newton (1995), drawing from other ethicists, discusses the moral duties incurred from telling a story and listening to one. In his poetic work *The Rime of the Ancient Mariner*, Samuel Coleridge looks at the need of the Mariner to tell his story:

> *O shrieve me, shrieve me, holy man!*
> *The Hermit crossed his brow.*
> *"Say quick," quoth he "I bid thee say—*
> *What manner of man art thou?"*

The Hermit and later the Wedding-Guest accrue an obligation to listen and absolve the Mariner at the expense of other demands. "Say quick . . . What manner of man art thou?" is an archaic form of the type of assessment question most social workers ask clients every day. What claims can clients make on workers as a result of their answering workers' questions and sharing the stories of their troubles? It is perhaps this deeper human obligation that places social workers in the position of having to cope with the dilemma of societal demands versus client loyalty. Narrative ethics does not suggest how people should think or act but is instead concerned with achieving communication between people on moral issues by relating their stories (Hugman, 2003).

In medicine, narrative is offering a new perspective on bioethics. Morris (2002) notes that in exploring medicine's failure to address the issue of pain,

> Narrative does not necessarily tell us who is right or wrong. In fact, it actively undermines false confidence—born of absolutist, objectivist theories of morality—that an ethical dilemma necessarily calls for or accommodates a single right action. What narrative offers to bioethics

are means to enhance understanding of the multiple values and conflicting perspectives at stake in medical action or inaction. It offers to situate moral thought within a form of understanding that finds stories as valuable, in their own way, as statistics. . . . Bioethics has long avoided the problem of medical under-treatment. Principles, it appears, are not enough. A bioethics that addresses the international failure to provide adequate relief for pain requires something like the resources of narrative to reveal both the suffering that statistics always conceal and the complexly interwoven texture of responsibility that makes adequate relief of pain so difficult to obtain. (p. 206)

Narrative workers, by taking a sociopolitical activist stance (Monk & Gehart, 2003), focus on the contextual nature of people's problems. For example, social workers can draw on Foucault's analytic approach to illuminate the ways in which the society's discourse marginalizes and silences some groups and privileges others (Chambon, 1999). This political viewpoint focuses on overt cultural problems, such as sexism, as well as covert ones, such as defining who is sick and who is healthy. Through deconstruction, workers extend and examine the assumptions behind such issues as the demand for normality and the oppression of women.

By looking at the oppressive nature of dominant discourses, the ethical focus in narrative work is on power and the desire to resurrect and honor the knowledge of oppressed peoples who have been silenced. Where the dominant discourse is seen as truth, what is known by those who are oppressed becomes invisible and beyond issues of fairness and justice. When one looks at the effects of the truths of previous generations, such as the benefits of eugenics, the superiority of formula-based nursing over breast feeding, and the neutral effect of tobacco smoke, it becomes easy to understand the politics of truth and whose interests such truths serve.

For example, a dominant discourse about women was (and some would argue still is) that they are too emotional and irrational to be full participants in society. That discourse overwhelmed the voices of women who pointed out there were few opportunities for them to find meaning and power in their lives. Or consider the following: Hiring and promotion by merit seem objectively right and fair. Yet are merit-based schemes actually based on merit when some groups in a society have been given few or no resources to achieve their potential and others have been given a great deal to do so? Focusing on the fairness of merit allows members of dominant groups to ignore the long history of political decisions that have been made in their favor.

Narrative workers' attitudes toward clients, as seen in their collaborative stance and externalizing of problems, arise from their belief that clients' subjective experiences of problems is a valuable story, often more so than the scientific one. This belief requires the worker to take an open and respectful stance, though not one that says that any story is the equivalent of any other. Some stories lead to oppression, death, and torture; a completely relativist, amoral stance would be disastrous. Discourses around pathology, gender, race, and culture are examined in narrative practice so that room can be made for the client's lived experience. The narrative approach considers social and economic power and the consequent hierarchical structuring of relationships as factors that maintain people's problems. A narrative perspective, therefore, is well suited for examining issues of abuse, domestic violence, gender, and the oppression of minorities and populations with special needs (Lyle & Gehart, 2000). A narrative approach to ethics (and to practice) is well suited to social work.

Narrative therapy can be criticized on the basis that constructionism sees many stories as true, and some of the stories propagated by society leave people vulnerable to problems. If nothing is true, and some stories cause pain, does that mean that anything goes and narrative social work is value neutral? No, because narrative workers recognize that cultural discourses can cause problems and will bring them forth to examine with clients in the context of the clients' lives. For example, domestic violence has political overtones and is seen as arising from the dominance of patriarchal discourses in the culture. Dickerson and Zimmerman (1996) note:

> We see problems such as abuse and violence as actions taken by someone who is afforded a position of power by the dominant culture against persons with less power, again supported by the dominant culture. Those given positions of power by the culture (we have focused on gender, but this could be race, class, or point of view) justify what they do based on these privileging cultural narratives, but they will readily admit that these actions do not lead to preferred outcomes or outcomes they want. The cultural narratives are the problem, and our stance is clearly *against* any subjugating narratives that specify how persons should be or that have harmful effects on others. (p. 80, emphasis in the original)

Narrative social workers understand the importance to their practice of values and of acting on the basis of those values.

## Transparency and Informed Consent in Narrative Social Work

When developing practices involving audiences for new stories, it is very important to get informed consent, as workers' enthusiasm can blind them to the possible reservations clients may have about these practices. *Circulation practices* (Lobovits et al., 1995, p. 224), in which clients' struggles and strengths are made known to appreciative others, can turn private pain into public policy, meeting the social work ethical obligation to turn to the public arena to right injustices. However, Lobovits et al. (p. 235) caution that clients may simply "comply rather than agree" to being involved in such practices. They recommend exploring in detail with clients the possible positive and negative effects of involving others and the potential futures to which such practices may lead. An important question is, "If you didn't really want to circulate this information, is there anything that would prevent you from letting me know that?" (p. 235).

When social workers expose their values to others and open them up to comment, others can see how the workers' values influence what they do, the hierarchy in the worker-client relationship is diminished, and workers are made more accountable because others can scrutinize their work. When social workers make stories of their work public, they receive in return a great diversity of accounts of problems' strategies and ways of influencing people, far more than obtained by traditional practice approaches (Lobovits et al., 1995).

Too often, however, informed consent means the right kind of paperwork being signed, not making sure the client has received (and understands) information sufficient to allow him or her to make an informed decision about treatment. To consent to treatment, a person should know what will happen, what, if any, alternatives are available, what the potential risks are, and what business arrangements will be necessary. To consent to a release of information, a client should know what information will be used, how it will be used, how it will be disguised, and how long it will be used. Recounting these facts alone is inadequate if the discussion of consent is treated in a pro forma fashion instead of as a real discussion that respects the client's position of power to refuse consent.

Issues of consent can be taken up in the classroom. Sometimes I use anecdotes in classes that are from work I did at another time in another state, and will do so without clients' permission. I have told my students that when I worked in an urban mental health clinic it was not uncommon for people to tell me about how they were approached on the street by dealers to buy drugs. A client once told me that if you invite these "old friends" to go with you to a Narcotics Anonymous meeting they will smile and walk away. I would not need consent in this case because it is not likely the client could be identified from my statement (although I did obtain consent to use the material for teaching, a process that validated the clients and let them know their wisdom was appreciated). However, if I were to describe an exact occurrence, telling the story of who said what and when, I would have to get permission because there is a possibility of connecting the person to the information.

Letting people know that you wish to convey their strategies to others facing the same situation is usually received as a compliment, as giving them credit for being experts on the problem. Epston, White, and "Ben," a client's chosen name, call this *consulting your consultants* (1995, p. 282). Consultants (clients) can share their wisdom and experiences in many ways. For instance, clients can give pictures and stories to workers to collect in an *archive* (Madigan & Epston, 1995, p. 261; see also Epston with Maisel, R., 2000). Epston started this approach by developing an archive of clients' depictions of their struggles and successes against problems; with their consent, he then shared their knowledge about standing up to problems with new clients. The knowledge of protesting against certain problems is more immediate when it comes from clients than from the professional literature, and it is frequently more creative, too. The possibility of a client participating in an archive could be broached in the following way:

**Worker:** You seem to have developed a real expertise in meeting Nervousness and standing up to it, not letting it take over your life.

**Client:** *I feel like it has been a tough road, but yes, I have made some big improvements.*

**Worker:** Would you like to share this knowledge with other people?

**Client:** *How do you mean?*

**Worker:** Sometimes people write down the story of how they stood up to a problem—beat Nervousness, in your case—so that other people who come to see me can have the benefit of their thoughts.

**Client:** *How would that work?*

**Worker:** Well you, or both of us, could write down how you learned not to be shoved around by Nervousness and what you learned in the process that worked for you. I would keep a copy here in what I call an archive. When a person comes in for help for a similar problem, I would offer to let that person read your story. You can disguise yourself as much as you wish. It would mean that other people may benefit from your experience, but also that people you don't know would be reading about your life.

**Client:** *Okay. Do you think it could help someone?*

**Worker:** Yes, I do, though of course I don't know for sure, but maybe seeing that people who aren't professionals can work on their own problems and succeed might help someone remember what he or she knows. But please understand that your story is *your* story, and I won't disclose it if you don't want me to. However, if you do want to share your story, you will choose what is put in the archive. And you can always phone or write and ask me to remove your story from the archive, and I will.

**Client:** *Okay.*

In this example, the idea of an archive and its function is presented. The client is informed of how it would work, what he or she would need to do, and of the option not to do anything. The process of what will be done with the materials is also made clear. This is all important information to convey to the client so that he or she can decide whether to give informed consent.

Consistent with narrative workers' emphasis on transparency, there are a number of professional and lay papers available on this subject on the Internet. Some of the papers and artwork that Epston has collected in an anti-anorexia and anti-bulimia archive can be found at http://www.narrativeapproaches.com.

## Negotiating Ethical Dilemmas

The following sections address dilemmas regarding confidentiality, medication, and assigning diagnoses.

### Confidentiality and Narrative Social Work

A form of treatment that places a premium on audience can run afoul of the strong confidentiality ethic in social work. Social work treatment has been traditionally seen as occurring in a protected and safe therapeutic relationship, and the profession's understanding of ethics reflects that view of the treatment relationship. In contrast to the fairly insular view of the treatment relationship found in most traditional therapeutic models, narrative practice focuses on the need to involve others as an audience for the new alternative story being coconstructed by the client and worker. It is important to keep in mind that when workers write letters to clients about their sessions, there is a possibility of breaching confidentiality should the wrong person read the letter. Informed consent in these situations will be discussed shortly.

As practice becomes more strengths-based and less focused on illness and deficits, the need for privacy diminishes. Most people are not ashamed and do not feel stigmatized by having strengths developed (Lobovits et al., 1995). Consequently, it may be that those settings where client secrets and privacy in treatment are most strongly emphasized may also be the breeding ground for "stigmatization, increased risk of exploitation by the therapists, and a lack of therapist accountability" (p. 224). Settings where social workers maintain authority and power over clients, engage in secret conversations in consultation behind clients' back, and make independent decisions on what the treatment plan should be and then have clients sign on to it are those where clients are vulnerable to having their power taken from them.

The narrative approach forces workers to look at the harm done in everyday "good" practices. When discussions of clients take place without the clients' presence, or even without their knowledge, the stage is set for objectifying people as their problems. Such practices make it easier for workers to talk about people being " 'manipulative,' 'attention-seeking,' 'personality disordered,' or just plain responsible for" their own problems (Simblett, 1997, p. 154). Such practices not only make it difficult to separate clients from their problems, but often also disempower clients, who then become less able to stand up to their problems.

Much of the NASW *Code of Ethics* defines ethical standards about relationships, be they with clients, other workers, employers, the profession, or the community (NASW, 1999). The social work code is quite clear about separating personal from professional relationships, because professional relationships are for the benefit of the client.

The treatment alliance is managed based on theories that prescribe using the relationship as a tool. Does the requirement for such a deep division shift when the focus is on strengths, not deficits? When I have shown narrative letters to my classes, it is not unusual to have one or two of the MSW students comment that the letters seem to breach an important relationship barrier. What that barrier is exactly is not clear, just that they would never write such a letter. The sense is that if the language in a letter to a client is not stilted and does not use a passive voice or objective "eye of God" perspective, then the written communication is too personal and may breach professional ethics. If personal reactions to clients' struggles are described, then there is a risk of blending relationships by being too reciprocal. In fact, we often register our emotions in person, so a letter without a personal touch seems more like a simple report than an actual communication between people and is likely to have very little practical value.

You should always ask clients' permission as to whether you can send them a letter and you should let them know what it is likely to be about. You should ask who else is likely to see the letter and how this should be handled. For example:

**Worker:** Sometimes I write and mail letters between sessions to people I'm working with. Some people have told me that they often forget what happens here and a letter describing it helps them. And, like what happens with most people, some of my best questions come up after you're gone, and I like to put those in too so that we can talk about them when you return. Would that be all right with you?

**Client:** *Yes, though I've never had that happen before.*

**Worker:** The letters?

**Client:** *Right.*

**Worker:** Yes, this is a little different. Another thing about the letters: after you've had a chance to read each one, you can tell me what I got right and what I got wrong. Sort of like a quality control. Of course, you can always refuse to let me write to you and I will respect your decision.

**Client:** *No, it would be okay.*

**Worker:** If I address the letter to you at home, would that cause any problems?

**Client:** *Problems?*

**Worker:** Well, who else is likely to see it?

**Client:** *Oh, my wife.*

**Worker:** Would that be a problem?

**Client:** *No, I can tell her about it or just give her a story or something.*

**Worker:** Would getting the letter lead to more troubles between you two?

**Client:** *No, in fact I think I will share it with her, so keep that in mind.*

Here the worker has proposed the letter, described what would be in it, asked permission to send it, discussed its possible benefits, and showed concern about who else might see it. The client has a pretty good idea of what he or she is agreeing to if this is presented at the end of the session. The worker at that time also could provide more specifics about what might be in the letter, should the client request more information.

## Medication

Medical treatment is often seen as a given, based on science and without moral issues. Some problems have physical components, and, as a result, medication can be a beneficial tool. However, people must take their medication in order to benefit from it. They may require help monitoring their medications, and systems need to be in place to make medication affordable.

Medication is sometimes associated with locating the problem within the person's body instead of the societal discourses in which it arises. For this reason, some narrative workers have not been supporters of medication. Anyone who works in the area of mental health has a sense of the amount of medication given to people who live in miserable conditions, who are oppressed in their dreams and wishes, and who may feel constantly in danger. Medication may help people rally their abilities to cope with such troubles, but it is clear that someone living in these destructive circumstances may well be confronting primarily social miseries and only secondarily biological ones.

It is important to look at the impact of drug companies in shaping the definitions of clients' problems. Beyond the pens, Post-it notepads, dinners, and luncheons, drug companies are a major source of mental health education for working professionals. Through lectures, workshops, and the provision of large numbers of sample medications to doctors and mental health centers (needed in a system that leaves the working poor unprotected), the biochemical story has become entrenched in the field (and recently has gained prominence among the general public, as well, through television ads).

Medication is a valuable tool and clients should always be given the opportunity to explore it as such. Cutting off this opportunity by not providing a suitable psychiatric referral because of the worker's ideology puts the worker's needs above the client's. As one narrative psychiatrist notes, "The biological and biochemical are neither ignored nor overemphasized" (Simblett, 1997, p. 145). But this stance requires time to ensure that the client is clear about how a medication works, has all questions answered, and knows there is a contingency plan established if there are any problems. Only then can medication act as a tool in challenging the problem.

## Diagnoses

At the end of the last chapter I discussed some of the benefits and problems of making and using diagnoses. In addition to those considerations, there also is an ethical issue that arises when the diagnosis is tailored to reasons other than the actual behaviors and complaints of the client. Some workers have decided to give all their clients the minimum diagnosis that will be reimbursed by a third-party payer so that clients are not stigmatized, while still meeting the payer's requirement that a diagnosis be made. The impetus for this action is loyalty to the client over bureaucratic rules. Intentional misdiagnosis, however, constitutes a fraud against the payer and could potentially lead to ethical violations if the client shows up at a hospital or is seen by another practitioner for more serious problems. It is far better to provide an accurate diagnosis and explain it to the client than to give a false one. It is hubris to think that one worker has all the answers and can help the client handle any and every problem. Misdiagnosis makes it that much more difficult for the next practitioner to assist the client.

## Exercise: An Ethical Dilemma: Alternative Scenarios

An ethical issue is presented here both in a principlist and in a narrative account. Compare the two descriptions and use a deconstructive approach to examine the assumptions of all the parties in the situation.

You are seeing a gay couple for couple counseling. The complaints are lack of communication (Tim) and lack of sex (Joe). The couple has been together for three years and adopted their first baby about six months ago. The couple has agreed that they need to work together on making the relationship better, as it has recently fallen into being one of quiet distance. You tell them that as your clients you will work with them to improve their relationship. Both partners agree to this.

One afternoon you get a message on your voice mail from Tim, the partner described as being sexually reluctant, telling you he is questioning his sexual orientation now that his mother, who cut him off after he came out, is on her deathbed. He says he will need some time to figure things out. He says that although he has become attracted to a woman at work, he has not approached her in any way while he is coming to terms with his feelings. In his voice mail message, Tim asks you not to tell Joe because this would ruin the relationship given Joe's emotionality.

Based on the NASW *Code of Ethics* (1999), what do you do and why? Here are some options:

- Ignore the information.
- Contact Tim to encourage him to discuss this with Joe.
- End couple therapy during the next session, saying that some things

## Social Work Ethics, Postmodern Ethics, and Where the Twain Shall Meet   85

have come to your attention that you cannot discuss but that will sabotage the therapy.
- Offer individual therapy to Tim to help him cope with his issues and do so without telling Joe.
- Refer Tim to individual therapy without telling Joe.
- Tell Joe you have referred Tim to individual therapy without saying why.
- Discuss the information learned at the next conjoint session, indicating that your obligation is to the couple, not the individuals.
- Unilaterally decide to bring up the mother's illness as the block to treatment and have the session focus on coping with that.

Now let us look at this situation narratively and see if other options become available:

**Tim:** This has been a real mess. It took me so long to realize I was gay and come to terms with it. I have a lot to be thankful for in a guy as loving as Joe, who is understanding and has put up with a lot. These feelings of confusion are really upsetting. Joe is so sensitive, though, that if I told him of my feelings he would get upset, probably not sleep at night, and maybe even start drinking again. I've seen things do that to him in the past. Parenting is more difficult than either of us thought, and though we love this little guy I'm not sure either of us could parent alone in an adequate way. That scares me, too. Joe is so loving, yet here I am turning away from him when we both need each other for the baby's sake. I hate myself sometimes. Now I have to struggle with my mother. Her stroke has really knocked her down and the doctor doesn't give her much time. She is very religious and hated me when I came out. She was so close to me before that, but then, though she said she still loved me, she told me I wasn't her son anymore if I wouldn't give up gay lovers. That crushed me. She doesn't want to go to her grave with me being gay; she says she wants to make sure I get to heaven and says I can still be forgiven. She can't talk much anymore, but whenever I visit her she sees Joe's ring on my hand and begins crying. It makes me feel so bad for being who I am. Then this woman at work, Marge, has been very nice to me and seems to be the only person I can really talk to. I don't tell her all my problems, but I really have been enjoying her company, and I've started to wonder what this is about. Maybe I'm bisexual or something. Would my mother not cry if she knew I was bisexual? Probably not. I don't know what I am. I can't talk to friends about this because they're all Joe's friends, too. I probably shouldn't talk to the social worker about my problems because the worker is working with Joe and me together, but I don't know whom to turn to. Also, I think that the social worker is frustrated with me for not being more open to Joe despite all his hard work. I just need to let the worker know that I'm not being an idiot about this, that I'm doing the best I can under the circumstances, but without knowing some of those circumstances, it doesn't make sense. I just pray the social worker keeps my secret. It could ruin my relationship with Joe, my baby's life, and my chance for a good future if the worker talks about me to Joe. I hope the social worker has got the sense to know that.

**Worker:** I can't believe Tim did this—leaving me to figure out what I should do under these circumstances. He left me information that could be very important and might explain why treatment isn't moving forward. My commitment is to work with the couple, and now he has given me information that puts me between them. I feel so caught over what to do. I like both of these people, and now they have a baby depending on them. I guess Tim was aggravating me when he seemed unable to move on the sex issue without being able to give his ideas of what was behind it. Joe was getting aggravated, too, and I wondered how long our work together could continue at that rate. On one hand, Tim knew that this was couple therapy, but I can't remember if I told them about the lack of confidentiality in any individual side conversations. I suppose I could just request that Tim tell Joe and refuse to go any further if he doesn't, but that secret really makes the treatment frustrating. I'm not sure how much further we can progress without some honesty here, even if there are fireworks as a result. If Tim leaves, I guess Joe could refuse him access to the little boy because there is no gay marriage law in this state, though whose name is on the adoption papers will affect that. This is really complicated.

**Joe:** I can't figure out what more to do to help Tim get this relationship back together. It seems that between the adoption and then his mother's stroke, he has been unreachable. He's really important to me and I am terrified that this could be the end of our relationship. The worker seems okay. But after seeing all I am trying to do to salvage this thing, I don't understand why the social worker won't just talk to Tim alone and tell him to shape up. Tim knows how much I love him and care about him, but eight months of just hearing "I'm not interested" is hard. I wonder if his mother's guilt-tripping him has turned him against me? God, does he blame me for her illness or something? I just hate all this uncertainty. What am I supposed to do?

CHAPTER 4

# Problem Definition as a Tool of Power: Externalization

Why do some things go from being seen as taken-for-granted, intractable, natural conditions to being considered problems? That is, what makes a problem "a problem"? What does it mean "to have a problem"? According to whom?

I begin this chapter by discussing how societal discourses shape problem definitions and how, as a consequence, definitions not only can convey an understanding of a problem's likely causes and possible solutions but can also reinforce the power of dominant groups. I then examine what can happen when problems are viewed as attributes of individuals and why it is therapeutically important to distinguish the person from the problem. Next, I discuss the narrative technique of externalization, wherein a problem is explicitly defined as being separate from and outside of the person. I offer a variety of examples to illustrate how this technique can be used, the ways in which it is compatible with more traditional assessment approaches, and how it can empower clients by encouraging them to stand up to their problems. Finally, I end the chapter with a description of social workers' responsibilities when working with clients to externalize problems.

## Locating the Societal Definition of the Problems Affects the Outcome

Events are defined by giving them unique meanings, which are influenced by societal discourses, and those meanings create reality for the perceiver. Getting married can be seen as the opportunity to love and grow with another person. Getting married also can mean being shackled to another person, having to consider his or her desires, and giving up your choice of other possible partners. How you think about marriage will have an impact on whether you get married and what that marriage will be like. The reality of marriage for one person is different from the reality of marriage for someone who has a different worldview of the institution. The same relationship will be a quite different experience for a person who is looking for evidence of love and compromise versus one who is seeing shackles.

How problems are defined creates a reality in the same manner. Family therapist Jay Haley (1976) notes the different response given to people who are defined as "mad" versus "bad" based on the same behavior. If a problem is seen as based in madness, then treatment is the response; for a problem caused by badness, punishment is appropriate. Problems seen as temporary or as part of a developmental phase are looked at and treated differently from those seen as either chronic or acute. Vivid imaginary friends are different phenomena from hallucinations, though both are in the sphere of distorted reality. Although many differences can be pointed to between these two phenomena, such as their friendliness and intrusiveness, it is also easy to see that the developmental and, hence, temporary nature of imaginary friends makes it appear the less worrisome of the two.

Madsen (2007) gives an example of two psychiatric teams working with the same woman. The first team identified the client as having a borderline personality disorder, which led them to distrust her and suspect she might not get much from treatment because she was "borderline." Their distrust of the client, in turn, intensified her distrust of the team. By contrast, the second team identified the client as a survivor of serious abuse who was desperate for help but who was distrustful of helpers, given multiple negative experiences. The differences between what the two teams saw in the same woman and how they interpreted her behavior were enormous; these differences also directly influenced how this woman saw herself through the eyes of the team.

A problem's definition will affect how a social worker sees a "wee patch of blue" in the currently dark sky of the client's life—that is, how hopeful the worker feels about change. How we assess clients and their problems puts us in different relationships with them. Some assumptions help us connect more closely to them; others require us to distance ourselves from them.

The reasons given by experts for problems have changed over time in the social work profession (Weick & Chamberlain, 2002). When friendly visitors of the late 1800s engaged in early forms of social casework, problems such as poverty were seen as indications of moral and constitutional defects. Problem definitions in the 1920s were derived from psychiatry and required greater expert knowledge, which not only necessitated the use of definitions familiar to other experts but also catapulted social work forward in its quest for professionalization. Problems were seen as symptoms of neuroses and developmental crises that led to stable character traits. More recent social work definitions of problems have attempted to include environmental aspects (Germain & Gitterman, 1996). Yet even when the assumptions are more clearly based on person-environment interactions, the focus of care rarely goes beyond the family system.

Medical explanations conceptualize problems as personal pathology, and the range of behaviors and emotions that fall within the psychiatric gaze keeps getting larger. Formerly nonexistent psychiatric pathologies are continuously constructed. An example is how expressions of loss and mourning have now been categorized as either "uncomplicated" or normal grief, or "complicated" or abnormal or troubled grief (Foote & Frank, 1999). As Weick and Chamberlain (2002) note:

> The redefinition of human problems has been a lasting legacy of psychologically oriented practice. What had been universal aspects of human experience throughout history evolved into new classes of behaviors, isolated from their context and viewed through the lens of pathology. Because these behaviors are removed from their larger social context, they appear to be unique failures and dangerous symptoms instead of pervasive, if frightening and puzzling, parts of human life. (p. 97)

Redefining problems as psychological has had the effect of focusing resources on the causes of problems rather than on potential solutions.

Even in those areas where medical knowledge has expanded to provide some relief to human problems, such as schizophrenia, epilepsy, diabetes, asthma, bipolar disorder, depression, and other forms of mood disorders, management of problems requires more from the person than just taking medication, although this in itself is a major task for many. Generally, the problem itself would prefer not being medicated and seeks reasons and excuses for the person to not take the medication. If you have ever not taken your complete prescription for antibiotics after feeling better, despite warnings, you have some sense of how this thinking can invade a person's life.

Current thinking in the United States places personal problems within the realm of the individual's body and/or choices. Compare the image of the poor during the Depression with the image of the poor today. The symbols around those in need have moved from individual failure (President Herbert Hoover, though approving aid to farmers' livestock, refused to provide any support to the farmers themselves), to unfortunate victims of structural conditions (seen as causing the stock market crash and the collapse of financial markets and giving us Social Security), to contemporary characterizations of unmotivated, manipulative, amoral women manipulating a dysfunctional public benefits system (bringing us Temporary Assistance to Needy Families). As a result, approaches to poverty have changed from very carefully portioned-out charity and small, state-level welfare programs, to larger federal initiatives that attempted to respond to structural issues beyond the control or influence of individuals, to agencies that now fashion themselves as job training and employment centers to overcome the evils of welfare dependency and laziness.

Locating problems within the person obscures the influences of cultural and societal forces. It minimizes the impact of oppression and discrimination. It is easier to label a child as having attention-deficit disorder and medicate the child if he or she has difficulty sitting still in an underfunded classroom with 30 students who also struggle with the problems of poverty than it is to look at the entire context.

The focus on pathology and individual responsibility makes the person the problem. Poverty is no longer the problem; conniving, greedy recipients are the problem, although a recent twist has cast the system of welfare entitlements itself as the primary problem, exacerbating recipients' other problems. Internalizing the problem leads to speaking in ways that ignore larger societal contexts and avoid broader issues supporting the problem. Such talk leads to locating the problem in the person's character or personality and pathologizes who he or she is and what he or she does. To fit in, people wind up colluding in the ways their own lives are governed and engaging in self-censure (i.e., "I'm not like those other welfare recipients"; Parton & O'Byrne, 2000).

Drawing on the work of Foucault, Freedman and Combs (1996) say that the most politically powerful views seem to divide us from each other and encourage us to treat ourselves and our bodies as objects and sources of problems. These politically dominant ideas and the institutions developed to promulgate and enforce them encourage *internalizing discourses* (p. 48), wherein people internalize dominant discourses to their own detriment (e.g., if you do not have a good job, you are a failure and an inadequate person).

Problem definitions affect social work practice by suggesting specific causes, focusing treatment in certain directions, and conveying either hope or despair. In addition, how a problem is defined informs the outcome desired from treatment—what is defined as success will depend on what someone sees as the problem. And all these problem-related assumptions influence the social worker–client relationship.

## Locating Problems Outside People: Externalizing Internalized Problems

A key concept in narrative work advanced by Michael White is that "the person is not the problem, the problem is the problem" (as cited in Abels & Abels, 2001, p. 54). To the extent that the person is seen as the problem, social workers are engaged in changing the person, a mostly frustrating and usually confrontational approach to working with people. Skilled workers can, of course, help clients see what is in their best interests and point out how they can achieve that with the gentle pressure of "demand for work" (Shulman, 1999, p.16).

Externalization, or seeing the problem as something different from or outside of the person, is an antidote to the worldview that locates problems within the individual. Through externalization someone who is depressed or who has a major depressive disorder (American Psychiatric Association, 2000, pp. 369–376) is now a person struggling against, or in some sort of relationship with, depression (or sadness or energy loss). Depression influences the person's life, perhaps strongly and frequently, but it is not the entirety of the person's life. The person is something different from and other than depression. Believing this distinction is something real and not just a word game can make a dramatic difference in how the person is dealt with, how help is conceived, and how resistance to change is avoided.

Carlson (1998) explores a client-generated metaphor for externalization that can be a helpful tool for understanding the process. Using the image of a computer virus, he describes how the virus requires an active agent to be written, gets into the computer unexpectedly, and changes the computer's operating commands, thereby leading to damage to the operating system and usually a loss of data. To protect against viruses, a detector program must be introduced that recognizes viruses and repairs the damage to the executive commands that run the computer. Because computer hackers are always trying to circulate new viruses, the detector must stay alert and be modified to meet new threats.

In narrative treatment, problems are considered to be outside forces that enter people's lives and rewrite the basic text of who they are. This process usually starts small and accumulates over time. As a problem gains more influence in a person's life, a dominant story is created of who the person is, and those parts of a person's experience that are different from that story are often lost, like data through a virus. When the person's problem is discovered, externalized, and its strategies for influencing the person are explored, the person can then act as a virus detector, rewriting his or her identity and counteracting the problem's strategies. Because problems are embedded in the dominant culture's discourses, the problem often over time will attempt to find other ways to reintroduce itself into the person's life. Narrative treatment can help people consider their future and how they will stand up to problems when they occur in novel ways.

As a cancer resister, I recently picked up a small plaque, whose author is unknown, from the local hospital's cancer center. It reads:

> *Cancer is so limited . . .*
> *It cannot cripple love,*
> *It cannot shatter hope,*
> *It cannot corrode faith,*
> *It cannot take away peace,*
> *It cannot destroy confidence,*
> *It cannot kill friendship,*
> *It cannot shut out memories,*
> *It cannot silence courage,*
> *It cannot invade the soul.*

Cancer, though certainly an important factor in resisters' lives, is not their whole lives. They can still have relationships with many different qualities outside the cancer; they can still experience love, hope, and faith, among other emotions. Those qualities will make life worth living even in the face of a life-threatening disease, though in fact cancer can affect people in all the ways mentioned in the plaque if they give in to its strategies. The real point is that you can secure an array of gifts even in the face of cancer.

## Why Externalize Problems?

White and Epston (1990) see numerous advantages to externalizing problems. First, externalization can reduce conflict in families and communities by not attributing blame to individuals. In social work, a systemic view also attempts to do this by broadening the definition of the problem and attempting to see it as a function of the ecology of the situation. The system perspective emphasizes families functioning in their environment (Hartman & Laird, 1983). Unfortunately, families then can be left with the sense of being broken or dysfunctional, of needing to learn how to fight fairly, for instance. Externalization, by contrast, encourages people to look at how fighting enters the family and ensnares family members.

Second, externalization can reduce the sense of failure that people experience with chronic problems. Some problems are very cunning and all pervasive; they ally with other problems to make changing one's relationship with them tricky and challenging. When you look at all the strategies that addiction uses to get into people's lives and to stay there, you have to be impressed that people have been able to quit drug abuse at all.

Third, externalization allows people to cooperate with each other to reduce problems rather than struggle against each other. By making the problem an independent entity, it can be excluded from, or triangled out of, the relationships of family members who are affected by it and who can work together to try to overcome it. Bowen family system therapists also often look at how "triangulation" can function to ease problems in families (Nichols, 2006, pp. 117–118); however, the emphasis of work is quite different.

Fourth, externalization opens up the possibility for people to take new and different actions against the problem, to do something other than what they might have considered when they thought of the problem as part of themselves. Externalization allows the person to create a more descriptive story of the problem with a beginning, periods of respite, and continuing conflict. The richer or "thicker" the story, the more it comes alive and becomes real. By seeing the problem as one in which the person's better judgment is being undermined, new possibilities are opened up.

Fifth, externalization allows people to take a lighter, more relaxed stance toward working with problems. Rather than conceiving of oneself as having an internal defect in need of correction, the relationship between the person and the problem is now seen as a competitive gaming one in which the person is attempting to outsmart an opponent. What will be addictive thinking's next move? Where will I see its next opportunity and my maximum vulnerability? What must I do to counter that move?

Finally, externalization presents the possibility of people having dialogues about the problem instead of monologues about what is the true cause or most effective solution. When clients provide information about their experience of "nerves" and the ways they have attempted to take their life back from their "nerves," their efforts are given the dignity they deserve. Through the externalization, the client, it is hoped, will realize that he or she and the problem are not the same thing.

When social workers see themselves as experts on problems and yet cannot get the results they desire with clients, they become frustrated. The seeming insolvability of poverty can lead to anger at its victims. Similarly, it is not uncommon for workers to get angry at clients for their repeated "stupid" behavior. People sense that they are being blamed for behavior that either made sense to them at the time or that they were convinced to do by the problem. Rather than blame the problem it is easier to blame the client, and there is a whole rather morbid humor built up in agencies and institutions around client problems and behaviors. This is not coincidental.

Western culture, particularly as lived out in the United States, places a high value on individualism. People are thought to succeed or fail of their own accord. If people are not able to succeed, it is because they either are lazy or lack willpower. If they are overweight, it is because they have not shown enough self-control around carbohydrates and fats and have not exercised enough. If they are poor, it is because they have not had the gumption to pull themselves up by their bootstraps and work harder. If they have cancer, it is because they did not eat the right vegetables. If children have emotional problems, it means their mothers are at fault. Environment contributes little to the equation because there are always anecdotes of people from poor environments who succeed, as almost any copy of *Reader's Digest* shows. If one person can succeed and do well in life despite poor schools, high-crime communities, discrimination, abuse, neglect, and suffering, then everyone should be able to do so. This ethic is deeply ingrained in most people in this country.

Externalizing lets the social worker be *for* the client. This is different from being *with* the client. Workers can advocate on the side of the person against the problem and express their outrage at what the problem is doing to the person. Workers' anger or sarcasm toward clients, usually expressed with other workers, is often attributed to workers' need to vent emotions or relieve anxiety. Yet such behaviors can also be seen as outrage at the suffering with which clients struggle. The philosopher Emmanuel Levinas (as cited in Frank, 1995) argues that unjustified suffering causes justified suffering for its witnesses. Those who bear witness also suffer and, as a result, experience outrage.

Social workers have a right to be justifiably outraged at the suffering they see. For example, depression has ruined many lives, destroyed marriages, and even devastated the lives of the children of those experiencing depression, not to mention the many times that it has convinced people that dying is a better choice than living. Poverty, racism, and sexism have given rise to a whole host of problems that play vicious games with those caught in their webs. Schizophrenia cuts into people's lives in their teens and twenties, destroying their dreams. Think of the toll that this problem alone has taken on people!

Social workers have a right to be angry, but that anger, as with clients' anger, is better directed at the problems that take over clients' lives than at the clients themselves. If workers truly see problems as separate from people, then anger can more easily be channeled toward problems. In turn, workers' need to present always with clinical detachment can be reduced.

People should be angry at what a problem can do. The following extensive letter by Ann Epston (as cited in Maisel, Epston, & Borden, 2004, pp. 160–162) to a 13-year-old client under the influence of anorexia, a deadly problem, provides an excellent example of how outrage can be directed in a helpful manner:

> Dear Emma, Sandra, and Brian [parents of Emma],
>
> It was good to meet you all last night and make a start on getting to know you. Thank you, Emma, for your frankness and bravery in talking and in answering so many questions asked by a stranger.
>
> I woke up at midnight and couldn't get back to sleep for hours; my mind was boiling with a furious anger against anorexia. I thought, "Here we go again, anorexia! So you have sneaked into the life of yet another innocent young girl, pretending to befriend her at a time of big changes. How cunning of you to detect Emma's uneasiness with her developing body, and how unscrupulous of you to offer her an 'easy' solution—dieting! How neatly you insinuated yourself into her uncertainty, her longing for friends and boyfriends, promising her that thinness would ensure attractiveness and popularity, would win her admiration and make her the envy of all who know her. Anorexia, did you tell her the price she'd have to pay? Did you warn her you'd eventually steal even her soul in exchange? I heard you actually convinced Emma she's your only victim, in a school of 1,200 girls!
>
> "You vampire, anorexia, haven't you taken enough already? Aren't you satisfied with the stream of young girls you've preyed upon, stealing their fat, then their flesh, their strength, their energy, their enthusiasm, their sparkle, their humor, opinions, sports, games, friendships, social times, confidence, trust, creativity, originality, individuality—their very lives?
>
> "I suppose Emma was an attractive choice: intelligent, friendly, humorous, a lover of animals, responsible, ambitious, prepared to study hard and train to be a vet. What a delightful tall poppy to cut down at the threshold of adolescence! What pleasure you must be taking in draining her energy, blurring her concentration, and alienating her from her own body.

"How did you do it, anorexia? How did you train Emma to criticize and reject her body instead of loving herself? How did you make her believe that some imaginary school boy's opinion was worth starvation? What vulnerabilities did you seize upon to convince her that thin, weak conformists are more desirable than strong individuals?

"I suppose you have lots of help: the movies, magazines, TV soaps, advertising, school girl culture—they all tell the same story, that less is best for girls' bodies and minds. Did you use your usual trick of comparing? Making Emma compare herself against friends and declare herself the loser, then offer your services in consolation, the perfect solution? Did you use the old drug dealers' trick of just a little bit at first? Did you slip smoothly from oh-so-reasonable 'no junk food' to gradually defining all food as junk? Did you use secrecy and the pretense of 'specialness' to isolate Emma in subtle ways from the loving concern of family and friends? And of course I know you used fear, that despicable technique favored by tyrants and bullies the world over. Yes, you terrorized this 13-year-old into accepting your lie—that you offer 'control' and without you, Emma will lose all control and her hunger will be insatiable.

"If it weren't so vicious and evil it would be laughable, your threat that a healthy, active young woman will become the size of a whale just by the simple fact of eating ordinary nourishing food. This fear has tormented and tortured countless thousands upon thousands of young women into submitting to your hateful rule.

"But, anorexia, we will not stand for it. Emma has wise and loving parents who will not allow you to prey upon their beloved daughter. They have chosen me as their anti-anorexia therapist, and with the help of Dr.___ and her dietitian and everyone who cares about Emma, we will fight anorexia and fear and drive you out of this family's life. We do this because we are perfectly clear about what is right and what is wrong. Take notice, anorexia, we will do everything in our power to free Emma from the spell you have cast over her. We are guided by two principles: unwavering support and love for Emma and unwavering hatred for anorexia and the harm it does."

Yours anti-anorexically,

Ann Epston

This letter was written to a client family after a first session. As it makes clear, the emotion is directed not at Emma, a child starving herself to death, but at the problem itself in support of Emma. The reader can sense the worker's hope and determination and can begin to understand what might be maintaining the behavior. The family is offered the opportunity to confront an adversary, not change a "sick" child or its "dysfunctional" family dynamics. In no way is the family held responsible for the problem; rather, it is supported and seen as a critical ally. Emma, the client, is told she is fighting an adversary who is taking advantage of her; she is also told she is not alone in this struggle. Her family and the professionals working with her are committed to her. She is reminded there likely are a number of people in her school who are struggling with the same problem. The letter conveys a sense of seriousness in the anger of the professional, who is prepared to fight alongside this girl as she struggles to reclaim her life. The girl also knows that like every other real relationship, the one with this worker is not a 50-minute-a-week one. The worker worries and thinks about this girl because she is important, important enough to take the time to write such a letter to her.

## Cautions in Externalizing

Narrative workers do not always work with clients to externalize problems, though they do consider problems and people to be different and separate. When clients are not feeling oppressed or overburdened by their problems or when they can still find different meanings in their lives despite the problem story, then direct externalization may not be necessary (White, 1995). White talks about a response to an exception in the following manner:

> Hey, wait a minute. This doesn't seem to fit with these other things that you've been talking about. Tell me more about these. How did you take that step? Would you say that this is a positive development or a negative development? What do you think are the foundations for this step? As we reflect on this development, what does this tell you about how you really want things to be? (p. 25)

White terms such exceptions *unique outcomes* (1995, p. 15). When clients have exceptions easily available and bring them into the therapeutic conversation without difficulty, they can be explored directly without the need to externalize.

Externalization carries the risk of sounding unusual and, therefore, could be discounted by clients. If it is just used as a technique, then any challenge to the approach by a client will likely pressure the worker to go back to traditional thinking. Unless workers come to see the narrative value of externalization, it will remain merely a technique, and not necessarily a highly successful one at that.

Externalization with perpetrators of violence can be tricky. There are strong societal messages, particularly among men, that encourage violence. White (1995) is emphatic that the focus needs to be beyond mere contrition on the part of the perpetrator. A man who is violent must work to change his very ways of being; he must become, in essence, a "new" man.

Although it may not be appropriate to directly externalize the story of the violence, the discourse around what it means to be a man toward others can and should be externalized and examined. Otherwise, contrition under pressure can occur as a concession to being caught rather than because the inherent wrongness of abuse has been accepted. If a perpetrator truly believes, based on his experience and the messages he receives, that men have to keep control over their family and that women and children must be made to understand this by whatever means necessary, then helping him to cope differently with his anger toward family members will go only so far. A narrative social worker can help him examine what he thinks he is entitled to in his relationships and what he believes he is entitled to do to accomplish those ends. He can look at where and how he learned these ideas and what effect they have on his relationships and the people he cares about. Whole different ways of being beyond a patriarchic worldview need to be considered.

## How to Externalize

It is not desirable to externalize too quickly or go too far ahead of the client. Talking about problems as independent entities is initially awkward for both the worker and the client. Some clients do not understand externalization and, consequently, see it as a gimmick. Talking about "it" or "this problem" in the beginning may make externalization more palatable (McKenzie & Monk, 1997, p. 100). This type of talk maintains the worker's need to see the problem and person as different and keeps open the possibility of a future transition to more explicit expressions of externalization. Specific language, however, is less important than the worker's attitude.

Workers can externalize problems by simply changing to nouns the adjectives that clients use to describe themselves. When clients say they are feeling depressed or are depressed, the reply might be to ask what depression is doing to them. In this way, the problem—depression—is gently distinguished from the clients' personhood.

Freedman and Combs (1996) provide an exercise, initially developed by Freedman, to encourage distinguishing between the concepts of people as problems and people as separate from problems. To begin, take a moment to think of something that describes you, a trait or emotion that you or other people think you have too much of: anger, being a procrastinator, being hard to get along with, or being lazy, for instance. Then ask yourself the following questions, which come directly from Freedman and Combs's exercise (pp. 48–49). I have inserted *lazy* and offer some possible responses.

> *How did you become lazy?* I don't know, maybe it's in my genes or maybe the things I do just aren't very interesting. I don't like to waste a lot of energy on stupid things.
>
> *What are you most lazy about?* Oh, housekeeping, getting my laundry done, paying attention to my diet and exercise, keeping up at work and trying to get ahead.
>
> *What kinds of things happen that lead to you being lazy?* Well, when something goes wrong I kind of feel like what's the use.
>
> *When you are lazy, what do you do that you won't do if you weren't lazy?* Well, I guess I spend more time watching TV and reading junky novels. I also just feel bad about myself because my house is such a mess, I'm such a mess, and I don't think people respect me at work.

Here is a more externalized approach, in which I turn the adjective *lazy* into the noun *laziness*. Again, ask yourself these questions based on the characteristic you selected.

> *What made you vulnerable to the laziness, so that it was able to dominate your life?* I guess growing up people told me I couldn't do much right and when I feel like this I say what's the use and just don't try.
>
> *In what contexts is the laziness most likely to take over?* When I come home after a hard day at work, or else when I planned so much to do that I think I can't really get it done and instead just get stuck. I plan to eat less and exercise more, but I am exhausted when I get back from work and just want to rest. Then I feel bad and don't want to do anything. So I guess at home, but also during weekly staff meetings, I never volunteer to do anything.
>
> *What kinds of things happen that typically lead to the laziness taking over?* If I don't sleep well because I am worried about things or if I feel disrespected at work, I get really down and begin feeling lazy. Like it is hard to just move. Like yesterday, at work I handed in my case notes to my supervisor like I'm supposed to. She just looked

at them and grunted. I was miserable when I got home. I ate ice cream and went to bed and watched TV until 1:00 in the morning.

*What has the laziness gotten you to do that is against your better judgment?* I overeat; now I go buy quarts of ice cream each week. I never go to the gym anymore, when I used to before. I also seem to just spend a lot of time watching the science fiction channel on cable. I hate to see the mess in my house so much that I just stay in bed, watch TV, and avoid getting up as much as possible so I don't have to look at my house. I don't try to go out with my friends much anymore and would rather just talk to them on the phone. I don't really want things to be like this and it bothers me that I do these things—wasting time on junk food, junk entertainment, and just living in junk. I know I could do better.

Did you notice any difference in how you felt when asking yourself the first set of questions versus the second? Does one set seem to open up more possibilities than the other? Externalization often provides people with the opportunity to be active participants in their life stories and creates the real possibility of resistance to the problem, not the worker.

Another way to externalize, which is more often done with children, is to make the problem into a person. Temper tantrums can become Mr. Trouble or Ms. Wildgirl, attention-deficit/hyperactivity disorder can become Mr. Jumpy or Ms. Firecracker. The name is not as important as the idea behind it. By personifying the problem directly, the problem is externalized that much more explicitly; as a result, the threat to the child of discussing a problem behavior is reduced. It also makes it possible to develop a game to outwit Mr. Trouble or Ms. Wildgirl, adding lightheartedness to serious problems.

## The Strategies of Problems

With the problem viewed as an alien entity distinct from the person it has influenced, the ways in which the client sees how the problem gains control can be teased out in the interview. Madigan (2003) looks at types of strategies that problems use to extend their influence into people's lives. He describes eight major strategies, or what he calls "conversational habits of highly effective problems" (p. 1). Understanding the ways these strategies operate suggests how cognitive "self-talk" can be an important factor in narrative work. Madigan's ideas and some of the questions he developed to explore each habit are discussed next.

Drawing heavily on the work of Michel Foucault, Madigan's first identified problem strategy is *surveillance/audience*. He suggests that without an internalized audience that supports a problem's negative assertions about the person, the problem cannot survive. People get recruited into internalized dialogues in which only those reactions in others that support the problem's definition of the person's negative identity get told and privileged. For instance: "Molly, my supervisor, didn't say hi to me today when I came in to work. She must be reacting to that terrible job I did presenting that case in yesterday's conference. She must be thinking that I am such a loser and shouldn't be in this field." Cognitive/behavioral practitioners term this *negative mind reading,* and it can result in a form of shame. Some possible questions to help bring this strategy out are as follows:

> Has the problem created a campaign of gossip about your life?
>
> What are your thoughts on gossip and gossipers?
>
> If you were alone to speak up for yourself what might you say on behalf of yourself? (Madigan, 2003, p. 4)

The second problem habit is *legitimacy*, or as Madigan asks, "Who has the rights to your story being told?" He says, "We can come to experience ourselves as 'refugees' (or fraudulent) in our own lives, with nowhere to belong or feel safe" (2003, p. 4). For instance: "You know maybe if I didn't do so well in that case presentation it really shows that I don't have what it takes to be a social worker. Who am I kidding?" Even successful people struggle with this strategy. I once met an internationally known scholar who, although widely acclaimed by his colleagues, would occasionally tell his wife that he must be a fraud and wondered when "they" would come and take back his PhD. Questions that might draw out this habit are as follows:

> Do you have a sense of who is backing up this story that you do not belong?
>
> Are there any views that society holds that make you feel like being considered a legitimate citizen would be difficult to achieve?
>
> Where [sic] there ever times when you questioned someone's illegitimate view of you as illegitimate?
>
> If so, what made that possible? And what did it make possible? (pp. 4–5)

The third strategy of internalized problem conversations is *escalating fear*. Escalating fear occurs when problems harness our greatest fears about disconnectedness and loneliness. For instance: "If I don't have what it takes, think of all the trouble I am causing the people who come to see me. They are in difficult straits in their lives and all they get is me. Of course Molly doesn't want anything to do with me; probably no one in this agency does. What will happen to me?" Possible questions are as follows:

> Do you have a sense that fear has launched a terror campaign against your life?
>
> How does fear manage to wreak havoc on your imagination?
>
> Are there ideas common to all of us that fear takes advantage of (e.g., job loss, death, disease, loneliness)?
>
> Do you ever catch fear exaggerating?
>
> If you are fearful, does this mean that there is something in your life worth protecting?
>
> What is it in your life that you feel is worth protecting? (Madigan, 2003, p. 5)

*Negative imagination/negative comparison*, the fourth problem habit, involves characterizing and evaluating oneself negatively, which leads the person to feel that he or she never quite measures up to cultural expectations. Negative imagination draws on the negative ideas from people's history to justify the negative story being told about them. For instance: "I often think of all the clients I've seen at this agency who left after one session and never returned. It's clear that my ineptness scared them off. If I was a great therapist like Mary Magdalene, the person who gave the last workshop I went to, I would have helped those people; now they just have to live with their pain because of me." Possible questions to elicit this strategy are as follows:

> Are there any popular ideas that assist in persons feeling bad about themselves as parents, employees, partners, children [or social workers]?
>
> What ideas assist us in believing that we are never quite doing enough?
>
> What has taught us to believe that everyone else has a right to be treated properly except us? (Madigan, 2003, p. 6)

The fifth problem strategy, *internalized bickering*, involves incessant worrying and second-guessing and continually practicing debates in one's head with individuals from the present or the past. This bickering restricts the ability to imagine different possibilities and leads a person to debate both sides of an issue with himself or herself over and over. For instance: "Maybe I should talk to Molly about how I'm feeling. But if I do, she will see me as a bigger loser. What if she really doesn't see me as a loser? Won't I sound like one then? Why doesn't she talk to me? If she was a real friend, she would discuss this with me; she should know I have been feeling upset about the case presentation. But maybe she's just giving me time to think about it so I can get my act together. What if she really tells me that I am a bad social worker? I would be crushed. But would she really tell me if she felt that way? How can I talk to her?" Questions that might be posed about this habit are as follows:

> Of what institutional and cultural standards does internalized bickering thrive upon?
>
> Are there any moral codes or rules that you have internalized regarding specific ways of behaving that bickering draws upon?
>
> I've heard we speak internally at approximately 1200 words a minute. Are there ever times that you can look back and address how much of your day was spent bickering with yourself?
>
> Do you ever stop to notice the calm you experience when the internal bickering quiets down? (Madigan, 2003, p. 6)

*Hopelessness*, the sixth problem habit, involves surrendering to the belief that all experience and stories outside the problem are meaningless and that all help and connection is pointless. For instance: "I often think about all those clients who could have been helped if they'd seen someone else. Even though I've finished my MSW program and have gotten my license, I am still worthless to those people. It all lets me know that this is just a colossal waste of time. I'm never going to get better if the talent isn't in me and it all just seems so pointless." Developing and recognizing alternative stories can be helpful here. Possible questions to draw out this strategy are as follows:

> What is the history of hopelessness in your life?
>
> Was there a time when it first entered your life?
>
> Is there a particular belief or any one person that most assists a hopeless view of yourself?

Was there ever a time when you experienced a little bit of hope for yourself? When was this?

Would anyone else know about this time? If so, who? (Madigan, 2003, pp. 6–7)

The seventh problem strategy is *the demand for perfection*, a goal that, according to Madigan (2003), is impossible to attain. This strategy involves a person in a never-ending pursuit of perfection, with increasingly rigorous efforts expended to achieve this elusive and ultimately unattainable goal. Madigan developed his understanding of the strategy through his years of working with women struggling with anorexia and bulimia. For instance: "You know what bothers me the most about that case presentation is that I put in so much time to make it just right, yet it wasn't. It means that spending two hours wasn't enough, so if I stay in this field I will need to spend at least six hours going over work so that it comes out just right and making sure that I have all the possible information that the team members might ask about the case." Possible questions are as follows:

Can you recall the ways you have been trained and pressured into ideas of perfection even though perfection is not possible?

Do you think it is a matter of perfection that is creating all this pressure and compelling thoughts?

Has the idea of perfection given you anything less than a worthy idea of yourself?

In what ways does perfection negate your ability to listen to another's praise of you? (Madigan, 2003, p. 7)

Finally, the eighth problem habit, *paralyzing guilt*, often is the product of cultural training received in religious, scientific, and academic institutions. This problem habit is also fostered by familial and cultural injunctions that link who we "should be" with dominant cultural expectations related to gender, class, sexual preference, race, and so on. For instance: "I have done wrong by my clients who haven't returned. They come from difficult backgrounds and are a different race from me and I have managed to let them know that yet again White helpers don't really care about them. As a woman, I should have some sensitivity to people's problems; it makes me wonder what's wrong with me, why I'm not a regular woman." Guilt is not bad in and of itself; it can function to make people accountable for behavior that is inappropriate. However, problems sometimes use guilt as a way to devastate people and convince them they are bad. Guilt might force people to not stand up for themselves or to not get out of a destructive relationship because of the pain it might cause others. Possible questions to explore this habit include the following:

> When you look at history, what conversations of guilt have been used as instruments of social control?
>
> Do you think men and women are equally trained up in guilt?
>
> Are there experiences in your life when you have wrongly been made to feel guilty?
>
> Has guilt ever been helpful or important to you? If so, how? Why?
>
> What might your feelings of guilt represent? Do they mean that you stand for something?
>
> What is this that you stand for, that you believe in?
>
> Why is this important to you?
>
> What is the history of this importance? (Madigan, 2003, p. 8)

Madigan's (2003) work is presented to show the kinds of strategies problems can use, but, of course, the first place you would go to hear about a problem's strategy would be the client you are interviewing. Consistent with the narrative concept of externalization, the idea of strategies makes the problem into an active, malevolent force capable of finding a variety of vulnerabilities in people and using them to take over their lives. These strategies, or habits, of problems and the questions to draw them out are offered merely as ways to stimulate conversations with clients who seem stuck.

## Getting Started

Doing narrative social work with clients requires that workers be aware of engagement issues, collaborative practices, problem stories and externalization, alternative stories and what people would prefer to have more of in their lives, and the challenges of doing postmodern narrative work in a modernist agency context. As in other practice approaches, narrative social work also begins with engagement and identification of the client's problem, strengths, and potential resources, although the meaning of these terms is different within the narrative framework. I discuss each of these processes here.

## Engagement

Narrative authors' focus on the politics of the treatment relationship has implications for involving clients in treatment. A less authoritarian stance acts to engage clients in strong treatment relationships that allow them to feel secure. If the social worker keeps the interview focused solely on the problem brought into treatment, then much of the session will be about the person's weaknesses, not his or her strengths. A balance must be struck between discussing the client's presenting problem and his or her life (and strengths) outside the problem's sphere. Delaying discussion of a problem too long will increase a client's anxiety. As new topics are introduced, the person should be informed about what the worker is doing.

Madsen (2007, p. 123) identifies three steps in engaging clients: "get to know clients outside the influence of the problem," "honor before helping," and "keep the problem on the table." Getting to know clients outside the problem's influence encourages the social worker to learn about clients as people, not just as problem categories. Madsen argues that "beginning with a focus on problems may have the inadvertent effect of amplifying those problems, further entrenching clients in a problematic identity, and constraining them from developing a sense that 'things could be different' " (p. 125). Especially when people have been coerced by others to see a social worker, starting the interview on a more positive note can make the rest of the session more helpful and less punitive.

Honor before helping means obtaining clients' consent before attempting to address the problem. Madsen suggests that a worker will be better able to garner consent by respecting those aspects of the person's life that are not necessarily part of the problem before dealing with the problem. This idea can be enacted not only through looking at people's positive activities but also by respecting their suffering and their attempts to cope with the problem. Wondering about how someone has been able to maintain some functioning in the face of difficult problems taking over his or her life honors the person, who is separate from the problem.

Keeping the problem on the table implies that engagement is a means to an end, not an end in itself. The problem, not the engagement process, should remain the social worker's focus. The purpose of the therapeutic encounter needs to be kept firmly in the forefront of the worker's thinking and should be continually checked and renegotiated with the client. What does the client see as the problem? What is he or she seeking that would be different in his or her life?

Taking a collaborative stance in the relationship should begin immediately. One way to do this is to seek permission to discuss different topics. We rarely do this in sessions because the interview is seen as the "worker's show." In typical sessions, collecting data that allow the social worker to use his or her expertise is what is important. By contrast, when the interaction is the "client's show," the client has a say in where the conversation goes. Morgan (2000) provides nice examples of how this can be done:

- How is this conversation going for you?
- Should we keep talking about this or would you be more interested in . . . ?
- Is this interesting to you? Is this what we should spend our time talking about?
- I was wondering if you would be more interested in me asking you some more about this or whether we should focus on X, Y or Z? [X, Y, Z being options] (pp. 3–4)

These types of questions respect the fact that giving information about oneself and being led into different topics of conversation can be intrusive. The attitude behind these questions also indicates that clients have some idea of what they want in treatment and what is important to them. Spending a good deal of energy forcing interviews into areas clients do not currently think important can lead to considerable frustration. What is seen as important by the client and the worker can change as stories are developed in more detail.

## Naming the Problem(s)

From a narrative perspective, naming the problem is one of the first steps in externalizing it. In relationships in which we are trying to give clients the maximum control and recognize their expertise in their own problems, what problems are called is important. Oftentimes people come to see social workers after others have told them what their problems are or what their diagnosis is. It is the clients who should determine the problems to be worked on and the names to be given to those problems unless they are coerced into coming. In that case, clients still get to name the problem, but they need to be warned that if they are trying to satisfy the requirements of coercive figures, such as a probation officer, a child welfare worker, or an employer, the problem's name should be such that working on it will satisfy those external requirements.

The name of the problem needs to be the client's so that the client can assume responsibility for his or her relationship to it. For example, a client may come in saying, "I'm depressed," or "I'm a borderline," or "I have an anxiety disorder." The social worker could ask if that is the client's name for the problem or someone else's. If it is someone else's, does the client think of it by another name? The name should be whatever the client uses to refer to the problem, not simply what an expert has called it, because it is important to stay with the person's actual experience. Depression can be experienced differently by different people, and an individual may find some aspects more salient than others. Boredom or tiredness may describe one person's experience of depression, whereas restlessness or hopelessness may be another's description. An expert might see all of these as symptoms of a single underlying disorder—depression—but a person's experience may be focused on one area, and that one area will be the problem for that person.

The first problem named may not be the problem that is discussed each week. Sometimes a different problem is named and discussed at each session. Problems often work as allies to each other in influencing people's lives. In the example of laziness given earlier, with further discussion it may be found that self-blame, overwhelmedness, and sadness all work as allies to laziness. At some point, the client may name one or more of these allies of laziness as a problem to which he or she would prefer a different relationship.

### Externalizing Strengths and Resources

Not only can problems be externalized, but it is also useful to see strengths and resources as externalizable. Few people are courageous or thoughtful or calm or loyal or industrious or hopeful all the time. When people are called such things ("Doesn't this mean you are a strong person?"), they often think of those situations when they were not strong (or courageous or loyal or so on) and they disregard or minimize the praise.

Just as it is unlikely for people to display a positive attribute all the time, it is also rare for people to have never shown behavior or thinking that corresponds with positive labels. Courage can enter people's lives just as laziness can, and people's relationship to courage can change over time and can be different in different contexts. By externalizing strengths, it may, ironically, be easier for people to see themselves as having a connection to them and derive a different meaning about who they are and what they stand for as a result. The following interchange exemplifies how this might occur:

**Client:** *Even though I knew my mother would be angry at me for saying it, I had to tell her that I needed to be in charge of my daughter, that she has been a great help, but it's high time I took over my responsibilities.*

**Worker:** Really! You did that—you told her where you stood despite your fear. Does this seem different from how you might typically have handled it?

**Client:** *Oh, yes! I would have just let her go and tell Tina that she could go out when I had already told Tina no, because it's her house and all. I would be too afraid of getting cut to pieces.*

**Worker:** Well, I really want to know how you were able to take this step. . . . I'm curious given how fear would always get between you and your mother around caring for your daughter, but you took the step you took anyway. What might have entered your life that could have accounted for you having these thoughts and taking this step?

**Client:** *I don't know what you mean.*

**Worker:** Well, could it be courage or defiance or independence or something like that?

**Client:** *Well, I guess you could say that it was my trying to become more independent.*

**Worker:** So independence was influencing you. Is independence something you see as a good or a bad thing?

**Client:** *Definitely a good thing!*

**Worker:** I'm curious, what makes you say that?

**Client:** *Well, in order to be the person I want to be I have to accept responsibility for my life and my daughter and grow up.*

**Worker:** Do you expect that independence will be making a greater presence in your life?

**Client:** *Well, even though the backlash from Mom was pretty hard, I can see this happening again in the future. I've got to do this if I am ever going to grow up.*

**Worker:** Is that what independence might tell you, that you might have to do difficult things sometimes in order to grow up? What do you think that says about you as a person who will be letting independence become a greater part of her life in the future?

**Client:** *I don't know, maybe that I can be strong sometimes?*

Externalization allows strengths to become something people can have a relationship with without a requirement that the strengths always be present. Externalization also diminishes the idea that people have resources that can be mined and exploited. If people do not see themselves as having any strengths or if they have not displayed them in the particular context of the problem, then are they without any access to those strengths? If young people are worried about getting hurt so they do not physically challenge themselves in sports, but stand up for unpopular views in their high school classes, are they cowards or are they courageous? Externalizing positives provides a person with some control over his or her relationship to the strength, the same as with problems. Although positives cannot be with anyone 100% of the time, there likely may be ways to increase the amount of time they are in a person's life.

## Maintaining Social Worker Responsibilities While Externalizing the Problem

Like it or not, clinical social workers in most agencies, because of regulation, funding sources, and licensing, must assess, diagnose, and develop goal-oriented treatment plans in line with the diagnosis of the client. Regardless of criticisms about whether social workers should use the DSM given its deficit focus and medical model (Kutchins & Kirk, 1997), the current modernist agency environment, which is where helping people primarily takes place, requires diagnosis.

There are legal and ethical restrictions on clinical social workers with regard to confidentiality, and clients need to be informed about what these are. Legal requirements typically dictate that the neglect and abuse of children, the elderly, and the disabled must be reported to the designated investigative agency. When a person discusses suicide or the intent to do violence to someone or something, there can be legal and ethical requirements concerning notification and taking action to prevent serous injury or loss of life. In addition, clinical notes routinely are reviewed by third-party payers, quality assurance committees, and/or supervisory staff.

Despite the initial impact on the relationship, the social worker should tell the client that what is said will stay between the two of them unless the worker believes someone is getting hurt or may get hurt, or the worker is subpoenaed. The client also should be told that the worker will share client information as part of routine office processes, such as supervision, case reviews, or quality assurance reviews. Clients should have an opportunity to ask questions about these rules before they talk about their problems.

## Assessment and Diagnosis in a Narrative Context

Madsen (2007) tries to create a compromise of modernist and postmodern principles by balancing the practices of assessment, diagnosis, and treatment planning against a narrative approach to looking at the client's situation. Before conducting an assessment, Madsen ensures that the family he is working with understands that they can review his assessment in draft form and make corrections if they desire. He believes this process increases the transparency of his work.

Madsen (2007) says he tells clients something like the following to introduce the assessment process:

> As you probably know, one of the things I'm required to do is write up an assessment of your situation. However, because this assessment is a story about your lives, I would like to propose that we do it together. What I would like to do is ask you a series of questions to get some information and write down much of what you say so I can make this assessment as close to your words as possible. After we are done here, I will write it up and we can go over it and see what you think. We can see what fits for you, what doesn't, and what you think we should add. How does that sound to you? (p. 84)

Madsen also expands the standard assessment categories in an attempt to thicken or enrich the description of the client. For instance, demographic information can provide the basis for the worker and the client to discuss whether factors such as race, ethnicity, and gender have a role in the problem. In describing the client, Madsen depicts the client's hopes and preferred futures, as well as his or her concerns and those of the referral source.

Madsen proposes that assessment also obtain a description of the individual's vision of life when the concerns are no longer a problem. He suggests gathering information about the problem's antecedents, possible cultural supports, and impacts; the client's beliefs about the problem; and the client's prior help-seeking experiences. To illuminate the client's current situation, his assessment model also obtains information about prior generations.

In addition, Madsen's assessment approach takes into account the client's physical health and its possible association with the current concern, as well as the individual's mental health, and whether the present situation is influencing his or her mental functioning. His assessment then explores various risk factors (i.e., suicide, violence, sexual and physical abuse, neglect, substance abuse) and individual, family, and community protective factors and resources that could be mobilized against the problem. As Madsen (2007) notes, "In our attempts to emphasize family resourcefulness, it is important that we not lose sight of risky situations and ensure that risk factors are always being adequately addressed" (p. 79). This is required of social workers both legally and ethically. I include the standard ways in which these risk assessments are conducted at the end of this chapter.

Madsen's assessment approach concludes with diagnosis and formulation, which entails using the information received to create a story from the worker's viewpoint that, it is hoped, can be of help to the client. Though some may disagree with the idea of making a diagnosis because of the conflict it can create, others have taken to formulating diagnoses with clients, showing them what the diagnosis means, and explaining why it is given. Keeping the process as transparent as possible is an important extension of minimizing the worker's power in the relationship.

In an agency that requires diagnoses be made using DSM nomenclature, social workers can discuss this with their clients, explain to them why it must be done, and offer them an opportunity to write a rejoinder, which will be retained in the file. When the social worker is ready to make a diagnosis, he or she can talk with the client about what has been written, the reasons for reaching that conclusion, and what it means to have a medical term for the problem. The social worker also can attempt to expand on how this is a very poor description of who the client is as a human being.

## Medication Compliance Issues

Diagnosis is especially important if the worker feels a psychiatric referral for medication might be appropriate. Although medication localizes the problem in clients' bodies, it can also be seen as a tool that can assist people in reaching their preferred outcomes. Medication is rarely the only intervention, and arriving at the correct prescription typically requires several psychiatric visits. Deciding on the type of medication and its dosage is not an exact science, and often a number of attempts need to be made before the right prescription is achieved. There can be a delay of as much as a month before the full effects of some medications are seen.

Even the best medication must be taken to have any effect. Medication noncompliance is a common topic in the literature as well as among clinicians. For example, in a recent study of more than 1,000 patients taking one of the newer atypical antipsychotics, more than 75% discontinued its use in less than 18 months (Lieberman et al., 2005).

Clients may need assistance in maintaining their medication regimen when the problem itself would rather they not take anything. When people are no longer experiencing symptoms, the side effects of medication may become oppressive and clients may decide they no longer need the medication. Discussing the complexities of medication is important to increasing the probability that it is seen as a tool, not a punishment, and that it is a tool over which the client always has control.

Given all of these contradictory pulls, it is not surprising that medication compliance is such a common issue in treatment and such a big source of worker frustration. It is better for clients to make a well-thought-out decision to discontinue medication as an experiment than to have them simply quit without the social workers' knowledge. In fact, medication does not work for everyone, and we all know that there are medications we just cannot take. Psychiatric medication should be no different and clients should be given choices.

## Risk Assessment in Narrative Practice

There are a number of points in social work treatment when the process itself may reduce the connection between the worker and the client. Arguably, assessment can be one of them. Another dividing point where the power of the social worker may be used against the client for societal good is in the assessment of risk.

### Assessing Suicide

The findings of large-scale research provide only the probability of a characteristic or an event appearing in a population, not the experience of the individual in front of you. However, findings from such studies can give some indication of the areas of concern workers need to be aware of. As clinical social workers, we have an obligation to assess for suicide and to attempt to intervene in most cases.

Research indicates that people who committed suicide within 1 year of being assessed for a major affective disorder typically had complaints of severe anxiety, panic attacks, severe anhedonia (loss of pleasure from usually pleasurable activities), and alcohol abuse (Clark & Fawcett, 1992). These are the concerns of many of the people who come to see clinical social workers. People with a history of suicidal ideation and/or attempts, as well as an extreme sense of hopelessness, were more likely to commit suicide in the longer term (Clark & Fawcett). It is not unusual for people in pain to want to end that pain, and in some cases self-destruction is a practice a problem might actively encourage, despite people's better judgment to the contrary.

Clients may feel put off when workers ask questions to assess for the risk of suicide. People frequently find it easier to say no when they are taken aback by a question than to think about how to answer it. Therefore, questions should be cushioned using externalization to reduce people's sense of failure in case they are having such thoughts. For the same reason, questions should lead gradually to the assessment of current risk of suicide. This is one of the places where the expert knowledge of the worker cannot be avoided.

The sequence for entering into this area of inquiry is through the concerns the client presents in the session. These types of concerns include being under the influence of overwhelming stress, depression, or negative voices (hallucinations). Substance use is a ready ally to these problems and makes a final action more probable. The social worker's questions should go from exploring passive ideas to more active ideas of wanting to kill oneself to finding out if there is a plan, including its concreteness and feasibility. Finally, the worker needs to know how far the person has gone in his or her plan, as well as the frequency and immediacy of the ideas (Carlat, 1999).

The following is an example of a suicide assessment:

**Client:** *I just get so upset. The shakes get to me and I feel like just blanking out; I can't cope anymore.*

**Worker:** When people are deeply under the influence of stress and sadness as you have described, it's not unusual for them to feel that they just want to give up and not go on. Have you ever experienced that?

**Client:** *Well, actually, yes, I have.*

**Worker:** Have you been convinced to think about suicide despite your better judgment?

**Client:** *Yes, I'm afraid I have. I can't take it sometimes.*

**Worker:** Well, you've described some very painful feelings and it would make sense that you would be open to hearing you did not have to endure them. If I may ask, what ways have you been influenced to try to kill yourself? Pills? Hanging? Weapons? Cutting? Heights? In a car? Any other possible ways I might have missed?

**Client:** *Well, I thought about taking pills a couple of times.*

**Worker:** Can you tell me about that?

**Client:** *Well, I have a bottle of antidepressants from when I saw a psychiatrist a couple of years ago. I didn't really take them then, and I have about 30 or so left. I keep them in my medicine cabinet as insurance for when it gets too tough.*

**Worker:** How close has it come to that?

**Client:** *Well, several days ago, I felt so bad I got drunk, not something I usually do, and took the pills out. I laid them on the table and counted them out. I really thought I was going to take them.*

**Worker:** I'm happy you didn't. I want to talk to you about how you were able to not take them, what went into that. But first, could you tell me if you put the pills in your hand, ready to put them into your mouth?

**Client:** *Yes, I did.*

**Worker:** And did you put any into your mouth?

**Client:** *No, I stopped myself before I could get them into my mouth.*

**Worker:** May I ask you how you were able to not take the pills?

**Client:** *I was torn; part of me said the hell with it and just wanted to end it, and another part said maybe there is a chance.*

**Worker:** I wonder what it was you saw of value that said there was a chance.

**Client:** *What do you mean?*

**Worker:** What about your life seems worth preserving? What convinced you to stay here?

**Client:** *That's a good question, but I don't really know the answer.*

**Worker:** Okay, let me switch a bit. Who supports you as a person worthy of life?

**Client:** *My children, I guess, but I'm not sure they would really miss me anyway. They have their own lives now.*

**Worker:** Although you have some doubts, what do they see in you that you might not be seeing now because the shakes have been getting in the way?

**Client:** *When I'm not messed up, they see me as a person who cares about them, I think.*

**Worker:** So when the shakes don't control you, you can be caring. I wonder if there were other ways in which this pain influenced you to consider ending it all with suicide.

**Client:** *Well, I had thought about buying razor blades and maybe cutting my wrists in the bath. The disposable ones I use don't cut.*

**Worker:** Did you buy the razor blades?

**Client:** *No, I never did. It seemed like too much work and I always had the pills.*

**Worker:** I'd like to know if you have been influenced to have these ideas more frequently now.

**Client:** Yes, every day. I'm really scared!

**Worker:** Well, because you are thinking about this a lot, have gotten the pills out, and almost took them, and because the support for you to live seems pretty weak right at this moment, I'm concerned, too. First, we need a backup in the same way that you have been pushed into thinking your pills are a backup. It seems to me that you need some time to consider your life in a setting where you will be protected from the effects of this problem. Would you be willing to go to a psychiatric hospital for a stay?

**Client:** *Would I only have to stay for a day or two? I'm a little freaked about going into a psych unit.*

**Worker:** I don't know. A hospital stay isn't my first choice unless someone really needs to be in a protected setting for a while, as the problem rages at them. The shakes are giving you a very bad time now, and you need to be safe before you fully deal with them. If you did go into the hospital, I would like us to plan for your return, for you to come back to a situation where you are feeling less stretched or pulled apart. Perhaps we could consider a celebration with those who would support you in life to see what can be done. Do you have any thoughts about it?

**Client:** *No. Maybe I could go in for a short time.*

**Worker:** Good. People rarely stay in psychiatric units for long periods of time anymore. The vast majority of people stay for only a short time, so your stay will likely be short, but that decision will be between you and the psychiatrist who treats you. Let's talk about how we can go about this.

In this transcript the social worker collected data on the intensity and frequency of the client's ideas about suicide, the existence of a suicide plan, and how far the client went in that plan. The social worker also checked for any other plans the person might have considered as well as what the influences against suicide were. Finally, the worker presented an assessment and began discussing what to do about the problem. If the client appeared desperate yet refused in-patient intervention and there were no community resources available for intensive out-patient protection, then the worker would have to consider involuntary commitment procedures. The worker's agency should have a procedure in place based on local laws that could be implemented to begin this process.

## Assessing Risk of Violence

The social worker's responsibility to assess risk does not stop with harm to self but extends to the client's current capacity for harm to others. As with the suicide assessment, talking about the client's current pain and stress can act as a transition to this discussion, perhaps by using the following questions:

> Given all the stress you are under it can be hard to keep things going. How has this affected how you get control of the children when they act up?
>
> Do you find yourself being pretty upset with them sometimes?
>
> Has this ever led you to strike them?
>
> Can you tell me what happened?

Another way to assess risk of violence is to ask clients about drug and alcohol use:

> Sometimes when people are experiencing a lot of stress, they drink or use drugs to help themselves feel better. Do you ever drink or use drugs to relieve your stress? Which drugs do you use?
>
> When you are feeling a little high, do you ever get into hassles with other people, such as your spouse or partner, your children, or people at a bar or a friend's house?
>
> Have those hassles ever led to fights? What happened during those fights?
>
> Were the police involved?
>
> Did anyone get hurt?

Exploring specific incidents in detail, including how long ago they took place and how frequently they occurred, should help to clarify the likelihood of immediate danger:

> How often have you gotten into fights with others because you had been drinking or doing drugs to relieve your stress?

Have there been any times recently when you have felt you could have really hurt someone?

Asking clients if they currently feel strongly about wanting to discipline or keep others in line or protect themselves from others creates an opening for discussing whether it is likely that they would hurt someone else.

## Questions to Assess Problems Rather Than Individuals or Families

Although Madsen's (2007) work is with multiproblem families, much of what he says is applicable to individuals. The assessment model that he developed is a case in point. Madsen (pp. 83–84) created the following questions to draw out information about client families and their presenting problems; these questions are clearly applicable for use with individuals, too:

Description of the [Individual/] Family

- Who are the important people in your lives?
- Can you tell me about your life together outside the immediate problems that bring you here?
- As I get to know you better, what do you think I might particularly appreciate about you?
- Where would you like to be headed in your life together?

Presenting Concern

- What is the referral source's biggest concern?
- What is your reaction to that?
- What concerns do you have (in rank order)?
- How will your life look different when these concerns are no longer problems?

Context of Presenting Concern

- In what situations is the problem most/least likely to occur?
- What is the effect of the problem on you and your relationships?
- How does this problem interfere with [your preferred life] your preferred life together?

- How do you explain the problem?
- How have you attempted to cope with the problem?
- What broader cultural support does the problem receive?

Family's Experience With Helpers

- What helpers are currently involved with you?
- What has been your past experience with helpers (good and bad)?
- What impact does that have on your view of helpers?
- How might that affect our work together?

Relevant History

- What is the history of the relationship between the problem and you?
- When has the problem been stronger/weaker in the history of that relationship?
- When have you been stronger/weaker throughout the history of that relationship?
- What has supported the problem's influence on you (family-of-origin level, family-helper level, broader sociocultural level)?
- What has supported your influence on the problem (family-of-origin level, family-helper level, broader sociocultural level)?

Medical Information and Risk Factors

- What effects has the problem had on your physical health? Has it exacerbated existing medical concerns for you or others?
- What, if any, interactions has the problem had with suicidal ideation, violence, substance misuse, sexual abuse, or neglect in your lives?

Formulation

- Where would you like to be headed in your life together?
- What constraints stand in the way of your getting there?
- What abilities, skills, and wisdom might you draw on to address those constraints?

## Exercise: Interviewing a Problem

A good way to begin to get a sense of how problems can be externalized is to interview someone who is role-playing a problem. (In the next chapter, your ability to externalize problems will be further developed by practicing with someone whose life is being influenced by a problem.) In developing the following exercise, I have drawn extensively on the general approach suggested by Roth and Epston (1996) and on the format and conceptual structure proposed by White (2005).

The class is divided into twosomes. Students in each twosome will reach an agreement on a problem that each will portray based on having some knowledge of it (through a client's or a personal experience) and a willingness to be interviewed about it. Preferably, each student in the twosome will present a different problem. For instance, if one person decides to use alcohol abuse or addictive thinking as the problem, the other might use depression, conflict, or procrastination.

In this exercise, each student in the pair will have a turn interviewing the other. For 20 minutes, the person being interviewed will respond as the actual problem personified. A short 5- to 10-minute debriefing will take place after the interview.

### Part One

The task of the interviewer is to interview the problem from a curious perspective to find out about its workings, influence, and shortcomings. White (2005, para. 1) recommends that the interviewer take the position of "an investigative reporter (a detective-type journalist who is good at exposing subterfuge and corruption)."

The trick is for the person role-playing the problem to stay in role as the problem and not role-play the more usual client position. If "the problem" begins talking about the problem as a third person—"Depression does this to people or to me"—the interviewer will have to gently correct the person by indicating, "Well, Depression, what do you do to people?" This might have to be done a number of times in the interview but should not detract from the exercise. The interviewer is not interested in why the problem exists or where it came from, but in how it operates. The first questions might be about what the problem does to people it selects:

> How do you affect the body of a person? The thinking of a person? The person's ability to enjoy life? The person's ability to work? How do you

affect the people around the person you have targeted? How do those other people react to your presence?

What strategies do you use to take over a person's life?

How do you undermine what a person knows so you can get control? How do you convince a person to doubt his or her abilities and skills? What ways do you have of speaking to a person that makes him or her think you are in charge?

Who and what stands in support of you against the person? Do other problems act as your allies?

What is it that other people do (even good-heartedly) that makes it easier for you to gain influence over the person you have targeted?

What is operating in the culture that makes it easier for you to have your way with people?

When you are challenged in a person's life, what do you do to get his or her life back under your control?

The interviewer then moves on to questions directed at the problem's weaknesses and failures. Problems always have weaknesses and failures, though one is often led to believe otherwise.

What areas of people's lives do you have the most difficulty taking control of?

What are the most difficult counterstrategies that you face when people try to get their lives back from your control?

Are there special types of "self-talk" you find most difficult to face?

In what ways do the people who support the person you have targeted make it difficult for you to gain a greater hold on that person's life?

How do people's values and beliefs get in the way of what you would desire for them?

What other ways do people have of reclaiming their lives from you?

## Part Two

Students take about 5–10 minutes to debrief on the process of doing the exercise. The person who has been playing the problem can talk about his or her experiences of the exercise, and what it was like to portray the problem. The interviewer can discuss how this interview seemed different from (and/or similar to) a traditional clinical interview. Both parties can then share their thoughts on proposals for action that might undermine the influence of the problem in people's lives.

## Parts Three and Four

For the third part of the exercise, the roles of interviewer (investigative reporter) and problem are reversed. Interviews are again conducted for 20 minutes. For the fourth part, students again debrief for 10–15 minutes.

CHAPTER 5

# The Effect of the Problem on the Person

In this chapter, I describe the impact of problems on people. I illustrate how social workers can secure clients' problem stories in interviews. I highlight the importance of listening to clients' stories as stories—that is, listening without preconceived notions about what is, or will be, important. I then discuss the importance of asking questions to deconstruct clients' narratives and demonstrate how questions can be used to draw out clients' knowledge of their lives. I show how the description and name of the problem can be developed through intent listening and questioning. I then discuss the value of identifying the problem's history in the client's life and illustrate how this can contribute to the development of alternative stories that point the way toward the client's preferred outcomes. Finally, I examine how problems, and their societal contexts, can impact those under their influence.

## Curious Listening

What you have probably learned about treatment so far in your education is that you should listen for the pieces of the client's story that make sense from your theoretical point of view, and when you find them you should develop those pieces. You will have then found the developmental cause, traumatic experience, negative or faulty cognition, family pattern of interaction, or reinforcing contingency that is most important in understanding the client's problem. Professional judgment requires sorting a large number of facts to find within them the pattern that contributes to causing or maintaining the problem and that suggests which intervention technique would be most suitable. Oftentimes clients do not recognize the pattern or its importance, understandings that rest upon the expertise of the worker and his or her theory.

Ambiguity and uncertainty are experienced as sources of anxiety for many social workers, who must find a theoretical niche in which to place the client's story's information. However, uncertainty is also the specialty of the professional, who quickly finds that no model totally explains the story a client tells without modifying the story in some way (Parton & O'Bryne, 2000). How the client's story is modified depends on the professional's theoretical orientation and expertise, which inform the questions asked and the interpretive reflections given.

Griffith and Griffith (1994) discuss how practitioners' "emotional postures can either open or close possibilities for therapeutic dialogue" (p. 66). They recommend that workers seek a calm and tranquil, rather than a "mobilized" (i.e., defensive, aggressive), response from clients (p. 66). They suggest three ways to achieve this: informing clients that they do not need to answer questions they do not feel comfortable with; respecting clients' integrity by asking their permission before delving into certain topics; and using clients' language, rather than the professional's, when discussing problems. In addition to these efforts to show respect for clients and to make storytelling easier, Griffith and Griffith recommend mirroring a client's outward behavior (i.e., shallow breathing, closed-off postures, leaning into the conversation) to stimulate a more authentic understanding of what the client is trying to convey.

Griffith and Griffith (1994) also suggest listening carefully for the metaphors in people's stories. Words such as *lazy, crazy,* or *successful* are open to many interpretations. Listening for statements such as "It's like . . ." or "It makes me feel like . . ." will make social workers more aware of the metaphors clients are using. Griffith and Griffith describe the use of this type of careful listening in their own practice with a female client:

> During the therapy, each metaphor was treated as if it were a label on a file drawer filled with life stories—stories of "artistic," stories of "weakness," stories of "crazy." Only as these stories were told did we come to a common understanding of the meaning of her words. (p. 84)

Narrative treatment requires an approach to listening that can best be described as curious or not knowing. When social workers take the position of giving clients credit for what they know about their own lives, then the workers do not have to have all the answers. Unfortunately, professional training and socialization make it difficult for most social workers to listen to clients' stories as stories; practitioners typically believe they have to "do something" (Freedman & Combs, 1996).

The narrative worker, through curiosity about the client's story, is always moving toward what, to the worker, is often an unknown conclusion. This is perhaps a more realistic appraisal of life in general given the uncertainty of life and of the consequences of life's events. At best, the predictive value of any theory of behavior is probabilistic; no theory can definitively predict future behavior.

The narrative social worker tries to understand the meaning of the story to the storyteller rather than the "meaning" of the story. Therefore, the worker explores any words that seem unusual, emotion laden, or not quite in sync with the story's development. This is not nearly as easy a task as it might appear. During workshop and classroom exercises, it is not uncommon to hear participants say, "This is so much harder than it looks!" Students generally find it a challenge to just curiously listen to and explore stories. They want to help, to solve problems, to develop solutions, not "just" listen.

The trick (and the challenge) of curious listening is to avoid thinking that people mean something other than what they say. Andersen (1995, p. 25) suggests workers look only at what is inside a word, not at what is "behind or under or over" it, which would require interpretation. According to Andersen, questions to try to keep the focus from shifting to interpretation include: "What do you see if you look into the word?" or "I noticed you said this or that" or "Can you say more what you were thinking when you said that?" (p. 25).

The focus of the worker is on getting information not yet known, not on asking questions to get data to fit a theory or to make a particular argument or point based on expertise. The difference is best laid out in an example:

A second interview in cognitive therapy might look like this:

> **Worker:** Linda, what about the automatic thoughts, all the need to know what to do? What do you notice as you think about them now?
>
> **Linda:** *Well, it's always the same thing. And it feels real urgent.*
>
> **Worker:** Do you notice anything missing?
>
> **Linda:** *Missing?*
>
> **Worker:** Missing compared to what others might think. You often mention your friend Gerri as being a logical thinker. What would Gerri say back to you, for example, if you were saying those thoughts out loud to her?
>
> **Linda:** *Ha. Well, she'd think I was crazy, but that's why I don't tell her, of course. Hmmm . . . I guess she'd point out that I don't know why he's late, it could be anything. Oh, that never occurs to me, does it?*

> **Worker:** *Right. Because people are late for all sorts of reasons, even super on-timers like you. (Both smile). So if it did occur to you, what might you come up with for Carl? Or whomever? (Cooper & Lesser, 2002, pp. 153, 155)*

In this interview fragment the social worker is making arguments to orient the client to healthier cognitions that would not foster or maintain anxiety about a partner who is often late. The client is helped to see the illogical nature of her cognitions, and how those illogical thoughts are a problem ("Oh, that never occurs to me, does it? . . . Right"). She is also encouraged to consider alternative cognitions through a reflection ("Because people are late for all sorts of reasons, even super on-timers like you") and a question ("So if it did occur to you, what might you come up with for Carl? Or whomever?").

A narrative interview might go this way in a second session:

> **Jill (*worker*):** Did the conversation we had last time leave you with any new thoughts or . . .
>
> **Hollie (*client*):** *I was just thinking . . . thinking about when I was little and growing up and, you know, how things were. And I had a discussion with my sister after I saw you. We were just talking about the family as a whole. You know, she said that she escaped, and she thinks I didn't. And I don't think it's just because my marriage is in bad shape, but she said to me, and this was very strange, because I said, you know, that you and I were talking about how I grew up in such a sexist situation all around, you know? And I'm not sure how it tied in, but she brought up a situation and I said to her, "I don't know why very often this particular scene pops into my mind." And she said the same thing. This one time, our family—there's three of us kids, my mother and father. . . . When I was getting dinner, putting it on the table, I can't remember what was going on at that minute. My brother, my little brother and I always would be verbally fighting at the table. And all I remember was that my father stood up at the table, took the entire table—food, dishes, everything, chairs—and knocked it over. Things were flying all over the place and there was broken glass everywhere. Everything was a wreck, and my mother just stood there and didn't say a word. And then, I don't know what happened. I guess she just cleaned everything up. It was just weird that we both said that we remembered this. What a scene.*

**Jill:** What significance did that have for you?

**Hollie:** *That my mother, when you think about it, she didn't like say anything, you know? She didn't take any stance, like say, "What the hell? What are you doing?" You know, "What's your problem? I know the kids are fighting" or whatever it was. But that was nothing. And it was like . . . it was bad. It was real bad. But she took it. She just tolerated it.*

**Jill:** What do you think must have been going on for her to just take it?

**Hollie:** *I guess, I don't know, she must have been scared. It was pretty scary.*

**Jill:** What do you think would have happened if she did take a stance?

**Hollie:** *I don't know. Maybe it would have been worse.* (Freedman & Combs, 1996, p. 159)

In this example the worker is not instructing the client, a woman whose husband has been caught giving expensive gifts to other women, on what to do, but instead is opening up discussion. The worker keeps expanding the story, not to find the truth, but to find its meaning for the client, where the client has provided a story of an upsetting and confusing event from her past ("What significance did that have for you?"). The worker asks the client to take her mother's perspective in the story to fill it out more completely ("What do you think must have been going on for her to just take it?"). The question is asked after the client's comments about being brought up in a sexist environment and how her mother just "took it." Notice how the focus could easily have shifted away from the client's story if the worker had inquired about how the client felt when telling this story or whether she felt unprotected by her mother in that situation, or if the worker had reflected that it must have been very difficult to be in that situation as a child.

The two examples of interview transcripts are given not only to show the difference between these approaches but also to suggest that without a conscious effort, narrative interviews can easily look like any other type of interview. If the values of client collaboration and client self-determination are not rigorously upheld, then narrative notions can be used as easily as those of any other model to convince people of a point of view. What if Jill's next comment had been: "Could it have been better, too?" or "Isn't it better to stand up for your rights in a relationship than to have someone abuse them?" A narrative perspective does not automatically take away a worker's issues with control or feelings of possessing the truth; it only sets up a structure in which these issues can be examined for what they are. It is just as easy to coerce clients into externalizing their problems as it is to label and challenge their cognitions.

*Deconstructive listening* (Freedman & Combs, 1996, pp. 46–47) is what is required. This involves appreciating the slipperiness of meaning and recognizing the likelihood that what the social worker understands is not what the client is intent on conveying. Every story will have gaps, and filling in the gaps can help expand the story and give it new meanings. Skills in summarizing and reflecting back to the client as well as exploring ambiguities in words or emotional reactions are required (Freedman & Combs, 1996). These skills are particularly important when the client's race, ethnicity, gender, sexual orientation, or other status is different from the worker's. For example:

**Client:** *I just needed it so bad. I went out and got some gear and copped some stuff on the street.*

**Worker:** So you went out and got some stuff. (*Summarizing*) What kind of drug was that? *(Clarifying)*

**Client:** *Heroin.*

**Worker:** So the gear then would be? *(Clarifying)*

**Client:** *Don't you know? Needles, syringe.*

**Worker:** Thanks for bearing with me, but I don't want to miss what you're telling me. How difficult was it to get your gear and stuff? *(Filling in a gap)*

**Client:** *Like buying candy. Pushers all know me and I know who'll treat me straight.*

**Worker:** I don't know anybody on my side of town who would know how to get stuff and gear. *(Commenting on own lived experience)*

**Client:** *That's because they all come to my part of town, all these young kids. We've got the stuff.*

**Worker:** What do you think it means that you can't find it in my part of town but it's all over your part of town?

**Client:** *'Cause we're poor and no one gives a damn about what we do.*

**Worker:** When you're poor no one cares if you kill yourself, but if you aren't poor all the stuff is pushed into the poor parts away from you. *(Clarifying)*

**Client:** *Yeah, that's right. The way the world works.*

**Worker:** Do you think that is good or bad? *(Asking for a value stance, evaluating)*

**Client:** *It sucks! My kid goes out to school and there are pushers all over the place.*

**Worker:** So why is that bad? *(Requesting justification of the evaluation)*

**Client:** *What do you mean! My kids got a right to grow up and be someone, just like your kids.*

**Worker:** So the current situation isn't good because it could keep kids—your kids—down, could keep them on the poor side of town. *(Summarizing)*

**Client:** *Yeah, it's damn unfair!*

Or:

**Client:** *I just needed it so bad. I went out and got some gear and copped some stuff on the street.*

**Worker:** I noticed when you talked about needing it so bad you looked like you shivered. May I ask you what it meant to you? *(Clarifying)*

**Client:** *It scares me to think of how much the stuff controls my life, like I'm a puppet sometimes.*

Simple listening and exploring can have an impact. Madsen (2007) describes a study in which he interviewed families around issues of medical noncompliance. At the follow-up 6 months after the initial family interview, seven of the nine patients being interviewed were managing their chronic medical condition for the first time in years. Through the research project, families had the opportunity during the interview to reflect upon their situation, and that seems to have changed their perspective.

Although helping people find alternative stories might be seen as the intervention in this form of work, it is critical not to rush and leave the problem too quickly. Moving away from the problem too fast can lead to a noncollaborative situation in which the client feels disrespected and disengaged and the social worker feels the need to try to force a solution. It can also result in the worker losing the opportunity to learn more from the client about what his or her life is all about.

From a narrative perspective, assessment means looking at the extent of the problem and the unique outcomes that are available. The problem story is important because alternatives and forms of protest against the problem arise from it. Moreover, the problem story is very important to the person sitting in front of you. Appreciating the full extent of the problem acknowledges the life story the client is presenting and constitutes "starting where the client is," a long-standing bit of social work practice wisdom.

Hearing of people's suffering is a privilege that social workers are given by society. Social workers bear witness to the plight of vulnerable people in society and the witnessing leads to greater truths for both the client and the worker. In his study of illness narratives, Frank (1995) talks about how the testimony, or story, of sufferers leads those who listen to consider what is important in life and how precious moments can be. It is not just the words but the life lived that conveys these messages. People who suffer know the value of life, health, and relationships through their loss (or threatened loss) of them. Respecting both the person's pain and the knowledge acquired from it conveys that the person is valued.

## Historicizing the Problem

When the client and the social worker have developed a description of a problem (or problems) and the client has named it (or them), it is then helpful to get a historical perspective on each problem. Historicizing the problem, which involves developing the problem's history (White & Epston, 1990), does several things.

First, it lets the client know that you appreciate the problem's significance to him or her. Not discussing the problem can leave a person feeling that he or she has not been taken seriously; by getting a history of the problem, the worker is displaying his or her interest in the client's perception of its frequency and impacts. Historicizing the problem recognizes people's sense of hopelessness about their troubles.

Second, tracing the history of the problem also allows the worker to look at the relative influence of the problem on the person's life over time. People may fashion their stories based on the assumption that problems start and get worse and worse until something is done about them. In fact, many problems do not operate that way and it may require some probing to find out how the client does experience the problem. Problems often wax and wane in a person's life, taking up more of his or her life at some times and less at others. Showing that the problem is not static affirms for the client that future changes are possible because examples exist of past changes (Morgan, 2000).

Third, historicizing the problem can lead to exploring the dominant discourses that are affecting the problem's development and maintenance (Freedman & Combs, 1996). For example, when looking at the abuse or exploitation of a female client by males, the following questions might be asked: Where did you learn that men should be in charge of women? Do you think this is something most people in this society learn? How do you think we are recruited into these beliefs? Do you remember any episodes of this happening? When? Any before that?

Looking at past episodes of a problem and the course it has run can help clarify the problem for the client as well as for the worker. It can extend empathy by spending time with the problem discussion; it can open up instances of resistance to the problem, which can lead to alternative stories; and it can lead to examination of societal discourses and how they function in the person's relationship to the problem. The intent of a worker's questions is to elicit a description of the problem and its impacts over time, not seek its psychological cause.

The following are examples of questions that can be used to historicize a problem and to look for differences over time:

> When did you first notice the problem? How long ago?
>
> What do you remember before the problem entered your life?
>
> When would you say the problem was strongest? When was it weakest? When did you feel stronger in the face of the problem?
>
> What was it like for you 6 months ago [3 months ago, 1 year ago, 4 years ago, 3 days ago]? What did you notice about the problem? How much of your life did it have at that time? (Morgan, 2000, p. 34)

Questions to expose dominant discourses that play a part in the problem include:

> Where did you learn this way of thinking about relationships?
>
> What models were there for these kinds of attitudes?
>
> How did fear so easily coach you to believe that? (Freedman & Combs, 1996, p. 70)

As you can see, these questions look at the life of the problem and the person's relationship with that problem, not the problem's possible causes.

## The Problem's Impact on the Person

Once a history of the problem has been developed, a rather extensive discussion can be started about the impact that the problem is having on the person and his or her relationships. This entails eliciting the client's evaluation of the problem's effects and his or her justification for that evaluation.

As with questions about the problem's history, those about its impact should keep the problem externalized to reduce possible feelings of hopelessness that can come from partializing out all the pain the problem has caused the person.

As motivational interviewing (Miller & Rollnick, 2002) recognizes, even problems can have good as well as bad aspects. If questions are focused only on the assumption that all the effects of the problem are bad, then a person who might be ambivalent about the problem is likely to pick up the other side (the benefits of the problem) in defense. For example, although drinking alcohol can lead someone to lose his or her family, friends, and job, as well as destroy the individual's liver, it also allows some people to unwind, relax, and talk to friends. Discussing only the negative effects on the client's family, job, or health might lead the client to defend his or her behavior on the basis of relaxation and recreation with friends. Or, a client simply might disregard the implications of the questions asked as being uninformed. The benefits and burdens of problems are true to the person's experience, and denying either side leads to a thinner story, one that is not as rich in detail and that ignores the person's lived experience. Letting people come to their own conclusions by asking about both sides of the problem encourages a more collaborative relationship.

Asking people to justify their evaluation is a way to have them look at what their preferences and values in life are, and whether the problem is in opposition to them. This involves repetitive questioning that can sound boring to the observer. Yet this process is far from boring; it is, in fact, an important part of the narrative social work process. Narrative social workers, as social constructionists, believe that it is through the process of the conversation that the worker and client develop new realizations about the problem's effects, new understandings of its impact on the client's life, and new appreciations about what is important and valued by each of them. In traditional forms of treatment, the assumptions that underlie clients' evaluations of problems' effects are rarely examined. In narrative work, doing so creates the opportunity to deconstruct, or unpack, what makes the problem so destructive to clients' lives and aspirations.

Morgan (2000, p. 39) lists 11 types of effects that problems can have, which I present here. For the first two effects I have included exemplar questions and interview examples with evaluation and justification questions to illustrate how these effects could be explored; I offer exemplar questions for the remaining nine effects.

"The person's sense of self: what they think of themselves as a person" [i.e., What does Depression tell you about who you are?]:

> **Client:** *I guess it makes me feel useless, like I can't get anything done.*
>
> **Worker:** Is not getting things done a good or bad thing?
>
> **Client:** *Well, bad, of course. Isn't that a silly question?*
>
> **Worker:** Sometimes I'm surprised. People can often see good and bad in many things, so I find it important to ask. What makes you say that this is a bad thing, not getting things done?
>
> **Client:** *Well, when I get things done I feel good about myself.*
>
> **Worker:** How do others feel about you?
>
> **Client:** *Well, they expect me to get things done.*
>
> **Worker:** Could you talk a bit about what some of those things are that people expect you to do and that make you feel more useful and good about yourself when you do them and that you would do if Depression wasn't in your life?

"Their views of themselves as a parent, partner, mother, wife, sister, brother, worker, etc." [i.e., What effect has Depression had on your view of yourself as a parent?]:

> **Client:** *It tells me I'm a lousy parent. When I get home from work, I don't cook or clean, I just go right to bed.*
>
> **Worker:** Is feeling this way good or bad for you?
>
> **Client:** *Bad. I see myself as someone who loves and protects my children, and I'm not acting like it now.*

"Their hopes, dreams, and sense of the future" [i.e., Has Depression changed how you see your future? In what way?]

"Their relationships with children, parents, partner, community members, colleagues, etc." [i.e., Has Depression affected your relationship with members of your church? Has it brought you closer to or taken you farther away from them?[

"Their work" [i.e., Has Depression affected your work in any way?]

"Their social life" [i.e., What effect has Depression had on your social life? Have you noticed any changes when Depression has a greater influence over you?]

"Their thoughts" [i.e., How has Depression affected your thinking? Does it tell you encouraging things or discouraging things? Does it make it easier or harder for you to make decisions?]

"Their physical health" [i.e., How has Depression affected your energy level? Does it help put you to sleep or does it keep you awake? Does it ever make you physically sick or even more healthy?]

"Their spirits" [i.e., Does Depression ever lift your spirits and help you appreciate life more? How does it do that?]

"Their moods or feelings" [i.e., How has Depression affected your moods?]

"Their everyday life" [i.e., How does Depression influence how your everyday life goes?]

Of course, not all of these types of questions need to be asked about each problem, but most social workers, feeling rushed to solve clients' problems, ask few of them. More questions would be better to draw out the problem's full impact on a person's life. Seeing the problem as something that affects many parts of a person's life is useful in at least two ways. First, when the problem is seen as affecting other people it can be easier to distinguish it as separate from the person. If it is depression's strategy to find ways to cut the client off from those who care about him or her, then depression, not the absence of others and their motivations, becomes the focus of consideration. What the client can do to outwit depression becomes more important than waiting for apologies from "disloyal" friends. Second, as people go into greater detail about how the problem has impacted them, they are likely to provide clues about where they have not let the problem take over their lives. This, in turn, suggests possible areas where they have protested against the problem, and these areas can be looked at in more detail to see if they could be the basis for an alternative story.

## Larger Societal Issues in Problem's Impacts

*Deconstructive questions* (Freedman & Combs, 1996, p. 56) take apart the dominant story of the problem's influence on the person and others around the person. It is easy to stay focused on the name the client gives the problem when it is first discussed and not look a little further at the possibility of societal oppression playing a part in its development and maintenance. Deconstructive questions help to unmask so-called truths and hidden biases behind disembodied ways of speaking (White, 1993c). Such questions make "visible the hidden, interpretative assumptions that give meaning to an idea" (Griffith & Griffith, 1994, p. 114).

On some level, we have become acclimated to impersonal language. Downsizing, which refers to the organization, ignores the trauma of unemployment to individuals, families, and communities. It is rarely upper-echelon executives who are downsized (and when that happens they often receive "golden parachutes" to cushion their landing), but rather those least likely to be able to pick themselves up. Patient management, as used in modern medicine, is a nice way of saying that it is now normative for the health care system to require people to sit for long periods of time in flimsy hospital gowns and often cold rooms while waiting for an expert to see them for a short period of time, make a pronouncement, and write a prescription. This is "the way things are" and, therefore, not open to question. Yet unless the assumptions behind these truths are examined, we are locked into whatever the social system requires, with only a limited number of options. Social work has a history, be it myth or not, that tells us we need not be satisfied with the way things are and should work for social justice and change.

When social work treatment happens in an office, the only conversation that takes place is what occurs between worker and client(s). These conversations can blithely ignore issues of inferior schools, dangerous neighborhoods, racism in everyday life, and sexism at home and at work. For example, the problem under discussion between a social worker and an adolescent client could be the young man's fighting with other students and teachers at school. The difficulty may be labeled as trouble, the discussion may be about how this young man seems to get into trouble at school, and the interaction may be simply focused on how he can get control of the trouble in his life. Trouble may be a problem, but the definitions of who this young man is—"a troublemaking Black kid" by the school principal; a tough, "won't-take-any-crap" guy by his peers; a troubled, deprived adolescent by the school counselor; or a "pain in the neck" by his family—will have a great impact on the way he sees trouble and whether he sees the problem as trouble or as one or more of trouble's allies (other problems). Anger can lead to trouble, which might be a preliminary description of the problem. Upon further discussion, however, it might be found that racism and discrimination at school or in the workplace may be allied to the young man's feelings of anger. The anger may be a protest against the oppression and may be useful, but the way in which the anger is expressed is through impulsive behaviors that are not focused on the sources of the oppression and that lead instead to trouble. Through deconstructive questioning the problem is revealed to encompass racism as well as trouble.

Freedman and Combs (1996) talk about exposing dominant discourses by looking at how context affects problems:

> What "feeds" the problem?
>
> What "starves" it?
>
> Who benefits from it?
>
> In what settings might the problematic attitude be useful?
>
> What sort of people would proudly advocate for the problem?
>
> What groups of people would definitely be opposed to it and its intentions? (p. 68)

According to Freedman and Combs (1996, p. 68), "questions such as these invite people to consider how the entire context of their lives affects the problem and vice versa."

To illustrate how these questions can be used to reveal the dominant discourses, I have applied them to the case just described—that of the problems presented by the young man in trouble supported by anger and racism:

> What "feeds" the problem? The young man feels disrespected, feels he is made to do things he will never need to do again and is not good at doing. He feels he is treated like he is stupid, and others are trying to run his life for no reason.
>
> What "starves" it? Respect. This helps him to do better, to see some value in what he is doing. It makes him feel like a person, not just some dumb Black kid.
>
> Who benefits from it? The young man may not have thought of it but several environmental systems may have a stake in, if not accruing actual benefits from, trouble and its allies. For instance, the public education system is under pressure to keep children in school and the state mandates attendance, and truant officers, school social workers, and in some cases juvenile magistrates are kept busy through young men like this one. Drug dealers, street gangs, variety stores, and theaters might benefit, depending on what the young man does with his time away from school. When adolescents from poor schools become truant and labeled as trouble, the broader society does not have to deal with inequities in the educational system based on class and race. The problem is solely that of irresponsible adolescents and their families.
>
> In what settings might the problematic attitude be useful? Being tough and defying the authorities are attitudes that hold currency in

the young man's peer group. Being tough may serve him well if he lives in a dangerous environment.

What sort of people would proudly advocate for the problem? A parent who feels that his or her child's schooling is inferior or even useless may be unlikely to support the child's school attendance, short of legal sanctions. Friends who wish to be truant may also support the young man missing school. Teachers who have this young man in class and find his attitude disruptive may support his nonattendance. Finally, racism is supported by the majority culture's attitude and by the way resources are distributed, so that those with power and class advantage receive a greater share of society's benefits.

What groups of people would definitely be opposed to it and its intentions? Family members and friends who believe in the young man and his future would definitely be opposed to the problem. Teachers who see his potential would be opposed to it. School authorities, such as the principal, school social worker, or counselor, might also be strongly opposed to the problem.

Looking at problems from this perspective allows the social worker to consider what societal discourses are at work. To the extent the problem is kept at the level of the young man's not attending school regularly, then poverty, racism, and oppression do not enter into consideration and are not discussed in relation to the young man's troubles. Although these societal issues are daunting, exploring them offers the opportunity for developing communities of students and families who band together to let their anger be known. Otherwise, the solitary protests of individual students can become lost in the juvenile justice and mental health systems.

Madsen (2007) notes another important question that helps to draw out the impact of problems and societal discourses on people: "What story might this problem try to tell you about what kind of person you are?" (p. 221). As with Freedman and Combs's (1996) questions, this question looks at how problems affect self-definition and how that definition is supported. In the example of the young man, the story told by the problem might be one of being beyond the control of a "useless" education system, of being independent and tough, and/or of being one's "own man." The problem's story might also tell the young man that he will never succeed according to the White, middle-class definition of success and that making it in his neighborhood may actually be based on whom he knows, not what he knows. It might inform him that he can make it his own way, not like some of the other "chumps" who put up with school. This is what trouble might tell him about who he is.

Standing up to problems, which sometimes can come to be defined as the problem, is made easier by taking a broader view, looking not just at how the problem is enacted in the person but also at how it is rooted in societal discourse. Unfortunately, it is far easier to see how past, compared to present-day, discourses have hurt people. But does that mean we are left with no choice except to accept today's common truths that voice hearers are damaged people; homosexuals are immoral; African Americans are incapable of positions of greatness but are suitable for easier, entry-level jobs; and women are too emotional for many of the tasks required by professional positions? Obviously not, but think of the pain and hate these truths have caused people for much of history by reducing the options available to them.

The clearer it is that a problem is supported by the truths of current societal discourses (poverty, illness, unemployment, hunger, homelessness), the more urgent it is to develop communities to support people in their struggles. It is not likely that people can cope with these truths on their own; to change them requires forming groups, taking action, engaging in advocacy, and encouraging mediation. The "boxes" that people struggle with are real in that they have very strong environmental supports. Imagining possible alternative stories can rescue a person's spirit.

## Exercise: A "Slowing Down" Interview: Interviewing on the Effects of Problems

Consider an event that has occurred in your life during the past week. This event should not be too emotionally trying, but something you think you could recover some details about. Examples might be taking a pet to the veterinarian or having an important conversation with a friend or family member, something with some emotional charge to it, but not anything extreme, such as being assaulted, witnessing a suicide, or having a difficult fight with a close friend or family member. Education and psychotherapy serve different purposes. Education should teach you to be a better social worker; psychotherapy should help you become a more satisfied person.

Break into pairs. Using the format for interviewing a problem laid out in chapter 4, repeat that exercise only this time instead of being the problem, the person being interviewed will have the problem.

The person who is the interviewer begins by asking the person who has the problem what he or she has been doing over the past week that he or she enjoys and feels proud about. Explore these topics in some detail before moving to the next step, which is to ask if anything occurred during the week that the person wishes to discuss. Help the person describe the problem situation and then ask if he or she can come up with a name to externalize it. Finally, go into detail about the incident and any historical precedents that can give it added depth and/or meaning. Interview the person about the externalized problem and its effect on him or her, including possible impacts on different aspects of the person's life and on the lives of others around him or her. Try to focus on making the interview as detailed and slow as possible.

After about 20 minutes, stop and take 5–10 minutes to debrief on the process of doing the exercise. Then, reverse roles so that the interviewer becomes the person who has the problem and the person who had the problem is now the interviewer. Again, conduct the interview for about 20 minutes and conclude by debriefing for 5–10 minutes.

CHAPTER 6

# The Effect of the Person on the Problem

When listening to problem stories it is often possible to hear the ways the person has taken a stand, no matter how slight, against the problem. Having looked at the problem's influence on the person, the social worker can then explore with the client what has been the client's influence on the problem. Times when the person has stood up to the problem and weakened or removed its influence from his or her life can provide the basis for developing alternative stories that may lead to preferred outcomes.

In this chapter I describe approaches to developing alternative stories with clients, who may see exploring an alternative story as frivolous or frightening, especially if they believe they have never been able to resist the problem's influence. I start, therefore, by discussing the various ways clients can stand up to problems and how these stances, if seen by clients as important, can provide the basis for an alternative story. I then describe how clues to clients' resistance to the problem can be found in the dominant problem story as well as in stories depicting other parts of clients' lives.

Following these discussions, I present examples of questions that can be used to probe for possible exceptions to the problem story and instances when the person may have influenced the problem. Looking at the person's influence on the problem requires tact because it takes the conversation in the direction opposite to what a client expects. I conclude the chapter by describing how to slow down an interview so as to elicit extensive details about clients' resistance to problems that can be used to enlarge and enrich the alternative story being developed.

## What Are Unique Outcomes?

Unique outcomes or *sparkling moments* (Monk, 1997, p. 13) are those times, events, or thoughts that do not fit with the problem story. Unique outcomes are exceptions to the problem and are not expected given the problem story. They represent the influence the person has had on how the problem influences his or her life.

Typically, it is not too difficult to imagine what a client's life would be like if the problem had total control over it. By carefully listening to the client's story, the social worker might note thoughts, actions, or events that do not fit the worker's image of complete problem domination; these are unique outcomes. For example, if a person is under the influence of exhaustion, a worker might wonder if exhaustion would want the person to stay in bed every day and not get up. If the answer is yes, then every time the client comes to see the worker is an exception, as is every time the person gets out of bed for any reason other than bodily functions. These events indicate that the person has protested against the problem's complete domination and has been able to influence the problem as a result. These unique outcomes are the basic building blocks of an alternative story to a preferred outcome.

The social worker may be first in evaluating the uniqueness of an event, but the event's final evaluation as a unique outcome rests with the client. Often these events are experienced as fragments of memory, and recovering them can be as difficult as recovering dreams the morning after. If the worker sees an event as unique and the client gives it little significance, then it simply is not unique and will provide little value to the client. Because meaning is developed within the context of conversation, the worker and client can explore in some detail the different facets of an event. The worker can then ask the client whether the event marks a difference in what the problem usually has him or her doing, thinking, or feeling. Such exploration can underline an event and bring out its significance. As a student once told me, "I didn't know I knew that until I was asked questions about it and had to explain it."

What are unique outcomes and what do they look like? Morgan (2000) has laid out how a unique outcome can be seen in "a plan, action, feeling, statement, quality, desire, dream, thought, belief, ability, or commitment" (p. 52). Examples best explain these categories:

> Jill has a *plan* to meet with a longtime friend for lunch, despite how Depression has told her to stay home because no one really likes her.
> After repeated attempts, Jack finally made an appointment and went to talk with a social worker about how Anxiety tells him he cannot leave the house. This *action* of leaving the house is a protest against Anxiety.
> Jill is feeling joy over finally graduating from her MSW program despite Inadequacy continually telling her that she could not do it and

that her being in graduate school was just a fluke. The *feeling*, as well as the action, is in opposition to Inadequacy.

Jack told the worker that he no longer wants to take heroin and is finally ready to begin a methadone treatment program. This is a *statement* that Addictive Thinking would rather that Jack had not made.

Jill treats her clients with caring and compassion despite the negative attitudes her coworkers seem to have toward them and appear to expect her to share. This *quality* of caring and compassion stands in opposition to the Disrespectful Beliefs of some members of her agency.

Jill's *desire* to build a strong relationship with her partner is a rebuke to Hopelessness's telling her that her relationships are doomed to fail.

It is Joe's hope to be back with his family and have a job when he gets on methadone. Joe's *dream* runs counter to what Addictive Thinking wants for him.

Jill thinks she is a good person even though Voices tell her she is evil. This is an example of a *thought* indicating protest against a problem.

Joe's *belief* that people could like him in the future goes against Self-destructive Thoughts that tell him no one could ever care for or love him.

Jill's *ability* to get to work every morning is a protest against Depression's trying to force her to stay in bed.

Joe's *commitment* to maintain a relationship with his mother despite her dementia conflicts with how Individualism wants him to take care of just himself.

Unique outcomes can be big or small, in the present or the past. It is generally better to start with those events that are closest in time to the present because it is easier to flesh them out in greater detail and clients are likely to find them more relevant to their current situation. An event that occurred 5 years ago, before the problem took hold, might seem irrelevant to the client, whereas a small attempt made last week to protest against the problem may seem more relevant to the current struggle, although the prior incident can prove valuable later in treatment in developing an alternative story.

Under the influence of optimism, the narrative social worker believes that no problem completely captures a person 24 hours a day, 365 days a year. Without this optimistic viewpoint, developing alternative stories in which the person at least considers taking a stand against the problem can be a challenge because people in trouble do not see their lives as being anything but troubled. However, further bolstering workers' optimism is the recognition that the focus of work is on changing clients' relationships to their problems, not the problems themselves, a small but important linguistic difference. Thus, although workers may not be able to make problems go away, clients can be assisted in finding ways to reduce their impact, which requires the clients to accept some responsibility for their relationship to the problems.

This optimistic view permits the social worker to recognize, for instance, that the couple who are seeking help with their relationship and who display intense conflict in the worker's office is not the couple who live together and get through the day with each other. The worker's belief that intense conflict is not the couple's only story requires him or her to explore the couple's willingness to separate themselves from the present turmoil and envision a story different from the two opposing ones being presented. There are times when the couple's tension is relieved, at least a little, in order to have the couple minimally function. These instances may represent unique outcomes and can provide the basis for developing an alternative story.

Social workers need to be cautious not to get too far ahead of clients. It can be very tempting to become the expert and drag clients along to a more optimistic view; however, that optimism may not be felt as authentic by clients. Getting clients' permission to look at these nonproblem areas is important and reduces the likelihood of workers persuading clients to be where the workers think they should be, rather than where they want to be.

There are two ways to explore clients' ability to push against the influence of a problem. One way is by using clues in the problem story. The other involves directly questioning clients about the existence of such examples.

## Clues to Unique Outcomes

Unique outcomes are often trivialized or dismissed, seen by clients as aberrations or instances of luck because they do not fit the dominant problem story. These hints of another story can come in the form of outright exceptions (i.e., I am completely isolated except that I go to church every Sunday) or in the use of such qualifiers as "almost always," "nearly every time," or "it seems like always." Noting these exceptions and referring to them later after the problem story has been developed can lead to discussing alternative stories and to a fuller story of the client. Although it may be tempting to focus on unique outcomes as soon as they become evident, it is important to make sure that the client is ready to leave the problem story and is interested in exploring whether these events are pointing to an alternative story.

Any alternative story is really just an expansion of the problem story, not a negation of it. For example, a story in which nervousness has taken over a person's life can run side by side with an ignored story of strength involving getting up each morning and going to work or having a relationship with another person. The problem story is real and the alternative story, which occurs at the same time as the problem story, is also real.

It is up to the client to choose which story is more useful for him or her. If the client wishes to consider the new direction suggested by the alternative story, then two stories are on the table: the problem story and the alternative story, which is a story of the person having taken stands against the problem (Smith, 1997). In this way, the approach is different from reframing (giving a different meaning to an event) or simply cheerleading (pointing out the positives and admiring them).

## Questions for Examining the Influence of the Person on the Problem

Clues to unique outcomes can be challenging to find because such outcomes have, by definition, not become prominent factors in the client's dominant story. A firm belief in the client's ability is needed in order to persevere. Stories containing clues may be incomplete or only fragments of memory, and clients may consider these clues to be insignificant. The best way to approach unique outcomes is to work from the information the client provides in his or her description of the problem story. Less desirable is to use what Morgan (2000) calls "back-up questions" (p. 57), because they can evoke superficial responses if the worker does not probe. However, at times such more direct questions may be needed; examples of back-up questions are:

- How have you managed to stop the problem from getting worse?
- Are there times when the problem is not as bad as usual? Are there times when it is less dominating and bossy?
- Can you think of a time when the problem could have stopped you or got in the way, but didn't? What happened?
- Is there a story you could tell me about a time when you resisted the problem and did what you wanted to do instead? (pp. 57–58)

Morgan (2000, p. 34) also recommends using "relative influence questions." These questions attempt to get people to consider the relative severity or impact of their troubles. For instance, a client could be asked to rate his or her problem in the following way: At this moment where would you put yourself on a scale of 1 to 10, with 1 being *the voices completely silent and having no impact on your life* and 10 *the voices raging and having complete control over your life*? If the client says "5" (or, in fact, anything other than 10), the social worker could ask how the client has been able to keep the influence of the voices from totally dominating his or her life.

There are still other ways to try to draw out unique outcomes. For instance, if back-up and relative influence questions do not elicit any instances of protest against the problem, a worker could try using "smalling questions" (McKenzie & Monk, 1997, p. 89), which direct attention to small details of experience, to gently give voice to the worker's persistence. Examples of smalling questions are as follows:

- Can you recall a brief moment when the problem was not influencing your thoughts?
- Have there been times during our conversation when the problem hasn't totally controlled or dominated our time together?
- Are there small areas of your life that the problem hasn't yet occupied?
- Have you had any dreams recently that have not been tainted by the problem? (p. 89)

These types of questions can help to broach and develop those aspects of a person's life in which he or she has taken stands against the problem. However, there are not always easily recalled or memorable instances of unique outcomes, and this may be especially true with children. With soiling or bed-wetting problems, for example, it may be difficult for a child to identify times he or she has stood up to the problem. In such cases, social workers can help clients look at strengths that, although not directly related to resisting the problem, they can harness to protest against it. Discovering that the child can find the courage to skateboard can give the practitioner faith in the child's ability to find the courage to stand up to bed-wetting. Developing that story of courage can give hope to a child who feels defeated by the problem.

## Slowing Down the Story of Each Instance of Resistance

Seeing a possible unique outcome does not automatically make it so; unique outcomes are unique only if the client identifies them as such. Morgan (2000) notes that exploring the context of an event plays an important part in helping the client decide whether the event is significant. To develop the context of an event that may represent a unique outcome, a social worker might have the following discussion with a young man under the influence of depression:

**Worker:** Barry, you mentioned that you go to church each week. Could you tell me how you do that?

**Client:** *I guess I just get up and go. I've always done it.*

**Worker:** Does Depression ever tell you that you don't need to go or that you should just stay in bed?

**Client:** *Well, often I would rather just stay in bed but I know I have to do it.*

**Worker:** How do you know you have to do it?

**Client:** *Well, my relationship with God is very important to me as a person.*

**Worker:** In what way?

**Client:** *I think we owe God something for what He has done for us.*

**Worker:** And this desire is stronger than Depression's pull on you to stay home, to stay in bed.

**Client:** *Yes.*

**Worker:** Do you go to church on weeks when Depression has convinced you to stay away from people and stay home?

**Client:** *Yes.*

**Worker:** Barry, would it be okay if I asked a few more questions about this?

**Client:** *Sure.*

**Worker:** On those Sunday mornings when Depression tells you or makes you feel you shouldn't go to church, how does it do that?

**Client:** *I just don't feel like getting up. It feels like such work. And I think no one will notice or care if I'm not there. And then I think maybe I just won't go to church.*

**Worker:** So how do you fight against it?

**Client:** *Well, not going to church would be a sin and I don't believe that going would be bad in any way. I simply stay determined to go and push myself to do it.*

**Worker:** What do you do to push yourself?

**Client:** *I just get up, slowly. Take my shower and eat my breakfast. I tell myself I will feel good about going—it's the right thing. I take it one step at a time. I guess I see how far I've come and realize I can keep going.*

**Worker:** I wonder if you see this as important in some way that you are able to stand up to Depression where your faith in God is concerned?

**Client:** *I guess so. I hadn't thought of it that way, but no matter what, I still go to church.*

In this conversation the worker has asked the client to set a context for the event that is different from the story of depression keeping the young man at home and away from others. By recognizing that the action taken was done in the presence of depression and exploring in some detail the ways in which the client has pushed himself to go to church, the worker and client have explored briefly the client's values and the way he has motivated himself to break depression's hold. When the client is then asked about the possible significance of this event, he is prepared to consider it not only as "something I do," but also as something requiring determination that he has chosen to do. It can be seen as significant, as a protest against depression, and as an indication that the young man has agency. Yet, he might not have paid much mind to this behavior if the worker had asked about its significance as soon as it was mentioned.

It is important for social workers to remember that unique outcomes can be found in people's action, thoughts, feelings, beliefs, and commitments (Morgan, 2000). Questions can be directed at exploring these various facets of an event, thus offering multiple vantages from which to assess the significance of an outcome. In the example given, the worker might be curious about what the churchgoing behavior says about the man's commitment to his faith and to standing up to depression. Does his churchgoing behavior also represent an ability to push away depression when he absolutely has to? Does the ability to tell himself that he can get to church represent a new belief about depression's influence in his life?

Again, the more detail people give to their stories, the more likely they are to experience them in the telling. This is evident when people discuss incidents of problems in their lives and become overwrought. Both the social worker and the client need to have patience and persistence if the client is to reexperience the unique outcomes that represent resistance to the problem. But such patience and persistence are critical to developing an alternative story that points to the client's preferred outcomes.

## Exercises

### Exercise 1: Spotting Resistance Against the Problem in an Interview Transcript

Break up into four-person groups and read the following interview transcript either individually or, if possible, out loud to each other.

Here is some background information about the situation: You are a social worker in a community mental health agency. You have the following information about the person you are about to see: The client is a 64-year-old African American man who has never been married and is retired from a longtime position with a large company. He was a tool and die inspector and had seniority in his small work unit. He lives with his parents, who are in their eighties and whose health is beginning to fail. His mother is confined to a wheelchair. He sees his retirement as caring for his parents. He is seeing you after an extended stay in a state psychiatric hospital for severe depression. He has been through several months of partial hospitalization elsewhere in your agency, and outpatient treatment with medication is the next level of care.

As you read the transcript, point out where you see opportunities to pick up on possible unique outcomes in this problem description. Note the specific client comments that suggest these opportunities. Where might you go back to explore possible unique outcomes? What further questions might you ask to bring out these outcomes in more detail?

Remaining within the narrative framework of this interview, how might you have handled the interview differently? Where might the worker have been more collaborative? How might you handle this differently from another perspective?

> **Worker:** Mr. Keene, I will be asking you some questions today. My hope is that we can talk about the problem you are being referred here for in a way that will be helpful to you. But before we do that, it might help if I know a little about you outside the problem. Do you think you could tell me what you enjoy doing?
>
> **Client:** *Enjoy? Been a long time since I really enjoyed anything. I used to like to go fishing.*
>
> **Worker:** What did you like to fish?
>
> **Client:** *Well, flounder, and cod when I could get out in a boat.*
>
> **Worker:** So you're a saltwater fisherman. When was the last time you were out?

**Client:** *About 2 years ago. We used to eat fresh fish every week when they were running.*

**Worker:** Store bought can't hold a candle to it, can it?

**Client:** *No, your store-bought fish is at least several days old. Even in ice it doesn't taste right.*

**Worker:** Relaxing when you don't have to fight for a spot.

**Client:** *Yeah, you have to be kind of clear on keeping people away when you start catching something. Everybody thinks it's all right to drop their line on top of yours.*

**Worker:** I can see that sometimes you have had to be strong when others have pushed in on you.

**Client:** *You have to!*

**Worker:** I agree. You have to be able to stand up for yourself, which you can do. I wonder if we might switch to the problem that brings you here?

**Client:** *Okay.*

**Worker:** Sir, based on the information I have, my understanding is that you are seeing me because you have had some trouble in the past year that was different from anything you had faced previously. You have been in the hospital for a while and in partial hospitalization. You are here now to get back on track with your life. Does that seem right? Or do you have some other thoughts?

**Client:** *Actually, no. That's right, I want to get back to my old self. I don't really know what happened to me. I'm hoping you can tell me so I can get on with my life.*

**Worker:** You would like me to tell you why it happened. I probably won't be able to do that, but you may come up with some ideas yourself as we talk. Would you talk to me a bit about what the problem was that led you to be in the hospital?

**Client:** *Depression.*

**Worker:** Depression?

**Client:** *Right.*

**Worker:** Is that your name for it?

**Client:** *My name? It was what the doctors called it and I guess it's what I have always called it.*

**Worker:** Did you have a name for what you were going through before the doctors called it depression?

**Client:** *Hell!*

**Worker:** I'm sure it was, but I'm wondering what your name is for it? Does "hell" work?

**Client:** *No, I have always called it depression.*

**Worker:** Okay. Could you tell when this depression first hit you?

**Client:** *About a year ago. I started crying at night. I had lost a good girlfriend after 10 years and I was having trouble at work. I started to drink, something I hadn't done before. Pretty soon I couldn't get out of bed and just sort of froze. I heard voices telling me life wasn't worth it and all. It was bad.*

**Worker:** It sounds terrible. Was it the crying or the drinking that let you know depression was in your life?

**Client:** *The crying. I never do that.*

**Worker:** So it started by making you cry at night. When was it at its worst?

**Client:** *Just before and just after I got to the hospital. I wasn't eating and I only slept. I hadn't taken a bath for a month. I can't figure out what happened to me.*

**Worker:** What do you think depression convinced you of that led you to act that way?

**Client:** *I don't know, maybe that I was a failure and that life wasn't worth it for failures like me.*

**Worker:** That's a pretty strong message. Do you think it had a hard time convincing you of that?

**Client:** *Pretty easy after my girl, Shelia, left. Like I said, work wasn't going too well. It was like, why bother anymore.*

**Worker:** Do you think many people would be convinced they were a failure if their work and relationships weren't going well?

**Client:** *Probably.*

**Worker:** Where do you think we learned that?

**Client:** *I guess everyone, when they get to my age, they expect their life to be easy. They figure they'd have a person and a good job.*

**Worker:** And if you don't?

**Client:** *You are a failure! Pure and simple.*

**Worker:** Where do you think we learned that a person is somehow a failure if he doesn't have a partner and a great job?

**Client:** *I don't know; I guess you see it on TV. People expect it of you; you see a lot of people like that.*

**Worker:** I would like to get back to this a bit later because I think it might be helpful to discuss. Is that okay?

**Client:** *Sure.*

**Worker:** Since the time you were in the hospital—that was when you say the depression's influence on your life was strongest—when has it been the weakest?

**Client:** *I guess over the past three months, since I've been in the partial program. It's a little harder now because my day isn't as scheduled and I have more time to think.*

**Worker:** When have you felt at least a little strong against the problem?

**Client:** *I guess I'm feeling stronger now. The medicine finally seems to be working.*

**Worker:** Do you think your ability to stand up to depression is entirely because of the medicine?

**Client:** *Well, no. It hasn't been easy even with the medicine. But getting the right medicine seems to make a big difference.*

**Worker:** Getting the right medicine can be very important. What percentage of the change do you think comes from the medicine and what percentage do you think comes from what you have done to push depression away?

**Client:** *I guess the medicine is at least half, if not more.*

**Worker:** Okay, so some of what has happened has depended on you, it seems, as well as on finding the right medicine for you. You have not entirely fallen under the influence of depression again.

**Client:** *Yeah, that's true.*

**Worker:** I wonder if I could change the topic a bit and ask about what depression's done to you?

**Client:** *That's fine.*

**Worker:** Well, maybe we could start by looking at what this depression has made you think about yourself. You already said something about being a failure.

**Client:** *Yeah, when I couldn't get things done on time at work anymore and my girl decided she wanted someone more interesting, it felt like I was a failure.*

**Worker:** It had you thinking that you were a failure. Did it tell you anything else about yourself?

**Client:** *That I was worthless, that my life was a waste, that I was just a burden.*

**Worker:** So it told you that you were a failure and worthless. And you would say that was good or bad?

**Client:** *Well, bad, of course. Who wants to be a failure?*

**Worker:** Everybody has different takes on their lives.

**Client:** *Oh.*

**Worker:** What about being a failure and worthless is so bad?

**Client:** *Well, you are here to get things done, to be someone. If you can't do anything or have anyone care about you, then you are nothing.*

**Worker:** So accomplishing things and being someone who could be cared about are important to you.

**Client:** *Right.*

**Worker:** Did depression change the way you looked at yourself?

**Client:** *What do you mean?*

**Worker:** Since depression entered your life, what change did it make in how you see yourself as a partner to your girlfriend?

**Client:** *It made me feel like I couldn't make anyone happy.*

**Worker:** Anything else?

**Client:** *No.*

**Worker:** So depression convinced you that you couldn't make anyone happy. Do you think this is a bad or good thing?

**Client:** *Bad.*

**Worker:** Why so?

**Client:** *Because I want to make people I care about happy.*

**Worker:** What makes that important?

**Client:** *Because it is important to love people and making them happy is a way to do that.*

**Worker:** So loving people and making them happy are ways of living that are important to you.

**Client:** *Yeah.*

## Exercise 2: Practicing Spotting Resistance Against the Problem in an Interview

This exercise is designed to give you experience in narrative questioning. Divide the same four-person groups as in the first exercise so that one member is now the client and the other three are a team of social workers. Have all of the group members read the following scenario:

> Client: Assume the person you are portraying has your own characteristics (race, class, ethnicity, orientation, age, ability). You are having a very difficult time with procrastination. You are a graduate student and often find yourself skimming your reading the day of the class and finishing (sometimes starting) your papers the night before. You do not have enough time in your life for everything you do, and schoolwork falls to the wayside because you are not crazy about it. You know you are not producing the best work you could. You are representing yourself in a way you do not prefer, but you cannot seem to push away the thoughts that minimize the importance of what is happening with your schooling. You are also aware that your graduate education is not cheap and that this is your only opportunity to take full advantage of it. So you are talking to a social worker at the university counseling services after you get a D on a paper, which you wrote the night before it was due.
>
> Worker Team: Begin with getting to know the person. Then develop the story using questions that look at the problem in some detail, externalize it using the client's language, and have the client evaluate and justify the effect of each impact. Notice points where the client provides clues to unique outcomes. Conclude the interview (after asking the client's permission) by exploring these possibilities, either by probing about prior clues or by asking directly about unique outcomes.
>
> Remember, you do not want to be like a police interrogator, so work to keep up an attitude of curiosity. Avoid leading questions in developing the story. You can choose one designated interviewer or all members of the team can be interviewers. If the team gets stuck, members can call a time-out to hold a conference about other questions or about the direction of the interview.

Have the teams conduct the interviews for 20 minutes. Then have them process the interview experience for 5 to 10 minutes using the following questions:

What did you learn?

When did the interview shift from curiosity toward finding an underlying cause or a solution? How did that happen?

When did the interview begin to feel a bit like an interrogation? How did that happen?

Did you pick up clues about unique outcomes? What were they?

How did the client experience the questions about unique outcomes?

Would anything else have been more helpful?

CHAPTER 7

# Richer Alternative Stories Along With Problem Stories

In this chapter I examine how unique outcomes can be found in the ways people stand up to their problems. I discuss how unique outcomes open up opportunities to describe alternative stories about oneself and the world and how these alternative stories, compared with the dominant problem stories, point to more desirable outcomes. The importance of an alternative story, which can run parallel to the problem story, is emphasized as a way to develop hope for continued change in the future. Transcript examples are used to illustrate the difference between the two forms of story.

I begin this chapter by discussing how stories must connect two broad levels of description and meaning, which are known as landscapes. I then consider the importance of these landscapes in treatment and how elements of these landscapes contribute to a narrative's coherence. Next, I describe how unique outcomes can be used to develop alternative stories and how the meanings of alternative stories to clients can be drawn out. I conclude the chapter by looking at how different instances from a client's life can be strung together to enrich an alternative story by both rooting it in the client's history and projecting it into his or her future.

## Landscapes Created by Stories

Jerome Bruner (1986), a noted psychologist, discusses the differences between narrative and scientific/logical thinking. Whereas narrative is

> built upon concern for the human condition . . . while theoretical arguments are simply conclusive or inconclusive. . . . [A] story must construct two landscapes simultaneously. One is the *landscape of action*, where the constituents are the arguments of action: agent, intention or

goal, situation, instrument, something corresponding to a "story grammar." The other landscape is the *landscape of consciousness*: what those involved in the action know, think, or feel, or do not know, think, or feel. The two landscapes are essential and distinct: it is the difference between Oedipus sharing Jocasta's bed before and after he learns from the messenger that she is his mother. (p. 14, emphasis added)

The degree of coherence in a narrative is influenced by several of its characteristics, including setting, characterization, plot, theme, fictional goal, point of view, and voice (Neimeyer, 2000). Eliciting and extending clients' thoughts about the landscape of action (what happened) and the landscape of consciousness (what it may mean) is important to developing the story, and questions should be directed at the two landscapes as well as interwoven to foster rich description. Landscape of action questions help clients understand that they have some control over their problems, which they may not previously have realized they had because the control was incomplete or not in line with the dominant story of the problem as something overwhelming and endless. Landscape of consciousness questions help clients become aware of their competence as problem solvers, and it is always more powerful for clients to discover their own self-efficacy than for workers to simply cheerlead with praise (Wetchler, 1999). (Or as one young person reacting to my cheerleading said, "Drop the damn pom-poms and give me a hand; this is hard.")

The landscape of action is the description of the who, what, where, when, and how of the story (Freedman & Combs, 1996). It represents the sequences of events over time and is best if enriched by different viewpoints on the story, such as those that could be provided by family members, for instance. The more detail the better in helping the person experience the event as much as possible.

The "how" is particularly important because we, as social workers, seek to emphasize personal agency (what did the client do, think, and feel to make something happen) as much as possible. If something the client believes is good happened, what, according to the client, did he or she do to make it happen? Often when people have problem-saturated stories they see the bad as something they are responsible for and the good as something attributable to outside forces.

How questions (e.g., What did you do that led you to this new feeling?) are also important in developing a static event into a story. For example, "I didn't wet my bed last night" is a statement of an event. It answers who (me) did what (I didn't wet the bed) where (the bed) and when (last night). A how question allows the statement "I didn't wet my bed last night" to be expanded into a story with a protagonist (me). Consider the following interaction between a social worker and a young man under the influence of bed-wetting.

**Worker:** What did you do to avoid wetting the bed?

**Client:** *I don't know!*

**Worker:** Did you notice that you thought something a little bit differently?

**Client:** *Well, I was thinking about wetting my bed before going to bed. I made sure that I went to the bathroom for a little longer to get it all out.*

**Worker:** How did you get yourself to feel any differently about Bed-wetting?

**Client:** *I remembered how well I did earlier in my gym class and how the teacher said I was getting stronger. I was thinking about that and it made me feel strong.*

**Worker:** I'm wondering how long you prepared for this move?

**Client:** *I've been thinking about how to do it for a day or two. I couldn't go over for my friend's birthday sleepover.*

**Worker:** So you decided to try to make a change, you recognized your strength, the problem was on your mind, and you tried to attend to it before going to bed. Did you do anything different during the night?

**Client:** *You know, actually, I set the alarm clock for midnight and got up and went to the bathroom.*

**Worker:** So you thought about how strong you are, felt that you could make a stand against this problem, were careful about preparing before you went to bed by spending more time in the bathroom and setting your alarm clock for midnight, and you ended up outsmarting Bed-wetting. Did I get it right?

**Client:** *Yes.*

**Worker:** Does this seem of interest to you?

**Client:** *I guess so. I guess I hadn't thought about all I did to get to a dry bed at the end of the night.*

Now there is a story with a character, a sequence of events, and a plot. The story can be further dramatized by treating bed-wetting as a character. How did bed-wetting try to get the client to forget his preparations? Did bed-wetting try to get him to stay in bed when the alarm went off? How did he get up despite that? What does he think bed-wetting thinks about his protest against it, his refusal to give it control? How will bed-wetting try to regain control? What does he think he can do to stay in the driver's seat?

Externalizing the problem, and in some cases personifying it, allows the story to include conflict and struggle. Of great importance is that it is the clients who are taking the actions, that they are exercising agency in their lives. In cases in which direct social oppression is involved (i.e., racism, sexism, and the like), rather than oppression by an identified problem, agency is more complicated; I discuss this later in this chapter.

The setting of the narrative is the "when" and "where" of it—its context. The richness of physical details in the story influences the extent to which the audience or the teller can be drawn into the story. Consider the following:

> A young male client is being interviewed about the people who had seen potential in him. One of the young man's elementary school teachers was interested in Japan, and this teacher sometimes wore a kimono to class and had the students make different Japanese crafts. In response to being asked about the color of the teacher's kimono, a look of surprise, then recognition crosses the client's face, and he excitedly says, "Blue!" It is clear from his facial expression and tone that the connection with the teacher is being reexperienced.

As this short example illustrates, verbalizing and clarifying the setting so that it becomes what is in the mind's eye can result in an emotional reexperiencing of the event.

Characterization involves the people, or the "who," in the story, what roles they play and how fully those roles are developed. Narrative therapists often get to this by specifically asking who is in each scene in the story and what the person's thoughts, feelings, and behaviors are. For example:

**Worker:** When you think of your teacher in the blue kimono, was there anything about her that led you to believe that you were special and had potential?

**Client:** *Oh yes! I remember her saying that a drawing I did of a dragon let her know I somehow knew about dragons.*

**Worker:** Really! What did you make of that?

**Client:** *That I was special, that I knew about fierce things. I wasn't feeling very fierce at that time, with everyone hurting me and all.*

**Worker:** Was she the kind of person who would say nice things to everyone?

**Client:** *I think that's true; she did say nice things a lot. Not like anyone in my family or neighborhood. But when she looked at me, and smiled, and touched* *my shoulder to tell me how good my drawing was, I just shook all over. It was so different.*

**Worker:** Were there other ways she had a role in your life?

**Client:** *Yes, I learned that year that people could be good by watching her.*

The plot is what exactly happens in a story. What action is occurring? As the action unfolds, the social worker can help the client to fill in blanks and gaps by questioning what happened when there are "jumps" in the plot. Various practitioners have developed a variety of ways to do this. The most common approach is to have the client assume that he or she is in a movie. The client then is encouraged to describe everything the camera picks up (Guidano, 1991; Walter & Peller, 1992). A similar approach used in family therapy entails securing information about all aspects of a family system during an event (Penn, 1982).

For example, a family is referred to a social worker because of the daughter's truancy and repeated curfew violations. During the first session the parents and their daughter, Suzy, discuss the most recent occasion of Suzy's coming home well after curfew:

**Worker:** So who would like to tell me what happened Friday night?

**Mrs. Tell:** *I will. Suzy was mouthing off to us as usual and Jim here smacked her. Something's got to change.*

**Worker:** Let's start from the beginning. Suzy, when did you go out?

**Suzy:** *I guess about 6:30 or so. I went out to Burger King with a friend for supper. Can I bring charges against my father? He slapped me!*

**Worker:** Let's take this one step at a time. What was going on when you left? Were there any hard feelings then?

**Suzy:** *There are always hard feelings when I go out with my friends; these parents of mine would like to treat me like I'm 5 years old.*

**Worker:** Okay, so what was said?

**Suzy:** *I was getting ready to leave and mom just kept asking me where I was going and what I was going to do and who I would be with. Then dad came home and she (turns to mother) got him all worked up and they both got angry at me, yelling, so I just left the house.*

**Worker:** What were you thinking when you left?

**Suzy:** *How much I hate them. How much I hate living at home with all the hassle.*

**Worker (*turns to mother*):** So, Mrs. Tell, is that how you saw what happened just before Suzy left?

**Mrs. Tell:** *Well, I think I have a right to know where my daughter's going and with who. You should see the kids she hangs around with! I was very angry and worried about her. I let Jim know about it as soon as he walked in.*

**Worker:** What did you tell him when he got home?

**Mrs. Tell:** *I just told him the truth, that Suzy is out of control, that if she isn't sleeping around and taking drugs by now it would be a miracle.*

**Suzy:** *I don't have to hear this crap!*

**Worker:** Let's see if we can just pull this apart. Everyone has a different version of what happened, so getting everyone's story should make it clearer how things went the way they did. So, Mr. Tell, what were you thinking on the drive home?

**Mr. Tell:** *How tired I am of the ride home. How life has become such a hassle. That the people I love all hate each other.*

Through asking questions that try to get to the actions, feelings, and thoughts of each person in the interaction, a clearer story can be developed that begins setting the stage for understanding. You can see in the dialogue how the plot of an adolescent daughter trying to assert her independence and of parents trying to assert authority over her behavior is developing and is heading toward conflict and violence. You can also begin to get a sense of the role each character plays and how the characters' mutual antagonism leads them to see each other as one-dimensional.

Whereas landscape of action questions ask about what happened, landscape of consciousness questions ask about the meaning of events in the landscape of action. Helping clients tease out what events mean or can mean to them constructs these events as an important and replicable reality. Aspects of the landscape of consciousness include theme, fictional goal, point of view, and voice. For some people the emotional nature of poetry gets at this dimension better than prose (Snyder, 1996).

The theme of the story is the way in which the characters' actions are explained; it is where clients look at what the story means to them. The theme of the story for Suzy and her parents could be parents trying to restrain a wayward daughter or a daughter trying to break free of restrictive parents. You can also see a young woman eager to grow up and parents who want to protect her along the way, a theme that offers more of an opportunity for reducing the conflict. If this family sees conflict as the problem, then the theme of the story could be looking at how conflict intrudes upon their lives or how they have been able to keep conflict from taking more of their lives.

The fictional goal is the projected end point of the story, or how the storyteller would like to see this section of the story end. However, although novels and short stories always have an end, stories in real life can continue and keep evolving long after the deaths of the characters. Life stories do not necessarily end when the teller is finished recounting them.

The fictional goal is particularly important in alternative stories because it reveals the client's preferred future. Social work treatment not only should assist the client with his or her present situation but also should help the client to project into his or her future. It is through this future projection that action to change is taken. What does recognizing a story in which people have stood up to certain problems mean for their continued ability to do so in the future? How can the current social work interaction contribute to clients' ability to resist problems' influences in the future?

The point of view relates to the form of the story—to the "type" of story the storyteller is recounting (Neimeyer, 2000). Some stories are narrated from a third person or omniscient author viewpoint; others are told in the first person, with a character telling the story from his or her vantage. Points of view range from an internal stream of consciousness of the teller to the more organized, formal writing of a biographical statement. Each point of view has its purpose. A stream of consciousness narrative of a unique outcome elicited in a session may be needed for the client to recognize its importance and to remember those times when he or she was in touch with strengths. On the other hand, the clarity that comes with detachment can be used by workers to celebrate clients' work through certificates or by clients themselves to proclaim their own "declarations of independence" (White & Epston, 1990, p. 192).

Voice is the tone that is taken by the storyteller. Neimeyer (2000) notes that a narrator's voice, or tone, can convey "a clear note of protest, a bid for understanding, an attempt at problem-solving, or a quest for objectivity" (p. 229). Listening for the tone and asking what it means deepens the exploration of the story. Voice can also reveal a sense of empowerment and a finding of unique selfhood, particularly for oppressed clients. It is the difference between noting that anger allied with feelings of discrimination leads to having trouble enter your life and having it lead you to standing up against being treated as less than other people because of who you represent. The position of the former voice might be helpful to people who are in chronic rage to their own detriment, whereas the latter might be useful to those who have ignored their experiences of discrimination to their own detriment. Through the questions asked, these aspects of consciousness can be explored to anchor the importance of unique outcomes, elucidating their meaning and impact on the identity of the client.

## Exploring Meaning in Stories

When people attempt to derive meaning from their actions it requires them to step back and reflect on their motivations, values, hopes, and desires, as well as on their actions' implications (Freedman & Combs, 1996). Through such reflection stories can obtain a significance they might not normally have. Morgan (2000) provides some excellent examples of questions designed to explore stories' meanings.

- Desires, wishes, preferences:

    When you agreed to go out with your friends for dinner, what do you think this says about what you want for your life?

    Staying in contact with your lecturer in your course—what does that say about what is important for your life?

    What do you think that says about the hopes you have for your relationship with your daughter?

- Personal values:

    What personal values is this course of action based upon?

    When you rang [called] your grandmother after the argument, what did that mean for what you value in your relationship? What personal values does this show?

- Relationship qualities:

    When that happened, how would you describe your relationship with John at that time?

- Personal skills and abilities:

    What went into doing this at this point in your life?

    What did it take to do this?

- Intentions, motives, plans, purposes:

    When you took this step what were you intending for your life?

What does it say about what you were planning?

What does it say about you as a person that you would do this?

- Beliefs and values:

  Managing to stay working in a pathologising setting, using respectful ideas—what does that say about what you think is important?

  Can you help me understand more about what that says you believe in or value?

- Personal qualities:

  What does it say about you as a person that you would do this?

  What did it take for you to do that?

  What do you think that says about your abilities/skills/knowledges? (pp. 62–63)

In the bed-wetting situation introduced earlier, sensitive questioning is used to draw out the event's meaning:

**Worker:** What has Bed-wetting been telling you about yourself?

**Client:** *That I'm weak and that no one can ever like me.*

**Worker:** What does it mean about who you are that you were able to put Bed-wetting in its place that night?

**Client:** *That I'm not weak. That I can stand up for myself and people can like me.*

**Worker:** If you continue to put Bed-wetting in its place, what would those around you think?

**Client:** *That I'm okay to be around, that I could stay over at people's houses, that I wouldn't be stuck at home.*

**Worker:** Is this a good thing or a bad thing?

**Client:** *That's a good thing, of course!*

**Worker:** Why?

**Client:** *I have to grow up and be more like other kids. I would like to stay with my friends. I hate the stink in the morning. I want to wake up happy.*

**Worker:** What do you think this might say about what you want for your life?

**Client:** *I want to grow up and be happy. I want to have friends and have fun with them.*

**Worker:** If you can continue to stand up to Bed-wetting, what does it mean about you as a person?

**Client:** *I can do anything I need to do. I can be strong.*

**Worker:** Is strength something you would like to have a closer relationship with in your life?

**Client:** *Yes!*

This conversation about bed-wetting has been developed to get more detail and to explore the meaning of the unique outcome (i.e., a night of successfully standing up to bed-wetting). Both the worker and the client are beginning to get a sense of what the client values in his life and what he hopes for it. From this one incident of protesting bed-wetting, which the worker was lucky to find although there may well be other incidents, he or she can now begin to explore the foundations of this achievement by looking at the client's relationship to strength and to being strong. It is in this alternative story, which occurs parallel to the dominant story of bed-wetting, that the young man is likely to "grow up and be happy," as well as put bed-wetting in its place.

## Stringing Instances Together

Looking at the foundation for a current unique outcome indicates that the outcome is not just a fluke but a new story that the current dominant story cannot account for entirely. If this new story is more desirable and is more in line with the person's values and desired outcomes, then further description and historical exploration are ways to root it in the person's life. Constructing a history of the alternative story, or historicizing it, requires that the worker persistently, though not coercively, seek earlier incidents in the person's life that serve as a foundation for the unique outcome seen in the present or near present (last several weeks).

Discovering an alternative story requires the social worker to remain optimistic and positive about the existence of such stories. Workers who are most successful in this approach have an unshakable belief that somewhere in a client's history, either recently or in the past, there are "life experiences manifesting fragments of ability, competence, or talent that the client is not presently able to notice or apply to [his or] her concerns" (McKenzie & Monk, 1997, p. 89). The worker tries to help the client excavate story fragments, inspect them, appreciate their significance, and begin constructing a new story that these fit into. Again, this alternative story is equal and parallel to the problem story; however, in contrast to the problem story, it can provide the person with the hope and confidence to continue making changes in his or her life.

In some stories, finding instances of direct change may be difficult. Taking what the problem tells the client about who he or she is and developing a story in contradiction to that image can be useful when it is hard to find exceptions to the problem story. In developing an alternative story that contradicts the problem's image of the client, the person does not directly connect with strengths to stand up to the influence of the problem. Instead, the focus is on other areas of the client's life, and strengths shown in those areas are identified, strengths that the problem has convinced the client he or she cannot possibly have. Helping the client to name this alternative story can be useful. When the alternative story is named, the worker can ask in later sessions whether an incident is more in line with the problem story (bed-wetting) or the alternative story (strength).

In the bed-wetting scenario, if closer friends, happier mornings, and growing up like other kids are what the young man values, then helping him search for a story to support these outcomes will help him attain them. He becomes a person who can stand up to bed-wetting rather than a person who is shoved around by bed-wetting. This is an issue of identity. The historicizing of unique outcomes into alternative stories helps the person see that the recent attempts to have some impact on the problem are built on abilities learned earlier and are not simply matters of luck or coincidence. In essence, this process allows the person to redescribe (Monk, 1997) himself or herself and become reacquainted with his or her ability to stand up to challenges.

The conversation between the social worker and the young man continues like this:

**Worker:** What do you think are the foundations of this relationship to strength in your life?

**Client:** *Huh?*

**Worker:** Can you think of other times you were able to show your strength?

**Client:** *No, not really.*

**Worker:** Is there any time you can remember where you might have shown a little strength or strength showed up to help you out?

**Client:** *Baseball! I stole home once.*

**Worker:** Really? Tell me about it.

**Client:** *It was the end of the game and we were in the last inning and our team was behind. I had hit a double and the next guy struck out, and the next guy hit a pop-up, and it was caught for another out. Joey, my friend, was up and he hit a single, so I got to third. Billy's not a good batter and he was up next. I told myself I was going to go for it. My third base coach said I should do it, too, but I'd never stolen a base, let alone home. Billy's hit was sort of a bunt, and the ball just sort of dribbled in front of the pitcher, who was running toward it. I just blasted away and didn't look at anything but home plate. I slid in and got the run in before they could get me out. We still didn't win, but I felt I didn't let anyone down.*

**Worker:** Wow! That's great. How did you do it?

**Client:** *Like I said, I just decided I needed to and ran and didn't look at anyone, just the plate.*

**Worker:** When was this?

**Client:** *Last year.*

**Worker:** Did it seem like you decided you were going to connect with strength and just keep going? I wonder if this says something about what is important to you?

**Client:** *Yeah. You need to help your friends and do your best, even when you don't think you can.*

**Worker:** So you are the kind of person who is loyal in helping his friends and will try as hard as he can, even harder?

**Client:** *Yes, friends are very important.*

**Worker:** What makes friends so important for you?

**Client:** *They just are. They keep you from getting lonely. They are fun to hang around with and talk with. They mean other people know you are an okay person.*

**Worker:** I called this strength, these times when you have done things that would surprise someone who believed Bed-wetting. What would be your name for it?

**Client:** *Hhhhmmm. Actually, I like strength. I hadn't thought of it like that before and I like it.*

**Worker:** I was wondering where you had found strength before that would make sense of how you were able to find it that night you put Bed-wetting in its place. This makes sense to me now. You had already had this experience. Can you think of any other times that you connected with strength? Let's first think about any times between when you stole home and now.

A little later the conversation continues:

**Worker:** What does it say about you that you are able to do what you've told me?

**Client:** *I can be a strong person sometimes.*

**Worker:** What do you think you have to do to connect with this strength?

**Client:** *I have to remember that I can.*

**Worker:** What might help you remember?

**Client:** *I guess to remember when I've been strong in the past and that I can be strong later?*

**Worker:** So you can be a strong person. Are there other people in your life who have seen you as a strong person?

**Client:** *I don't think so.*

**Worker:** No one? Anybody no longer with you, but who saw this strength in the past?

**Client:** *Well, my grandmother, maybe.*

**Worker:** What did she see to lead her to believe you could be strong?

**Client:** *I think she was strong and maybe she assumed I would be, too.*

**Worker:** So you take your grandmother's strength with you?

**Client:** *Yes. She once told me I can be strong.*

**Worker:** Can you tell me about that time?

Now the worker has begun to discover a different story of this young man's life—his relationship to strength—and this new story runs counter to what bed-wetting has been telling the client about himself. Had there been not even an inkling of having stood up to bed-wetting, even when using smalling questions, the alternative story might have started with the story of the stolen base and then built up to the present.

History is important in developing alternative stories because it is through history that unique outcomes are fleshed out and become full narratives (White, 1995). The new story is thus rooted in the identity of the person telling the story, and its values can be clarified and more closely identified with the person's. Through history, the client can become involved in critical reflection: Is what the problem is telling me about who I am right? Am I just a weak bed wetter? Will no one ever care about me? Will I always have to stink and wash sheets in the morning?

The alternative story is further strengthened by developing an audience of supporters, which is discussed in chapter 9. At this point it is safe to say that the more people who recognize, or recognized, in the case of deceased members of a client's network, the alternative story and support it, the stronger the story and its implications become to the person who is the subject of it.

Questions about history are important, but as Monk (1997) points out, so too are questions that focus on the future: What does the development of this alternative story mean for the person's future? How can the person use this story to identify options available to him or her? To evaluate those options? How does the person plan to use the ability or knowledge that he or she has rediscovered to confront the problem in the future? What can the person say about his or her future with regard to the problem now that he or she has rediscovered this ability or knowledge? Will he or she draw upon this ability or knowledge all at once or little by little?

The conversation between the social worker and the young man resumes:

**Worker:** With this relationship to strength that you had, but that Bed-wetting had you forgetting, what do you think the future will hold for Bed-wetting? Will it get stronger or weaker?

**Client:** *Weaker.*

**Worker:** What makes you say that?

**Client:** *I think I can use my strength to not let Bed-wetting push me around all the time.*

**Worker:** How will you draw on strength?

**Client:** *I will remember how I have been strong in the past and the way my grandma believed in me and that I can keep doing it. I don't want to have messy beds anymore.*

**Worker:** How will Bed-wetting try to trick you into forgetting again?

**Client:** *It will try to tell me it can't be beat, but I will say no to it.*

As White and Epston (1990) note, "In striving to make sense of life, persons face the task of arranging their experiences of events in sequences across time in such a way as to arrive at a coherent account of themselves and the world around them" (p. 10). Stories are how we make sense of the world and of who we are, even though these stories reflect only some of the events of our daily life. These concepts are quite important to understanding the narrative approach, which sees discovering, reexperiencing, and putting meaning to an alternative story as important curative factors (Harper & Lantz, 1996). White (1997) nicely summarizes these ideas:

> It is through personal narrative that we take in and give meaning to our experiences of the events of our lives. It is through personal narrative that we link together the events of our lives in sequences that unfold through time according to specific themes. It is through this meaning-making process that we experience being in the flow of time, and that we experience our lives moving forward. And, in that action is significantly prefigured on the successful interpretation of the events of our lives, it is through this meaning-making process that new options become available for action in therapeutic practice. (p. 129)

## Exercises

### Exercise 1: Expanding a Possible Unique Outcome

The bed-wetting transcript in this chapter contains two unique outcomes: one is a non-bed-wetting night and the other involves stealing home base. Both of these unique outcomes are explored in some detail in the transcript; however, questions are inexhaustible when you are really interested in a story. Choose one of these unique outcomes and develop at least 10 landscape of action questions and 10 landscape of consciousness questions to expand the event.

### Exercise 2: Coconstructing an Alternative Story and Its Meaning

Further develop the two unique outcomes discussed in this chapter's bed-wetting transcript into an alternative story by carefully examining the foundations that make the alternative story consistent. Practice using the following format to develop further questions:

1. Pull together the two events and look for similarities.

   *What questions would you use to do this? (Guess at what those similarities might be in the exercise.)*

2. Explore in some detail these similarities and what they might mean.

   *What questions would you use to do this?*

3. Help the client develop a name for this element in the new story.

*What questions would you use to do this? (In the conversation with the social worker, the boy concurred with strength. Because you are curious about this, how would you explore if this is the same name he would give to his ability to plan and get up in the middle of the night?)*

4. Project into the future with regard to how this new story can have an impact on the problem.

   *What questions would you use to do this?*

CHAPTER 8

# Written Work to and for Clients

Written correspondence and documents are an important development of narrative practitioners. In their foundational text on a narrative approach to working with people, White and Epston (1990) devote nearly two thirds of it to correspondence and what they call *counter documents* (p. 188; e.g., awards, certificates, proclamations, and the like). Informal surveys of clients who received letters from narrative therapists have found that one letter is worth, on average, 3.2 (Nylund & Thomas, 1994) to 4.5 treatment sessions (White, 1995) in terms of its effect on a client's life. In this chapter I look at how written work can have such a powerful impact.

There are many different reasons for writing letters to clients and to others who are important in clients' lives. Like narrative work in general, letter writing should open up possibilities, not lead to rote, copybook procedures. Therefore, although letter writing may seem like merely a technique, it is really an expansion of a theory or worldview about working with people. Once some basic concepts are mastered and the unusual forms of language practiced, the full creativity offered by the use of written documents should become clear.

In this chapter I illustrate how letters and other documents can be incorporated into social work practice. I review the rationale for using written documents in clinical work and discuss ways to introduce these novel materials to clients. I present a variety of types of letters that can be used, strategies to improve letter-writing skills, and practical and ethical considerations associated with letter writing. I also touch on methods of in-session note taking and dictation.

Perhaps the best way to start this chapter is to have you write a letter that might be helpful to a client. Although this letter will not actually be mailed, compose it as you might normally write a letter to a client. Begin by thinking of a client at your practicum or work who might benefit from a little added attention or who poses a particular problem to you. Choose someone you would feel comfortable discussing with another classmate. Remember to disguise any information that could possibly identify the client.

Consider what you might say in the letter. Then draft it, making it no more than one page long. The next day do a quick edit for spelling, grammar, and content. Perhaps you will have time during your next class session to exchange letters with another student. When you read the other student's letter, imagine what it would be like to receive the letter if it were addressed to you at your home. Do you feel honored, concerned, interested, or worried? Do you get angry, pleased, embarrassed, or do you feel patronized? What strikes you as most helpful? Why? What changes might you make to remove parts that you are uncomfortable with? Even if you do not exchange letters, keep the one you have just prepared to compare to the others you will write in the exercises at the end of this chapter.

## Letter Writing: The Lost Art

Just as narrative treatment differs from traditional forms of treatment, narrative letters differ from other forms of professional letter writing. Professional social work correspondence is usually directed at other professionals. When letters are sent to clients, they are usually intended to clarify the contract, which means describing the expectations and responsibilities of both the client and the social worker. A typical letter might remind a client of the importance of coming to scheduled interviews if the person has missed one or more meetings, specify a homework assignment or task given during a session, or clarify what the worker has said he or she will do for the client.

A letter designed to clarify a contract might say: "I missed you during our last session. If you are still interested in coming in for an appointment, please contact me." Or, it might say: "This is to put in writing the following steps you agreed to take this week to reach your goal of having and keeping friends, as a way to reduce your feelings of isolation and loneliness. First, you said you would look through your address book, the phone book, and on the Internet to recover the numbers of at least three people who were previously your friends. You stated you would contact them and, if necessary, leave the following message on their answering machine. . . ." Yet another example is: "This is to remind you that I agreed to get you the application for the job-training program you were interested in, and we will look at the application together next week. You agreed to get the information you need for a résumé and will bring that to our session next week."

Letter writing to other professionals serves many purposes. The quality of correspondence and the appropriate use of professional language and labels not only provide information about the client to some other professional but also display the knowledge and credibility of the professional writing the letter. Other professionals will give considerable weight to what is said in a well-written professional letter or case record. Dictation, which serves a similar purpose, is discussed later in this chapter to illustrate how narrative thought can be fit into a structuralist framework.

Rarely do most professional letters take the client's abilities and understandings as their focus. Narrative-style letters, in contrast to typical professional correspondence, focus on telling a story rather than evaluating it. Letters offer the social worker an opportunity to give the client the benefit of another retelling of the story, to ask questions that are more rhetorical and that may need greater time to consider than is available in the session, and to develop more helpful alternative stories that might have an impact on the person's identity. Letters also offer a further opportunity to bear witness to the client's new version of self and to stand as a testament to his or her change, which can be repeatedly reviewed (Wetchler, 1999). Questions in letters can function as a sort of homework, keeping the work alive between sessions.

## Why Written Documents?

Written statements have great power in our society. Under federal law, courts in the United States presume written statements to be the true beliefs of a person and require a higher burden of evidence to refute than oral statements (Mueller & Kirkpatrick, 2007). White and Epston (1990) note that Western culture tends to give credence to knowledge acquired through the sense of sight, as the adage "seeing is believing" suggests. Writing can have the effect of legitimizing an idea or a story. Writing permits facts to be located in time and in relation to other facts. Writing allows the worker to carefully lay out facts so that the logic behind their pattern becomes evident. And writing permits the reader to return to a prior part of the story if he or she gets confused, thus ensuring the story's clarity and cohesiveness.

If you have ever read a transcript of a social work interview you will notice unless the transcript is greatly cleaned up that the conversation rarely takes a direct route. This is true even in court transcripts in which skilled attorneys are trying to get people to describe events in a clear order. In addition to guttural utterances, transcripts often show off-track answers, tangents, and revisiting of already covered material. In most cases, only when analyzed or edited do transcripts form a coherent story. In fact, the primary function of closing statements made by attorneys at the end of a trial is to form a coherent story that jurors can take to their deliberations.

Written statements have the benefit of being both concrete and correctable. According to White and Epston (1990), letters can serve as a way of expanding a person's short-term memory. A person can remember only so many things in a sequence, and written work allows the reader to capture and extend that sequence. Letters are easy to revise, and the reader can point out areas of confusion to be clarified or mistakes to be corrected.

Letters have a physical existence—they can be picked up, held, filed, and retrieved—and this can enhance their value. Compare the different feeling you get from reading a personal letter versus a personal e-mail. Clients recognize that letters require some special work and thought on the part of the social worker; consequently, receiving a letter can lead clients to feel valued by and more connected to the worker.

Letters have another very important attribute: They contain the writer's signature. Legally the importance given to one's signature on a contract, a will, or a check is clear. A signature represents a personal affirmation of responsibility (and, hence, is a source of some of the anxiety around therapeutic letter writing) as well as a very personal representation of the self. Think of the attraction of autograph collectors to the signatures of celebrities and how some forms of handwriting analysis claim to assess personality on the basis of a signature's characteristics.

Letters provide workers with a good way to apologize for the occasional errors they will make. For instance: "I realized that when I moved too quickly to thinking of ways in which you can fight against depression you could have felt I was ignoring some important parts of the pain in your life. I'm sorry for this and hope to have the opportunity at our next session to discuss what you desire."

Social workers write to clients in the context of a relationship. Not surprisingly, perhaps, letters seem to work best if they are in the voice of that relationship. The client will read and interpret a therapeutic letter in the context of the relationship that he or she has with the worker.

The worker's ability to write from the heart with sincerity and to craft a letter that can be of use to the client will impact the client's interpretation of it (Moules, 2003). If the letter sounds entirely different from the tone of the session it documents, as well as from the client's perception of the worker, then it will be seen as untrustworthy and confusing, and will be of little value.

Workers report that clients who have received letters often say to them: "I can't believe you took the time to write me a letter." Such comments indicate clients' appreciation of the work being done for them, and this can enhance the positive nature of the worker–client relationship, which is an important part of any treatment. Although a letter may deepen an existing relationship, it will not create one. If a relationship is not already established, then it is likely that the letter will be seen as inauthentic.

Practice is required to write good letters quickly. Reducing letter writing to an inflexible technique will defeat the purpose of the letter.

## Presenting the Idea of Letters to Clients

As any social worker knows, despite all the reasons why letters can be useful, they can also be ignored. As in task-centered social work, the narrative social worker must prepare the situation to increase the probability that the written material given to the client will have an impact.

Morgan (2000) suggests that a worker begin by consulting with the client and perhaps the client's family about the possibility of the client receiving letters from the worker. The worker would describe the purpose and possible content of the letters and offer different options for how the letters could be sent. If the idea appeals to the client, the worker would specifically ask whether the client is interested in receiving letters and inform him or her that the letters and the experience of receiving them would be topics of discussion at subsequent sessions.

Confidentiality is an important aspect of this work, and the worker should engage the client in a thorough discussion of where letters will be sent; who will most likely receive them at that location; and who, other than the client, might read them. The worker also may wish to explore whether the client tends to read letters more than once or throws them out after the first reading. If the client were to decide to keep the letters to read again, where might they be kept? Getting a client's consent in writing can be a helpful way to allay worker fears that he or she might be breaching confidentiality by sending such letters.

## Types of Letters to Clients and Others

White and Epston (1990) give examples of different types of therapeutic letters, some of which are written by workers and others by clients. *Letters of invitation* (p. 84) typically are sent by a worker to a family member who did not appear at an appointment. For example: "We were concerned about you and we wanted you to know we discussed this. We think your point of view would be invaluable, so we look forward to you coming in, but only when you feel ready and when you think the time is right."

*Letters of redundancy* (p. 90) are written by clients to release people in their lives from roles that have been a source of trouble to them, such as being "Mom's marriage counselor" or "my brother's keeper." A letter of redundancy might say: "This will inform you that you have been invaluable to me in helping me get through the hard times but I am now in a place where I can go it on my own. I want you to know that you no longer need to look out for me as you have done, and I will respond to your telephone calls by trying to tell you less about my troubles so that you don't feel the need to get involved. Therefore, because you have done such a good job in the past, I am formally retiring you from your role as the supportive big brother who saves me, and I will let you get on with your own life."

*Letters of prediction* (p. 94) are given to clients by workers at the termination of treatment. In these letters, workers offer their predictions about where clients will be in their journey six months forth. Clients commonly are instructed not to open the letter until a certain date. In this way, clients receive reassurance of the workers' confidence in their ability to proceed in the alternative story.

*Counter-referral letters* (p. 96) are positively focused letters sent by workers on behalf of clients to their referral source. The purpose is to counter the usual problem-saturated referral letter that is written about a client; the hope is to have the counter-referral letter placed in the client's record to document a different side of the person. Clients may collaborate in the creation of these letters, thus reinforcing the gains they have made with their alternative story.

*Letters of reference* (p. 98), addressed to "To Whom It May Concern" or to specific individuals, attest to people's accomplishments. Drafted by workers, they are given to clients, who may use them with others in their social networks. For instance, a letter of reference might say: "This is to say that Charles is fighting against addictive thinking and is pulling his life back from alcohol. He acknowledges he needs all the help he can get in this struggle. If you are a person whom Charles usually drank with, you may be tempted to take him out with you. Please think about whether this is helping or hindering him in his attempt to get his life back."

Finally, *letters for special occasions* (p. 103) are prepared by workers to acknowledge a particular event or achievement. Arguably every letter can be thought of as being for a special occasion, but these letters are intended for unique events, such as funerals, births, graduations, or an instance of severe trauma, and are more extensive than other letters, encapsulating a richer story.

## Note-Taking and Writing Therapeutic Letters

In narrative practice, the reason for taking in-session notes and the kind of notes taken differ from those for a traditional session. A major aspect of taking notes in a narrative-style session is to get down the exact words or phrases the client uses that seem important. The intent of this type of recording is to try to privilege clients' speech over workers' language as much as possible. Freedman and Combs (1996) discuss dividing a note-taking page into two columns. On the left-hand side, clients' words or phrases about the problem story are recorded (e.g., their name for the problem, how they see it controlling them, specific incidents); the right-hand column includes clients' quotes that seem to suggest the existence of an alternative story (e.g., unique outcomes, times when the problem was weaker, examples of standing up to the problem).

For example:

**Worker:** So when this fear takes over, one of the things you say it does is make you feel weak. Is there anything else?

**Sally:** *Yes, I not only feel weak, but I get sick to my stomach.*

**Worker:** And is this a good or bad thing?

**Sally:** *A bad one, of course. No one likes to feel sick!*

**Worker:** No one likes to feel sick. Is there any other reason this is bad?

**Sally:** *Yeah, I can't drive when I get sick like that. I end up staying home and missing out on things. I was supposed to go out with friends and I was really looking forward to it. But I got this feeling and figured I'd never graduate if I didn't stay home and study. Thinking about it got me sick.*

**Worker:** Did you study?

**Sally:** *No, I felt too sick.*

**Worker:** So you would like a life where you can get your homework done, drive, and go out with friends, but fear seems to get in the way of that.

**Sally:** *Yes. I'm really frustrated.*

**Worker:** No wonder. Are there times when you push fear aside and actually go out and get things done?

**Sally:** *Yes, sort of. I do go to my classes even when I don't feel up to it.*

**Worker:** How do you do that?

**Sally:** *I tell myself that I have to and that I will get a bad grade since attendance counts and that I will learn something by going.*

Figure 8.1 depicts an example of a note-taking page. Not only do the notes offer the worker a record of Sally's point of view, which is helpful for completing paperwork required by the agency, but they also provide meaningful quotes from which to develop a letter after the session. These notes are significant in that they reflect what Sally, the client, is thinking, not just those comments that indicate diagnostic material for an assessment, or identify general progress, or mark relapses in the problem at hand.

---

**Figure 1. Example note-taking page from interview between Sally and the social worker.**

| Problem Story (Fear) | Possible Alternative Story |
|---|---|
| Feel weak | Go to my classes even when I don't feel up to it |
| Get sick to my stomach | Tell myself that I have to |
| Because of being sick | Will learn something by going |
|    Can't drive | |
|    End up staying home | |
|    Don't go out with friends | |
|    Can't study | |
|    Figured I'll never graduate | |
| Really frustrated | |

---

After discussing the purpose of note taking, consent to take notes should be obtained from the client. Oftentimes notes are kept private during the session and clients are curious about what the worker sees as important enough to write down. Narrative workers frequently not only share what they are writing but ask clients if they recorded their words correctly and offer them a copy of the notes. For example, "You said that you tell yourself 'I have to go to class' and you do. Did I get it right?"

When writing a letter at the end of a session, the easiest format to use is to first give specific compliments to the person for coming; next sketch out the problem story, recognizing its impact on the person; then provide more specific details on the beginnings of an alternative story; and end with several reflective narrative questions that could be discussed during the next session.

An example of a letter summarizing the events of a session follows:

*Dear Mr. Doe,*

*It was a pleasure meeting you last Friday. It can be very difficult talking to a stranger about personal information and I appreciated having the opportunity to hear about all you have come through recently* [specific compliment for coming in]. *When you initially called this agency, you sounded like you were in the grip of hopelessness, yet now you say that you have more frequently found hope. As you had seen no one here during that time, you are 100% responsible for this remarkable turnaround* [beginnings of an alternative story].

*During our meeting, you discussed the loss of your sister last year and how that caused you to experience grief and depression* [recognition of problem story]. *You told me that as you have allowed yourself to remember more and more of the good times you had with your sister, you've been better able to face your challenges, even without her physical presence. You said that this was because you know she is "in your heart." Despite all the pain, you have again begun to see your strength, which the grief had hidden from you* [beginnings of an alternative story].

*You also discussed how "fear" and "distrust" had gotten between you and your wife despite all the remarkable work you have been doing to repair the rift between you and her after the affair* [recognition of problem story]. *Last, you talked about what you called your "lack of confidence" in yourself in meeting people and maintaining relationships with them. You said, "This isn't like me," given your history as a confident schoolteacher* [recognition of problem story]. *I saw this strength and confidence in you, especially in your decision to quickly pull away from a therapist you felt was hostile and in your making up your own mind to work on your marriage after being "flooded with advice" from others* [beginnings of an alternative story].

*After you left, a few questions occurred to me that I want to share.*

*Did you request the change in your wife, or was it all her idea? How has her change affected your ability to change?*

*Looking back, what did you do to bring hope back into your marriage? How did you know to do that?*

*Is staying with hope difficult now? If it is, how have you managed to maintain it?*

*Who would be the least surprised to see you work so hard in this relationship? What can or could they see in you that you might not see in yourself [narrative questions]?*

*I look forward to meeting with you again next week, when we can discuss any thoughts these questions might bring up. If you can, please bring this letter with you.*

*Sincerely,*

*Ms. Thompson*

The social worker has asked Mr. Doe to bring the letter to the next session so that he can read the letter out loud, thereby giving it another rehearing, before they discuss it.

The following longer therapeutic letter is a little different. Although it was written at the end of the first session with the client, it goes into greater detail, providing a history of the problem and the resistance the person had been showing to it. This letter was written by David Epston, a codeveloper of the narrative treatment approach. It is addressed to a woman who had been neglected and abused throughout her life. The woman came to the first session telling Epston that she was "bad." After the session, Epston wrote to her:

*Dear Marisa,[1]*

*I am writing a summary of our meeting as agreed. I do this for a number of good reasons: firstly I take it that telling me, a virtual stranger, your life story—which turned out to be a history of exploitation—frees you to some extent from it. To tell a story about your life turns it into a history, one that can be left behind and makes it easier for you to create a future of your own design. Secondly, your story needs to be documented so it isn't lost to you and is in a form available to others whom you might choose to inspire. They will come to understand, as I have, how you were, over time, strengthened by your adverse circumstances. Everyone's attempts to weaken you by turning you into a slave, paradoxically strengthened your resolve to be your own person. This, of course, is not to imply that you haven't paid dearly for this and haven't suffered. You almost accepted your family's attitude towards you and this accounted for the doormat life-style that you lived for some time.*

---

[1] The bracketed text offers background information about people and events mentioned in the letter. Most of these comments are summaries of statements footnoted in the original letter; those that were not previously footnoted, were suggested by David Epston in a personal communication in May 2008.

*You were born the twenty-first child to a woman worn out with child rearing and "an old man", aged 72, who fathered you and loved you for the five years that remained of his life.* [She learned later in her life that the neighborhood woodcutter, who went out of his way to be kind to her, was her father.] *You probably wondered why he loved you quite so much when your mother didn't want you and continually coached you into domestic skills so you would be of some use to others. She taught you a servant mentality; that is, to do for others and expect very little in return. For a mother to betray a child into servitude, she must have had to convince herself that you were bad. If she hadn't she would not*[2] *have been able to live with her guilt. She must have had to convince herself you were bad; otherwise she couldn't have been your Judas and betrayed you. You were turned into a Cinderella with other people in charge of you. Your mother did deals with your exploiters. She trained you into housework and made sure, as did others, that you did not discover who and what you really were and could be. You were beaten into submission. You probably believed that your family always did the best for you and you should be thankful for their efforts on your behalf. Your family did the worst for you and tried to have you believe that that was the best you could or should expect because you were 'bad'. They tried to convince you (and were undoubtedly successful for periods of time) that you deserved their punishments and cruelties. No wonder Carl* [her brother-in-law in the UK with whom she was sent to live at age 13 by her mother] *prevented you from attending school and your sister co-operated with him. They must have known that someone, sooner or later, would tell you the truth about yourself. And, sure enough, Mrs. Donnely* [her remedial reading teacher] *understood that you were not a slave serving time for some evil deed and probably guessed that you were paying for someone else's evil deeds. No wonder Carl put an end to a glimpse you had of a different future for yourself* [he prevented Marisa from having contact with Mrs. Donnely and withdrew her from school on her 15th birthday, when school attendance no longer was compulsory]. *Everyone tried to indebt you to them by convincing you that you were only worthy of the miserable treatment they handed out to you. There were some who refused to go along with your oppression—your brother, Luigi, 'the old man' who turned out to be your father, Mrs. Donnely, and Aldo* [a brother-in law who sexually interfered with Marisa], *who, despite his real appreciation of you, was tempted to exploit you too. Carl used his*

---

[2] Although not in the 1989 version, this word was added by David Epston in May 2008.

*guardianship to turn you into his slave while your sister sat by, and your family, by taking no interest in you whatsoever* [although she regularly wrote to her mother and family about her bondage in the UK and begged to be repatriated, none of her letters were ever answered], *made their contribution to your abuse. You even had to beg for what was rightfully yours. But even if you had returned to your family in Italy, they would have found more ways to degrade you. My guess is that they would have crushed you further to make sure you didn't have a self because, if you did, you might have borne witness against them for their injustices towards you.*

*Seeing that medium* [whom she consulted at the age of 30 and who advised her to take action in her relationships closest at hand] *who called you a 'doormat' was a turning point in your life and you started your revolution with your husband* [whom she wed after emigrating to New Zealand] *because he was closest at hand. When you were a slave, you no doubt chose a partner who would be your master and you could serve, grateful for crumbs from his table. You further submitted to your exploitation without being fully aware of it. You probably were grateful for what you got because it was without malice. Your husband must have been shocked by your demands for justice and equality in your relationship. You had not spent all your strength in your suffering and slavery. Instead, this marked the onset of your taking action in this family. And you started accepting and trusting your own experience. Your own power was being drawn upon to shape events in your life for the first time. You broke out of some of the things that were depressing you and keeping you down. You gave yourself evidence that your anger was righteous anger. I gather your appreciation of yourself gained you more respect in your husband's eyes. He had been waiting, knowing there was more to you than the doormat lifestyle you lived. No wonder you had sought out older women to dominate you while you tried to please them, much like your mother and older sisters. You tried to prove you were worthy of them by serving them more and more. This made them think less of you more and more.*

*In your 30's, your own power surfaced and was accepted by you. And no one could submerge it any longer. You had so much courage, in fact, that you decided to seek justice and put things right. By doing so, you drew a distinction between your history and your future. In your history, your life was defined by other peoples' attitudes and ideas about you; in your future, your life will be defined by your respect and appreciation of your self. You went back to England and renounced Carl and your sister, who, by now, had herself been turned into 'a zombie'. In New Zealand, you rid yourself of your domineering friends. In Italy, you confronted your mother with the truth about yourself and her. Your truth was more powerful than hers because she had been living a lie. Your mother's death finally freed you—you no longer had to search for a mother who could never be. You were released to go forwards in your life, believing in yourself. No wonder you feel dizzy with possibility. Remember being a prisoner can make you accommodate your prison. To be released from it is disconcerting and many return to it for refuge. However, I don't believe you ever totally surrendered yourself to anyone. I believe you always, always, had some sense that evil was being done to you and, for that reason, you were never made into a real slave. Rather, you were a prisoner of war, degraded, yes, but never broken. I base my assumption on some rather obvious observations: if you had been made into a real slave, you wouldn't or couldn't be the person you are now. You would not have revolted against your oppression and exploitation. You would not have recovered yourself.*

*I would be very interested to meet with you again to discuss the above. I think it is going to be a while before you fully appreciate the events in your life so far and the significance they hold for you as a person, a wife, a mother, and a woman. To my way of thinking, you are a heroine who doesn't know her heroism. I very much look forward to helping you rewrite your history and carve out for yourself a liberating future. If your husband would like to join us in this discussion, I, for one, would welcome his thoughts and contributions.* (Epston, 1989, pp. 129–131)

This letter was written in response to a session that was primarily historical and that focused on a problem story that justified why Marisa was "bad." Epston begins the letter by complimenting Marisa on coming in and telling him her story. He describes it as a story of survival, while recognizing it also as a story of slavery. All along the way he builds a dual story—one of suffering and one of strength—that culminates in her current situation and testifies to her unrecognized heroism. In the story he narrates, Marisa's current anxieties and outburst of anger are not signs of mental illness or nervous breakdown, but of a unique turning point. Epston did not ask any reflective questions in the letter, but implied is the question: "Now that your heroism is recognized, where will you go from here?"

Marisa is said to have read and reread the letter, particularly when experiencing flashbacks from her abuse. She is said to have destroyed it eventually, but by then she was on track to a new life (O'Hanlon, 1994). Even if Marisa never returned for a second session, the letter could help to increase her ability to cope.

## Letter Writing in an Age of Privacy

The Health Insurance Portability and Accountability Act offers a new level of patient protection and has forced a new appreciation of confidentiality among health care providers, a designation that often includes social workers. I have found some students get very anxious about the idea of sending letters to clients, and their concerns seem to center around three issues: lack of time, getting too personal (loss of boundaries), and potential legal liability. As with any other way of working with people, students need to look at what makes them anxious and decide if the anxiety would make them ineffective in using the tool or whether the value of the tool to the client outweighs the anxiety.

As mentioned earlier, the social worker should discuss the topic of letter writing with the client prior to sending him or her a letter. The client should be told that the letter can be marked confidential, if he or she prefers (Steinberg, 2000). The client's desire and possibly even formal consent to receive the letter should be affirmed. These issues could be introduced as follows:

> I sometimes send letters to clients when something happens in a session that has got me thinking and I have the time available to respond to it after we meet. People I see tell me the letters are helpful in pulling together things that were discussed in the session. Would you be interested in receiving such a letter? It would include a bit about what went on in the session, what impressed me, and some questions I had that you might want to give some thought to. Would anyone else be likely to see this letter if I sent it to you? Do you wish me to write "Confidential" on the envelope? Would that help or make things worse? If you want to keep the letter, do you have a place to keep it so others won't feel free to read it? Will the agency's name and address on the envelope cause a problem?
>
> Because confidentiality is a concern, would you be interested in signing a short form that indicates I mentioned I might be sending you treatment letters and that verifies the address you want me to send them to?
>
> I, _____, on this date _____ understand that _____, my social worker, wishes to have the option of sending me letters from time to time about my treatment. I agree to this, and I understand that the letters may contain personal information and that they will be sent to the following address:_____
> _____
> _____.

I may take back this consent at any time, understanding that once I do so no further letters will be sent to me.

Client's signature _____ Date _____

Worker's signature _____ Date _____

The other two concerns students raise, lack of time and getting too personal, are also worth examining. Letters take time and to do them right will initially take an hour or so apiece, one reason why a practicum is a good place to practice before one confronts the heightened service unit requirements faced by social work professionals. The amount of time needed to compose letters can be reduced with practice, but letters will always take time. It is possible to use some shortcuts, such as composing lists to indicate the influence of the problem on the person; short letters can be effective, too.

The suggestion that letters can be perceived as being too personal, and thus create boundary problems, is a legitimate concern. First, therapeutic letters and social letters between friends both arise from the relationship, serve to maintain connection, and extend a discussion in written form (Moules, 2003). However, in contrast to social letters, the purpose of a therapeutic letter is to benefit the client and the client's response is confined to the professional session.

Second, there is always a risk that words on a page can be interpreted, or misinterpreted, in ways that cannot be immediately remedied. Although this risk cannot be eliminated, attention to how letters are crafted and to discussing clients' responses to them can reduce the likelihood of misunderstandings.

Third, therapeutic letters require the social worker's honest reactions to life's constraints and traumas. This honesty ("I was shocked to hear," "I was thrilled to hear about," "I am amazed by," "I was so angry at how drinking inserted itself to try to destroy any caring between you and your children") conveys the worker's personal responses, and in the process the worker exposes himself or herself as a person. Although this can make workers feel vulnerable, it affirms the humanity we share with our clients.

Finally, letters are a written record in the possession of the client of what is going on in treatment, thus constituting a form of treatment documentation provided by the worker to the client. By contrast, in most traditional practice approaches, treatment is documented solely in the structured case file, which is written by the worker for other workers. Although exposing our work to clients' scrutiny may seem uncomfortable initially, sharing a written record of treatment with them demonstrates narrative therapy's commitment to trying to equalize power in the treatment relationship, respects clients' expertise, and makes practice as transparent as possible.

The best that can be done to reduce the concern that letters may be seen as too personal or as violating a boundary is to work at writing letters that you would not mind receiving, are tenuous enough to offer food for thought without in-depth worker analysis, stay away from labels and advice, and have a tone of hopefulness. To produce letters possessing these qualities requires the social worker to bring hopefulness more into his or her own life (Rombach, 2003).

## Common Errors in Letter Writing

There are several common errors that students make in writing their first letters. For example, given the way most social work practice theories are constructed, it is difficult to avoid assuming an expert stance, which leads to hierarchical attitudes coming out in letters. Letters also can be drafted to avoid all negatives and focus only on positives, which is not an accurate representation of how people see their lives. Alternatively, letters can be too specific about the negatives identified and can make the client feel endangered by having those negatives put in writing.

In the following sections, I discuss the pitfalls of using thank-yous and professional language.

### Be Careful of Thank-Yous

A very common error is to begin a letter by thanking the client for coming to see the worker: "First, I want to thank you for coming in to talk to me." This is a common opening because students want to recognize the humanity of the client and they struggle to find ways to indicate this. Unless the client has given the writer something he or she authentically recognizes as worthy of thanks, the thank-you can sound patronizing or merely polite and can confirm the power differential. Note the difference between the usual thank-you opening and the following:

> I was left thinking today after our first meeting of all the ways in which your trust in others has been used to misuse you. As I heard you say that "God still loves me" and that you always "knew something better would come" to you, I was taken aback by the power of your faith and courage and wanted to thank you for teaching me this.

Commending by recognizing the difficulty in coming to an appointment given all the barriers to that is different from a thank-you. Even clients who are coerced can have their reluctance to come in and the barriers they face recognized and affirmed.

> At our meeting today you told me that your probation officer would recommend jail unless you came in, that you really had no personal problems, that you didn't want to look crazy by seeing a social worker, that there were many more pressing issues you faced, and that coming in would take away time and resources from more important things. I appreciate how difficult it was for you to see me for all the reasons you gave and realize you made some sacrifices in doing so.

In fact, you are privileged to be hearing the stories of others, stories that, in some cases, people might not tell their family or most intimate friends. You are hearing clients' stories within a cultural context that says this conversation will develop into something that helps them face life. Because privilege to receive information also conveys power, it is important to think carefully how you convey this sense of privilege.

## Notice Professional Language

Professional language tends to distance people and treat them as objects or categories. Using such language in letters can accentuate clients' experience of themselves as categories, which would diminish the letters' benefits by reinforcing the "object" status of the person. Students are taught to communicate with other professionals through dictation, summaries, and case studies. They are rarely taught how to write to clients. Consequently, it is not uncommon to see first letters containing a great deal of professional jargon:

> "I was very pleased to meet with you and discuss your *family system* [versus: the people in your family] and *codependency* [instead of: showing love to someone who doesn't seem to help the client stand up to a problem]."

> "You did an excellent job of discussing your *resistance* to making changes in your *relationship* with your children."

> "I think you made great progress in *overcoming* your *denial* of your drinking."

I emphasized the term *jargon* because many students do not even see these words as jargon given their professional socialization. Identifying the word *relationship* as jargon in the second sentence may seem a bit extreme, but what actually is meant by "your relationship with your children"? Am I, as the worker, referring to the client's behavior toward his or her children? How the client thinks about his or her children? How the client feels toward his or her children? How the children respond to the client? The idea of "relationship problems" obscures the specificity of how people would like to see their life differently.

It also is not uncommon for certain labels to be used in letters and their use should be considered carefully. These include such phrases as "as my client" or "your case." These labels objectify the person, solidifying a hierarchical relationship. Their function is that of boundary setting and their use should be considered in that respect. If a client asked his or her social worker to go out on a date, then boundary setting would be appropriate; however, in many cases boundary setting operates as an unnecessary form of distancing from clients.

## Briefer Therapeutic Documents for Clients

In addition to the types of therapeutic letters mentioned so far, two other, briefer forms of documents can be useful. The first involves simply enumerating the knowledge recognized during an interview. The client can keep and reread this document, strengthening its influence with each rereading. This type of document can take the form of a simple "translation" of the session or a statement of position against the problem (White, 1995, p. 201). For example, with assistance, clients can write their own documents that express their knowledge in their own words:

Joe's Standing Up to Anger [*translation of understanding*]

1. I am tired of Anger pushing me around and taking away the people I care about.
2. I will turn my anger against Anger and use my understanding to get out from underneath it.
3. I know that when I take a deep breath and count to 10, I will calm down 75% of the time and Anger will have less of a hold on me. I will remember to do this.
4. I know that when I ask myself if this is more important than friends and family, Anger will often go away and I will try to work something out with the other person.

Anger Messes Up My Life [*statement of position*]

1. When Anger gets into my life it makes me do and say things I am ashamed of.
2. When Anger takes hold of me I get into trouble with people and they don't want to be around me.
3. When Anger gets hold of me I sit and think about it for a long time and sometimes stay up at night getting more and more upset.
4. If Anger continues to get the best of me, I will be thrown out of school, lose my friends, and be in trouble. I want to get Anger out of my life as much as possible. I want a different life from trouble and loneliness. I want a life where I can be happy and not be so upset by everything, where I can be upset about only those things that are worth being upset about.

The second type of brief document involves listing the rules that the problem instructs the client to obey (Rombach, 2003). This type of document can be used to strengthen the externalization of the problem. It illustrates and reinforces for the client how the problem is controlling and leading him or her to act against his or her better judgment. For example:

Anger's Rules

1. Anger tells me that the world is always unfair and people are out to get me.
2. Anger tells me that I am entitled to special privileges and no one has a right to take those away from me.
3. Anger tells me that if I am hurt or embarrassed, the best thing to do is to get angry at other people.
4. Anger tells me that if I yell and hit other people, they will treat me with respect.
5. Anger does not want me to talk things out or even tell someone that I am angry because of something.
6. Anger does not like it when I decide not to fight; it says I should always fight.
7. Anger tells me that being calm means I am "girly," so I have to yell, call people names, and hit people so I can be a "real boy."

These types of briefer documents increase clients' ability to consult their own knowledge of the problem and confirm their motivation for changing their relationship to it.

## Dictation You Would Be Proud to Show Your Client

Dictation serves the purpose of accountability to funding agencies. Most agencies use a dictation style that emphasizes problems and deficits. Agencies often require the dictation format to focus on treatment goals and accomplishment of those goals. For example, dictation on individual sessions may be set up in a format that requires the social worker to state what goals were worked on and what progress was made toward reaching those goals, with a small area left for general comments about the session. In some cases, tasks assigned are another category. The general dictation format used by many behavioral health agencies is initial summary, treatment plan, progress notes, quarterly summaries, and closing summary.

The intake summary, which needs to be completed after the first or second session, usually has sections for identifying information, presenting complaint or problem, history of significant issues and prior treatment, family and social information, suicide/homicide risk, child abuse history, and substance abuse and domestic violence evaluations. There also typically is an assessment section, where the worker conceptualizes what is "really" going on based on the facts deemed significant by virtue of a theory (which many workers, in fact, have difficulty identifying).

The intake summary often ends with an initial treatment contract that lays out the goals to be accomplished in treatment. In some agencies the treatment contract has a separate format that divides broad goals into specific objectives that are then divided into tasks to be carried out by the client and/or the worker within designated time frames. Both client and worker sign the treatment contract, an act designed to acknowledge its supposed collaborative development.

Each treatment session has a progress note, which may or may not follow a specific format. Most agencies require a quarterly review of progress (three-month summary) that addresses the extent to which the goals have been accomplished and changes or additions to the goal list because of new information. The last dictation is a closing summary, which typically looks at the goals accomplished and the course of the treatment. Because treatment is frequently unilaterally terminated by clients, closing summaries often end with an examination of client "resistance."

The NASW *Code of Ethics* says: "Social workers should provide clients with reasonable access to records concerning the clients" (NASW, 1999, Ethical Standards section, subsection 1.08[a] Access to Records). Yet despite this standard, most dictation is written not to clients, but to the omniscient file. It is not surprising, then, that the language of most dictation tends to treat the person as an object of consideration rather than as a partner in a cooperative venture.

Files can live on to define people long after a worker and a client have discontinued their association with an agency. Records, and the diagnoses contained in them, can impact clients' future treatment; health care; insurance; and, in some cases, employment opportunities. They can also affect decisions about child custody in divorce proceedings and in placement decisions in abuse, neglect, or dependency situations. Despite a recorder's intent, statements in files represent expert evaluations in the eyes of society and are accorded a special level of truth that can impact a person's life well beyond the treatment relationship.

Records, however, can be developed to be helpful to clients. Giving clients copies of all dictation ensures that what is written will be in support of, not in opposition to, them. This requires workers to consider carefully what they are thinking and saying about clients. Sharing difficult information with clients along the way allows for course corrections.

In contrast to how an assessment is usually done, a narrative approach to assessment initially focuses on the problem story and its impact on the client. Overlaying a narrative framework on traditional assessment categories leads a worker to assess how the problem influences the person (mental status), how it most recently (or currently) impacts the person (current complaint), what its history and strategies are (treatment history, social history, and risk factors), and what the client's preference is for a future (combined in the formulation). Including two more dimensions—how the client would like his or her life to be and what constraints (problems, discourses, oppression) get in the way of the person having that life—would create a more thorough assessment, one that clients could find helpful (Madsen, 2007).

In what follows I look at the various sections of an intake summary to see how each could be approached from a narrative perspective.

## Identifying Information

The information in this section is important in determining how a person is likely to be respected or disrespected by the dominant culture and what barriers to understanding might exist between the worker's and the client's worldviews. Here is an example of identifying information:

> Joe is a 17-year-old African American who looks to be about six feet tall and weighs about 185 pounds, who comes from a primarily African American neighborhood, and who shows his pride by wearing gold necklaces. He lives with his mother and she supports the family through housekeeping jobs and public assistance. The family is helped by Joe's "hustling money," some of which he contributes to them. He is proud of his ability to get along with most people and to earn their respect, being "tough" when necessary.

Think of how Joe's worldview might differ from that of the following young man:

> James is a 17-year-old White male who typically wears casual polo shirts and slacks and lives in a primarily White suburban neighborhood. He lives with his parents, both of whom practice law, and a younger sister. He is on the football team and is most proud of his ability to have so many friends at school.

In fact, both young men might prefer a similar lifestyle: no financial worries, a loving family, and a comfortable home in a safe neighborhood. However, the way in which they will be treated and how their actions will be interpreted by the dominant society are likely to be markedly different. Identifying information places the person in the context of the society's discourses.

## Presenting Complaint

The presenting problem, or complaint, should be recorded in the client's words. If there is a referral agent, then both the client's and the referral agent's depictions of the presenting problem should be included.

For instance, if Joe is referred by his probation officer for fighting (assault and battery), then what the probation officer said should be noted: "Joe is in trouble again for fighting with members of a rival gang. He put a 16-year-old boy in the hospital with a broken arm and two broken ribs. He needs to learn to control his anger or else he will end up in prison." Joe's response to his probation officer's description should be recorded, too: "He [the probation officer] has got it all wrong. That guy I hurt was coming after me with a knife and his friends got rid of it before the police came. I was just trying to defend myself." The referral agent sees the problems as anger and violence, whereas Joe sees the problem as the probation officer misunderstanding the situation. The probation officer's description also suggests that this is not the first time Joe has been in trouble and that trouble will inevitably lead him to prison—that a bad reputation may be a factor.

## History of the Presenting Complaint

Because most agencies' intake forms emphasize deficits and problems, the social worker will need to change the emphasis to context and constraints: When did the problem take hold of the person's life and how did it do so? What factors made it easier for the problem to gain such control? What strategies did it use to do that? What effects does the problem have on the person's general health, family, friends, work, school, and community?

These types of questions focus discussion of the presenting complaint's history on the influence of the problem on the person. Interspersed in this history may be unique outcomes, either explicitly mentioned or implied, that can suggest alternative stories. Included in this history, too, may be information about the client's prior experiences with helpers. For example:

> Joe has gotten into many fights in his life, beginning when he was about six years old. He says all his friends fight and he would be picked on if he didn't. He says that probably about 25% of the time he could get into a fight but chooses not to. He says he was able to avoid fighting because he "didn't really have to." Joe explains that when "people don't try to mess with you on your turf," even if they "ignore you or say nasty things to you, you don't always have to fight them to save your respect." He says that when he meets other people in the neighborhood who aren't part of his group, he has to evaluate whether they are "calling me out." He says this is very tiring and makes going out of the house "a drag" sometimes. He feels like a gunslinger in the old cowboy movies—the one who always goes out and shoots people who call him out. He doesn't see much future in this and thinks this reputation will land him in prison, just as the probation officer has said.
>
> Joe says his mother doesn't get along with him anymore because he now spends so much time on the streets. Until about five years ago they had a loving relationship. He now wonders if that caring is "almost gone" because of all the bad feelings.
>
> He has been going to an alternative school because of fighting. He says he likes two of the teachers and can talk to them. He says they see him as a person who might make it, "even if I can't see it."

> He has seen two counselors in the past. The first counselor was a White woman. He says she spent most of the time letting him know he would go to prison if he kept fighting and then put him on drugs for "being hyper." But he stopped taking them after a month because no one saw a difference. He refused to go back to see her. The second counselor was a Black man at the juvenile detention center who was "cool." This second counselor told him he could do better than he was doing and could make it in life despite how things had been going so far. Joe lost touch with this counselor when he was released from the detention center.
>
> Joe says his reputation has earned him some respect in the neighborhood. He has a steady female friend, only hangs out with people from his gang, and is not supposed to act too differently from them. He feels all this makes it a little "hard to breathe" sometimes. He seems interested in something else for his life.

## Family History

Some family information will show up in the history of presenting the complaint, as few problems will not affect close family members. Family is not just those who live in the household but includes extended family members who have an interest in the problem. For example:

> Joe lives with his mother and until a few years ago enjoyed cooking and going to church with her. He says his mother would be most proud of his determination to have a better future despite his reputation and troubles. He has not seen his father for about 11 years. He says he wishes his father could know how strong he has become and how he has been able to survive without him. His grandmother lives in the neighborhood and she worries about him. He has always done errands for her and still talks to her in a respectful way. He says she sees in him a determination to do things that he doesn't always see. She sees his helping her out as evidence of his kindness, and this kindness is something he would like to have more of in his life. His uncle and aunt live in another state and he rarely sees them, though his mother gets Christmas cards from them each year.

## Medical Condition

Constraints on people reaching the life they prefer can be physical as well as social or emotional. A number of medications have consequences for personal functioning, in addition to relieving or controlling the physical problems for which they were prescribed. Because the symptoms of many diseases and the side effects of medication can get labeled as mental health disorders, it is important to look carefully at this dimension. For example:

> Joe is seen at the local county health clinic for his school physicals and has had a history of chicken pox and measles. He says he briefly took Ritalin about five years ago. It was prescribed by a general practitioner at the clinic with the encouragement of his counselor, but it left him feeling "bummed out" and he did not think it changed his life in any way. He quit taking Ritalin after about a month. He currently has no physical problems, but upon further probing, he admits to frequent headaches and says he has trouble sleeping about twice a week. He treats these problems with marijuana and is quick to point out he does not, and will not, use anything "harder." He says he only gets high when he has a headache or cannot sleep. He says that seeing so many people who become "less than human" on "stuff like crack, heroin, and meth" has convinced him he does not want to go down that road. He says that he has a reputation for being a "straight arrow" like that, so people do not push it on him too much anymore. He also thinks his mother would throw him out of the house if she found out he had been doing anything stronger. He says he has about a six-pack of beer a week with his friends when the weather is hot but is not a big drinker, either.

I have included drug history here because people are more likely to discuss their drug use in terms of the purpose it serves in their life than simply as a habit. Using marijuana to self-medicate, for example, is more acceptable than saying it is being used because of dependence. Although the client may eventually see his or her substance use as a problem, it has not been identified as one yet.

There is, of course, the legal issue of mandated clients violating probation and the need to report such violations. This report may trigger drug screens and clients should be aware of the consequences. The worker's obligation to the referral agent should be clearly discussed with the client as well as the worker's social control function when he or she conducts risk assessments. Even with strengths-based approaches we cannot abdicate our responsibility to address risky situations, and richer descriptions of people's lives do not mean only positive descriptions of their lives (Madsen, 2007).

## Formulation

Traditional assessments are geared to discovering the problem and its cause so that the social worker, using expert knowledge, can select an appropriate (and empirically tested, best-practice) intervention. A narrative approach, instead, looks at the desires of clients and the constraints they face in meeting those desires. It also looks for potential building blocks of an alternative story that could point the way toward a more desirable outcome. Thus, from a narrative perspective, formulating a response to the problem involves a collaborative effort by the worker and the client, and through this collaboration both parties gain an understanding of what is involved in reducing the problem's influence on the person's life.

Madsen (2007) recommends that a narrative formulation address three specific areas:

- Where would the client/family members like to be at the end of our work together?
- What supports and constrains them in accomplishing this?
- What abilities, skills, and know-how might they draw on or develop to enhance those supports and address those constraints? (p. 82)

The following narrative formulation addresses these areas:

Joe would like a life where he works a job and has a family. He would like to live in a place with less trouble, drugs, and gangs. He is not sure that he can make any changes right now. He faces the problem that getting out of a gang could be dangerous, and he has never lived outside of his neighborhood. He says he is tired of always having to fight and always getting into trouble. He says trouble seems to find him wherever he goes. He would like a calm life; he could work and find someone to care about if things were calm. He also struggles with the idea that a man must fight to protect his reputation, because if "you aren't respected, you aren't nothing." He thinks his grandmother, mother, and teachers at school would support him becoming a "young man who can find calm in his life." He sees himself as strong, and it is this strength that can help him take his life back from trouble, complete school, and leave his gang. His grandmother sees his kindness, and he feels that this kindness would also carry him to find other friends outside the neighborhood. He realizes he will need a lot of self-respect to get respect back from people like his probation officer, who see him only as having a bad reputation. He thinks gaining respect from White people in general will be difficult because they are biased and seem scared of him. He sees himself as turning around people's ideas about him by showing more of his kindness, although he understands that old reputations die hard.

## DSM Diagnosis

The last part of most assessments is the development of the diagnosis. Despite arguments about reliability and validity and questions about whether social workers should be diagnosing clients, the fact is that until we change our social service, behavioral health, and mental health systems so that financing is not based on a medical model, we cannot avoid using the DSM in the United States. The DSM is what we have despite desires to the contrary (Saleebey, 2001). We practice in a modernist, structuralist, bureaucratic environment and we must accommodate to the requirements of this environment as best we can. If the diagnosis provides a story that we are concerned might be too thin and/or too focused on pathology, then we are obligated to expand that story by discussing the diagnosis with the client and documenting his or her response to it (Madsen, 2007).

# Exercises

## Exercise 1: Practicing Short Letters

Therapeutic letter writing is time-consuming; speed and creativity in therapeutic letters come only through practice. It is worth the effort to develop excellence in what is indeed a skill. Practicing with one or two letters will not be sufficient to fully appreciate what can be done with this medium. Once you develop some confidence in letter writing you will find that it is a place where you can show considerable creativity.

Take the letter you wrote at the beginning of this chapter and transform it into a therapeutic letter by using the following format. If you did not write the letter, select a client from your practicum or work and write this letter to him or her:

Dear _____,

Compliment:
_____
_____
_____

Problem story and effects of problem on the person:
_____
_____
_____
_____

Beginnings of an alternative story:
_____
_____
_____
_____

Introduction to your questions:
_____
_____
_____

Questions:
_____
_____
_____
_____
_____
_____

Closing:
_____
_____

Sincerely,

## Exercise 2: Creating Lists

Use Ann Epston's letter on eating disorders that appears in chapter 4 to come up with a list of rules about anorexia.

Rules Anorexia/Bulimia Imposes

1. _____
2. _____
3. _____
4. _____
5. _____
6. _____
7. _____
8. _____
9. _____

CHAPTER 9

# Teams: Audiences, Reflecting, and Ending With Pomp and Appreciation

Once an alternative story is coconstructed with a client, the social worker should locate people who will confirm and support the story, thereby strengthening it. The social constructionist perspective that underlies a narrative approach to social work gives great importance to people's social interactions in the wider environment. The environment provides opportunities as well as constraints to people developing their preferred identities and outcomes. Although social workers may be able to give people the narrative space needed to pull together a different story of who they are, if the environment continues to treat them as nonentities or as permanently defective, then the "new" story can last only so long. The environment's strong countervailing messages are likely to push clients back to the older problem story.

This chapter describes several methods that narrative workers have developed to assist people in getting their stories out to others, which allows stories to be expanded and enriched through their retelling. I discuss how individuals who saw earlier indications of the new identity in the client's life can be engaged to form a supportive team. I describe how possible members of a supportive team can be drawn from among those in the client's life who are no longer living, and how people in the client's present who are willing to stand by him or her during this time of transformation can become team members. I also consider the use of reflecting teams and how the professionals who make up these teams can act as appreciative audiences for the new story and enlarge it with each telling. I conclude the chapter with a discussion of termination from a narrative perspective. If entering a helpful conversation with a social worker is not considered a sign of failure but is instead seen as an attempt to stand up to a problem, what does successful termination look like?

## The Importance of Audiences

Audiences are helpful in solidifying the alternative story that leads to the client's preferred outcome. Audiences can support the person in telling this story. They can give their reactions to the story and describe how it affects them. More important, they can retell the story, and with each retelling the story's truth and richness increase as it becomes infused with each audience member's viewpoint. People's lives become more richly described when the stories of their preferred histories and identities are told and retold. A sense of community is created in this way, with the linking of people's lives through shared values, beliefs, and commitments (White, 1997).

Think for a moment about what it would be like to feel you were not part of a community. For example, if you were a member of a group where someone continually talked about all your failures, would you be likely to feel a sense of community with the group? If you did, what changes might occur in your behavior? How might you be seen by the group? What impact would this have on you? Or, have you ever been in a situation in which any story you told was countered with a conflicting story that reflected values at odds with yours? What was your experience of this like? Did it increase or decrease your sense of connection?

The point is that we have all had experiences of noncommunity, of times when we were disrespected. Given what we know from our own lives about the importance of community, what can we, as social workers, do to codevelop communities that are concerned about the people who are consulting us, so that their preferred identities and histories are enhanced, not diminished? The people who come and talk with social workers are often in great need of community.

Yet community can be a two-edged sword: On one hand, it can be a source of enormous support and strength; on the other, it can give rise to oppressive discourses. Workers and clients, therefore, need to consider carefully which communities are likely to be helpful and how the context for clients' participation is to be structured (Lobovits et al., 1995).

## Who Supported or Will Support the Alternative Story?

After an alternative story has been discussed, questions can be asked that focus on the story's portrayal of the client's reputation. For example: Who would be least surprised by your ability to stand up to this problem? Why would you say they would not be surprised? What did they see in you that the problem has prevented you from seeing? Can you think of a time when they showed you this support?

A social worker would probe for as many specifics as possible to enrich the alternative story and to identify additional potential members of the client's community. Questions the worker might ask the client to draw out this information include: What do you think this says about you as a person that this individual was able to see this in you? Can you think of someone else who would not be surprised at your ability to do this? Who do you think in your life now would be willing to support your bringing more self-care (or self-respect or any other project) into your life as opposed to self-hate (or self-denigration or any other problem)?

These types of questions lead to a sort of *re-membering*, a word coined by anthropologist Barbara Myerhoff (1982, p. 111) and taken up by Michael White (1989). Re-membering occurs on two levels: the events that support an alternative story are rediscovered in memory and the members of the person's community who are supportive of such a story are identified and connections with them are (re)established.

## Re-membering Practices

Re-membering practices start with the idea that memory is a group project. For instance, in the midst of divorce, a person looks back at the marriage, which was presumably happy at some time, and now sees only false betrayal. This negative remembrance is a contextualizing of the memory of the marriage that serves the person's current purposes. Support for this reinterpretation may come from the person's friends, family, and sometimes legal representatives.

Re-membering is often a collective remembering because remembering and forgetting are social activities (Madigan, 1997). Whether the who, what, where, when, how, and why of events are recalled and discussed are strongly influenced by cultural discourses about who can remember and what they can remember. For example, Freud's initial theory of infantile sexuality considered the possibility of widespread sexual exploitation of girls. However, Freud subsequently reconsidered and backed away from that position, changing his theory to one of sexual attractions that occur in fantasy (Miller, 1984).

Memories of events have political aspects, too. A night out drinking, for example, can be a source of shame, a badge of manhood (or maturity), a cultural tradition, or fond companionship (Madigan, 1997). After many years of where stories about these people, have stood for certain values. Again, the level of description desired requires going slowly with clients in order to fully elicit a rich story and their reactions to it. Once a deceased member, or a member heard about only in others' stories, is "resurrected," clients can begin considering what the person would likely say to them in their efforts to stand up to the problem. These words, and the image of the person saying them, can be retained by clients "in their heart" and can be called upon to help them contradict the negative self-talk they may be struggling against.

## Internalized Other Questioning

Epston (1993, p. 183) developed what has come to be called *internalized other questioning*, in which the social worker attempts to encourage the client to break from a negative pattern of thought or interaction by bringing into the conversation the perceptions of other people, particularly those who cannot be present. In this technique, the worker stops the conversation and asks the client what he or she thinks those identified as supportive might say. After asking and receiving permission, the worker then interviews the client as if he or she were the supportive person who is not present. This is done to expand the alternative story.

This conversation is different from Gestalt empty-chair procedures that attempt to recombine two voices or parts of the self through a dialogue or confrontation between them. Here the focus is simply on getting a new perspective on the client's story, as the following illustrates:

**Worker:** So, Joe, your grandmother was the person you feel would have recognized your ability to take your life back from anxiety, is that what you said?

**Joe:** *Yes, she would have seen me as someone strong enough to do that.*

**Worker:** What would she have told you?

**Joe:** *Stick with it! You can do anything you want to.*

**Worker:** I see. I wonder . . . I know this might sound silly, but you mentioned your grandmother died when you were 14. Do you think you remember your grandmother enough to answer in her stead?

**Joe:** *Well, I think so. We were very close.*

**Worker:** Would you be willing to try it?

**Joe:** *I guess.*

**Worker:** Her name was?

**Joe:** *Emma.*

**Worker:** Okay, Emma, I wonder if I can talk to you about your grandson, Joe?

**Joe as Grandma:** *Sure.*

**Worker:** Joe is regaining his life from anxiety and panic and he said you were the person who would most support him.

**Joe as Grandma:** *Nice of him to say that.*

**Worker:** What about the way you related to him would give him the idea that you would support him in this?

**Joe as Grandma:** *Well, she—I mean I—would always let him know that he was a good person.*

**Worker:** What about him did you see that led you to believe that he was a good person? Can you give a specific example?

**Joe as Grandma:** *Well, I remember when he was only seven and he asked if I would give his Christmas presents to poor kids who didn't get anything for Christmas.*

**Worker:** Do you remember where that took place?

**Joe as Grandma:** *Yes, in my living room. The whole family had come for dinner on Christmas Day. They would always do that.*

**Worker:** How did his comment about giving away his presents come up?

**Joe as Grandma:** *Everyone was talking about presents. I asked him what he got and he told me "lots of things." Then he said he wished he could give them to poor kids.*

**Worker:** So there were other family members around?

**Joe as Grandma:** *Yes.*

**Worker:** Who was there?

**Joe as Grandma:** *Well, there was me and Grandpa. Uncle Jim—I mean my son, Jim—and his wife and their two children, Rich and Jill, were there. Then there was my daughter and her husband, Joe's parents; and Joe's sisters, Mary and Margaret.*

**Worker:** So he said that in front of all those people?

**Joe as Grandma:** *Yes, I think everyone heard him.*

**Worker:** What did that mean to you?

**Joe as Grandma:** *I thought that it was sweet, that he was a very sensitive child who cared about others and had real compassion. I always knew he had a great capacity to love.*

**Worker:** What did you say in response to his comment?

**Joe as Grandma:** *I just kissed him and told him I loved him.*

**Worker:** Did he seem to get what you said?

**Joe as Grandma:** *Yes, because he hugged me and gave me a big kiss back.*

**Worker:** So you saw him as a person who was sensitive and compassionate.

**Joe as Grandma:** *Yes, I think I saw that in him very early on.*

**Worker:** Are those good things?

**Joe as Grandma:** *Yes, but very painful things, because the world can be very cruel.*

**Worker:** Did you see him as the kind of person who could suffer in order to keep sensitivity and compassion in his life?

**Joe as Grandma:** *Yes, he was pretty gutsy to say that in front of the family, even at that age.*

The worker could continue the conversation by asking questions such as the following:

Can you talk about any other times that supported these views of Joe?

What do you think you did for his life?

Why did you do that?

What would you say knowing him did for your life?

What did he give to you?

Is there anything else I should know about?

Is there any question you wished I had asked you but didn't?

This type of interchange is intended to further strengthen the client's alternative story by letting the client know that he or she is not alone in the interpretation. The benefits of using internalized other questioning are that it casts the recognition and praise for the client's positive characteristics as coming from "outside" the client—in another's voice—and that it allows the client to explore his or her positive attributes before taking responsibility for them. People who are experiencing their lives as hopeless and themselves as defeated or "not up to standard" are frequently reluctant to directly acknowledge and appreciate their own skills, abilities, and knowledge. Using the voice of another can help develop a richer story that the client can then use to support an alternative view of his or her life and identity.

This type of questioning, when somewhat modified, can be used to develop a sense of empathy for someone the client has victimized or to foster an understanding of the viewpoint of another when there is a conflict. These uses are explored in chapter 10, as part of a discussion of mediation, and in chapter 11, in relation to the prevention of violence.

## Communities of Concern

The old African saying that it takes a village to raise a child is true not only about raising children but also about constructing lives in general. From a narrative perspective, it takes a village to be recognized and seen as a person. Unfortunately, this village does not appear to exist for many of the people social workers see, clients who have little sense of community or who do not realize that they have a club of life whose members value them. Sometimes club members are estranged from the client because the problem's influence on the person gets in the way of a continued connection. Club members may have felt exhausted, thought they were being called upon for support too frequently, and been unaware that others might be available to assist. With older people and with individuals who live in oppressive conditions, many members of their club, and often the most important ones, may be dead from disease or violence.

Narrative practitioners have developed a number of ways to address the apparent lack of community felt by clients by offering them opportunities to increase their connection to others. *Communities of concern* (Madigan & Epston, 1995, p. 257) involve all those who share a client's concerns, such as family members, friends, involved professionals, others experiencing the same problems, and others who have an interest in the problems. The social worker can assist the client to tap into already existing communities through letter-writing campaigns; can encourage the client, as the expert on his or her own problems, to form or participate in a supportive and politically active league; and can arrange, with the client's consent, for other professionals to serve as a reflecting team to validate and expand the client's stories. Technology, such as the Internet, now makes it possible to create communities of concern in cyberspace among individuals who may never meet in person, but who nevertheless can give each other support, share strategies to overcome a problem, and act in concert to change oppressive societal discourses.

## Letter-Writing Campaigns

One way to help people develop a community of concern is through a letter-writing campaign, which attempts to help people be re-membered into their clubs of life from which they have been dis-membered by problems (Madigan, 1997). Madigan and Epston (1995) have been instrumental in developing letter-writing campaigns as a means to gather an audience for a client's preferred story and preferred identity. Letter-writing campaigns provide clients with a concrete product: letters from potential club members that they can consult in times of need. Some people carry these letters with them, tape them to their bedroom walls, or keep them secure in a scrapbook.

Like all narrative techniques there is considerable flexibility in how letter writing is carried out. Madigan (1997), for example, offers the following approach: While eliciting the client's preferences on how he or she wants to be seen differently, the worker begins to create a list of the people mentioned by the client who might support this different point of view. The worker then asks the client which of the people on the list would see the client as someone different from the problem's description and would support his or her efforts to realize the preferred description. Next, the worker and the client collaborate on drafting a letter that asks these individuals to provide information of a positive nature about the client, including anecdotes that make concrete this nonproblem version of the client's identity. The client needs to decide whether the return letters are to go to his or her home or to the worker's office, a valuable option if privacy is desired. Madigan says he supplies envelopes and stamps if necessary.

If a client is ambivalent about a full-scale campaign, he or she can start by sending out letters to only a few members of his or her club. It is not unusual for a client to become curious and wish to pursue the campaign after receiving the initial return letters from these members.

As the letters come in, they can be read and reread by the client and the worker in front of each other. The worker would read the letters aloud after the client has read them aloud, in order to emphasize the retelling of the client's story. If there is a sufficient number of letters, they can be reviewed for themes, which could give the client a better picture of the good things that others see in him or her. The product of the letter-writing campaign is extensive documentation of a richer narrative, which can help solidify for the client his or her nonproblem identity.

Madsen (2007) provides an example of a letter-writing campaign undertaken by an adolescent who had been involved in a variety of systems because of substance abuse issues, school and family problems, and multiple placements in foster care. With the support and encouragement of her worker, the teen asked a variety of people for letters. As a child of multiple systems, she sent almost two dozen of her initial letters to professionals she had found helpful. She then contacted each person who wrote back so that she could arrange a meeting. At each meeting, the adolescent and the respondent read the letter together and were photographed. Through this ritual, the client ended up with a letter, a photograph, and other mementos, all of which she placed in a scrapbook that she took wherever she went.

An illustration of the use of a letter-writing campaign for a different purpose comes from Decker and Buckley (2003), who describe its use by a couple in conflict. The couple sent letters to friends and family asking them to come to a celebration where they would create a time capsule of the couple's relationship. The invitees were asked to contribute poetry, letters, photos, collages, or other artifacts that would be interesting and relevant to the couple in 5 years' time when the capsule was to be opened. The items could reflect what the contributor had appreciated about either member of the couple or about the couple as a unit, what he or she appreciates now, or what he or she might appreciate in 5 years. Or, the contributor could donate something that reminded him or her of the couple's hopes and dreams. This ritual meant that the nonconflictual part of the couple's life was recognized by their community of concern and spoken of during the celebration. By implication, it also meant that the couple had made a 5-year commitment to each other.

This type of ritual can be compared in some way to a eulogy made on behalf of a person who is not dead (Madigan & Epston, 1995). Few eulogies focus on a person's faults or mistakes but instead look at the good parts of the person and his or her life. How many times have we been to a funeral or memorial services and thought, "If only the person could have heard this!" A letter-writing campaign has the effect of asking letter writers to re-member the memories of the person separate from the problem, of documenting alternative versions of the person's story, and of opening up the potential for new stories.

An example of an invitational letter, based on Madigan's (2003) ideas, follows:

*Dear Bessie,*

*My name is Gary Pasture and I am a social worker working with Johnnie Lee in his efforts to lead a life free from alcohol. He is writing this letter with me. As you may be aware, it has been a struggle for him and he mentioned you as someone who would understand that he can keep alcohol from taking over his life again. Alcohol has kept him from the people he loves and blinded him from the good things in his life. We are asking if you would consider sending him a letter through me at this clinic. In the letter we would ask that you keep a positive attitude, as alcohol has brought him great shame already, and answer the following:*

*Before alcohol entered Johnnie's life, what kind of person was he and what did your relationship with him mean to you?*

*Do you have any stories about Johnnie (outside his experience with alcohol) that indicate what is good about him?*

*When Johnnie is able to push alcohol out of his life, what kind of relationship do you see yourself as having with him?*

*Who else might be willing to write a letter in support of Johnnie taking his life back from alcohol?*

*If you choose to write a letter, please send it to Johnnie Lee c/o Gary Pasture, Exciting Mental Health Center, 1000 Healthy Blvd., Exciting, Wyoming 83456.*

*Sincerely,*

*Johnnie Lee*

*Gary Pasture*

The last two questions, however, might not be appropriate in all cases, especially if the person is a helping professional.

The questions in this letter touch on three important areas: what the client meant to the person before the problem dominated the client's life, specific anecdotal evidence of the client's better points, and what the relationship could look like in the future. These questions are designed to counteract three specific messages that are common tactics problems use to diminish people's resistance: "No one ever cared about you or thought you were special"; "You have no redeeming qualities"; "No one will care if you take your life back from the problem and you will be all alone." The letters should produce evidence that directly contradicts these strategies of problems. Different problems might use somewhat different strategies with different persons; the questions should be tailored to the beliefs of the individual client.

## Sharing Stories of Success With Others

In the narrative approach, clients are seen as the true experts on their problems; through their struggle to change their relationship to their problems, they acquire *local knowledges* (Madigan & Epston, 1995, p. 260), an understanding of problems and the strategies for standing up to problems that emerges from the clients' specific situations. Accordingly, clients may wish to have the opportunity to help others through their hard-won experience. And sharing their struggles, in turn, increases the value of these experiences to them.

Social workers can ask clients if they would be interested in having their methods of dealing with their problems shared with other clients who are struggling against similar problems, and if so, to give permission to use these stories of success. They also can inquire about whether clients would be interested in writing a letter or description, or in the case of children, drawing pictures, that would be included in a handbook for new clients. Clients might even be willing to serve as paid consultants (Lobovits et al., 1995). Lobovits et al. note the benefits of this process for clients, who report that their stories of hope and pain are validated by connecting with sympathetic others. Where clients were previously in a degraded position, the practice of sharing their expertise upgrades their status: They are not victims, but survivors. Helping clients connect with others who are standing up to similar problems is perhaps best exemplified by the development of client-run associations or leagues.

Epston and Madigan have been instrumental in instigating client-formed leagues that go beyond the usual support groups (Madigan & Epston, 1995). Leagues developed as Epston pulled "together a network of clients with the purpose of consultation, information, and mutual support" (p. 261). These people became Epston's colleagues and consultants. Madigan and Epston say, "Leagues are a gathering of persons who have a desire to protest the effects of a particular problem on people's lives.... A league's focus is directed toward combating a particular identified problem ... and the structures that support the problem" (pp. 261–262). These structures include cultural and professional institutions.

Leagues are different from 12-step programs because they take on political issues (e.g., the way the culture supports sexism or ageism), which is not part of the 12-step mandate. Examples of social change actions undertaken by the Vancouver, British Columbia, Anti-Anorexia/Anti-Bulimia League include the development of a media watch to publicly denounce what it sees as " 'pro-anorexic/bulimic' activities against women's bodies," the formation of a school action committee to conduct education in schools, and the creation of T-shirts and music with anti-anorexic/anti-bulimic messages to educate the public (Madigan & Epston, 1995, p. 267).

Leagues function to provide members with support and with ideas for standing up to the problems that confront them. They create a community that is specifically concerned with not letting certain types of problems take over people's lives, is not deficit oriented, and helps develop general awareness about the problem. Confidentiality rules and/or statutes in the United States, which emphasize privacy and secrecy, impede workers' ability to easily instigate leagues. These rules require explicit written permission to share specific information about a particular party with another identified party (in this case nonprofessionals) and, hence, maintain the individual, nonpolitical nature of problems.

## Reflecting Teams: Outsider-Witness Practices

Narrative social workers have refined and expanded the use of reflecting teams in treatment, a technique initially described by Andersen (1987, 1991, 1995). There is a long tradition in certain forms of family therapy to have teams of professionals watch the worker and family from behind one-way mirrors. The team members' observations lead them to develop hypotheses or to make suggestions that are conveyed to the worker in some fashion (e.g., a telephone call into the session, a team member walking into the session, or a team member rapping on the mirror to signal the worker to leave the session for a consultation). The worker is then informed of the team's decision or given instructions on what to present to the family in terms of a final observation or task. Thus, the team is used as a form of live supervision, with the worker being supervised within the session.

The opportunity to see family processes in action was critical for developing theory and training workers in structuralist methods. Students of the Milan approach to systemic family treatment have found this model of work particularly valuable (Nichols, 2006). However, from a narrative perspective, which stresses the importance of power relationships, this type of observation represents a top-down process that focuses on the specialized knowledge of the professionals and is done in secret, outside the view of the family. The notion of interventions being "done to" a family goes against the ethic of recognizing clients' expertise in their own lives.

Narrative-based social workers have developed a different notion of reflecting teams (White, 1995). In narrative therapy, reflecting teams are designed to keep the power as decentralized as possible. Social workers who are new to reflecting teams and narrative processes need to be aware of the privilege of trust bestowed on them by their clients. They also need to recognize their own privilege in terms of race, ethnicity, income, and gender, which may create options for them that are not available to the people who consult them. Workers have a great deal of power in the therapeutic endeavor and they should be aware of how they use it.

As part of narrative treatment's use of reflecting teams, social workers will be asked to interact in front of clients, and to do so with an awareness of how what they are doing is informed by their privilege. This process encourages workers to more honestly acknowledge, not discount, clients' experiences of and struggles against their problems. Workers also will be asked to become curious about those aspects of people's lives that may provide a point of departure from the stories of suffering and pain. Finally, and perhaps most important, they will be asked to bring to the discussion the context of their own lives from which their thoughts derive. Although the primary worker needs to be cautious about self-disclosure, even when considering the taking-it-back practices described in chapter 2, reflecting team members have somewhat more freedom in this realm.

Individuals as well as families can benefit from reflecting team meetings, which can provide them with input on standing up to the problem. However, before a reflecting team meeting is held, the process should be thoroughly explained to a client and his or her consent to participate elicited. If consent is obtained, the reflecting team process, as described by White (1995), moves forward as follows:

First, the team watches through a one-way mirror as the worker interviews the client in the interview room; team members remain quiet during this observational period. The client is given the option of meeting the team members either before the interview or during the second part of the process. When they do meet, team members tell the client who they are and what they do professionally.

Second, the team switches places with the client and worker. The client and worker go behind the one-way mirror and watch the discussion among the team members. There are some boundaries to the discussion to make sure it does not wander into diagnostic or other talk that would objectify the client.

Third, the client and worker again change places with the team. After reentering the interview room, the worker asks the client to talk about his or her experience of the first two parts of the process. The team members again quietly observe the interaction from behind the one-way mirror.

Finally, the team members join the client and worker in the interview room and all the parties debrief about the process itself: Where was it going? What was the thinking behind certain questions? Where could the team have been more helpful?

The development of the second stage of the process is worth exploring in more detail because it is perhaps the most nontraditional aspect of these reflecting teams. White (1995) provides some structure for this process. Before the client and worker leave the interview room to go behind the one-way mirror, the worker should describe to the team the circumstances that led to the reflecting team meeting being called and how the client has been experiencing those circumstances. The client can then clarify or add anything he or she believes would be important for the team to know.

If the team members did not introduce themselves to the client during the first stage, it is now time to do so. In addition to giving their names, team members should explain how it is that they became involved in the consultation and identify where they work or what their areas of clinical interest are. The team then begins to discuss those conversational developments they witnessed that could be leading to preferred outcomes, exploring them in some detail and looking at the possibilities offered by these developments.

The process is comparable to that used in a therapeutic conversation with the client: the questions first address the behaviors and thoughts and intentions of the person involved in making the changes and then consider possible meanings and significance. Simple cheerleading or applause is to be avoided; merely pumping out praise, without specificity or a sense of challenge, is of little value. A way to avoid this is for reflecting team members to interview each other about the comments they make so that they explore them in more depth and give them context. Thus, the members' comments are deconstructed; that is, the team members, either by themselves or through the questions of others, center the comment in their own experiences.

This structure for reflecting teams and the remarkable focus on transparency in the therapeutic process are unique to the narrative approach and can sometimes be jarring to professionals who are being asked to draw upon their subjective experience over acquired expertise. When most discussions of treatment take place in closed case consultation sessions, where clients are not present, it is easy for the discussions to degenerate into problem-focused and deficit-based language. By contrast, because narrative reflecting team meetings involve clients, they are not likely to devolve into problem-focused or deficit-based talk, and corrections can immediately be made if they do. Not surprisingly, these meetings can have a direct and powerful impact on clients.

When workers talk about why certain questions or ideas are important to them, based on their lives and thinking, and do so in front of "troubled people," it is hard not to realize the impact our lives have on the people we work with and the impact they have on our own lives. This connection runs counter to the application of objective principles to solve the problems of the "other." This type of exposure requires workers to be especially sensitive to boundary issues, which are less clear when the connection between worker and client is based more on basic humanity than professional distance. In these situations, the worker is required to remember at all times that the purpose of the meeting is to open up a conversation that gives the client more options and support and that encourages the client to stand up to the problem affecting his or her life.

Because reflecting teams function differently from case conferences or even live supervision, further discussion of how reflecting team members approach the task is warranted. Team members need to be aware that the client, and perhaps the client's family members, are listening to their comments; think about what they would want to hear if they were in the position of the client who is listening to their comments; keep in mind the damage that could be caused by pathology-centered remarks; and be willing to admit that being a professional doesn't mean one has the truth (White, 1995). Griffith and Griffith (1994) note, "Anyone who has accidentally overheard oneself discussed in a derogatory manner in another conversation knows the power of the reflecting position for magnifying hurt" (p. 161).

Although reflecting teams have the potential to cause hurt, they more often are a unique source of assistance and support. Reflecting team meetings can have an impressive impact on both clients and team members. Where there is a clear need for getting out of a "stuck" position in treatment, a reflecting team meeting can have remarkable effects, and client comments about it being the most important part of their treatment are not uncommon. Couples interviewed after experiencing reflecting teams have noted the helpfulness of being forced to listen to the team's comments without being able to interrupt or respond to them; interestingly, their therapists did not see this as important (Sells, Smith, Coe, Yoshioka, & Robbins, 1994).

Reflecting team members acknowledge the experiences of clients and the possible hidden presences of less-problematic possibilities. Responses are situated through members sharing something about what moved them, describing why they were moved by those particular things, and acknowledging the impact of that experience on their life. Reflecting team members are encouraged to engage in dialogue rather than individual monologues. They also attempt to present both sides of any dilemmas to encourage clients to see their options as not just narrow "either-or" alternatives, but as "both-and" possibilities (Lax, 1995).

Team members deconstruct each other's reflective comments—that is, expose the experience from which the reflector's comments arose—to show that the opinions stated come from lived experiences, not some ultimate truth or formal position. This lets clients see how the opinions are connected to the team member stating them and they can reach their own decision on how to interpret them. Reflecting team members, as helping professionals, are likely not to be the usual group of people most clients spend time with, unless they are helping professionals themselves. Thus, reflecting team members' comments and reflections can offer clients perspectives that differ from those encountered in their everyday life.

A team member who is affected by a comment or conversation should remember that boundaries remain important and that the focus of the reflecting team meeting is supposed to be on those seeking consultation, not on the consultants (White, 1997). A reflecting team member's comments are not to be merely cathartic, a self-disclosure with the idea of "letting it all hang out." Should this occur, the other members can ask questions to draw out the context of the statements and to refocus the member on the client's experiences.

The process used by the reflecting team attempts to ensure that all members of the group have a chance to respond. For example, after an interview with a mother (Jade) and child (Jimmy), Joe, a reflecting team member, begins to talk about how he and his mother had exactly the same problem and he starts to give the group and the family the benefit of his mother's wisdom in a very definitive manner:

**Team member Joe:** I noticed that when Jimmy started talking to his mom about how she didn't care about him, didn't understand him, and just needs to leave him alone, I guess I just got very angry because I remember doing the same thing to my mother and she was such a saint about it. She just used to shake her head and leave me to stew, and later I learned to really appreciate her for what she was able to do. I think my mother showed remarkable patience putting up with that stuff from me and letting me stew with it until I was able to quiet down. I can never repay her for what she has given me. I guess I wish Jade would do that; it would make all the difference.

Other team members, seeing that the discussion is becoming focused on Joe and his mother and shifting away from Jimmy and his mother, pick up and go further with Joe's comments:

**Team member Sharone:** What exactly was it that occurred that so powerfully evoked your mother's image?

**Joe:** Well, I guess it was when he talked so angrily to his mom and just seemed so frustrated; when he told her that she didn't understand. I was thinking of what my mother had done in reaction.

**Team member Sam:** Did you see reflections of your mother in Jade's ways of being with her son?

**Joe:** I guess I did see some of that. Although she eventually got angry back at him, there was that period of delay. It wasn't an automatic thing; she waited a bit first. I saw Jade's patience and caring in that delay and it reminded me of my mother.

**Sharone:** What was it like to have Jade evoke your mother's image in this way?

**Joe:** I guess I began to see a side of my own mother I had forgotten, and it also helped me to understand that despite all the current chaos, these things can pass.

**Sharone:** If you were to evoke your mother in your work with other women in this situation, the way Jade was able to evoke her for you, I wonder how it might affect your work?

**Joe:** Now that I think about it, I guess maybe Jade got me more in touch with my mother's patience and with how I can see the current problem, and maybe even parents and children in general, in a broader perspective.

**Sam:** I was wondering, Jean, what did you see in Jade and Jimmy's conversation that stood out for you?

**Team member Jean:** I was silenced by the pain of two people with a long history of loving concern for each other, and I was struck by how conflict had taken that from them. I wonder what their lives will be like in 5 years after conflict's influence has been diminished and they have seen that love between them again?

As the dialogue illustrates, the reflecting team discussion did not leave Jade feeling she did not meet the standards of perfect motherhood. If anything, it may have lessened those feelings in her by demonstrating how her experiences affected an outsider, who through his experience of her and the team's expansion of his story may use what happened to make a positive impact on the lives of other mothers. In addition, whereas Jade might previously have considered only a negative future for life with her son, she now might see herself on the road to patience and to a more positive future for her family.

## Definitional Ceremonies

Reflecting team meetings have been characterized as *definitional ceremonies*, to use a phrase first coined by Myerhoff (1986, p. 267). Definitional ceremonies deal with problems of invisibility and marginality; they "provide opportunities for being seen and in one's own terms, garnering witnesses to one's worth, vitality, and being" (p. 267).

A reflecting team meeting can be thought of as a definitional ceremony in that participation can give rise to new, publicly displayed self-definitions, just as traditional ceremonies can make someone visible and proclaim who one is (White, 1995). Witnesses who are not part of the community serve an important function by acknowledging clients' stories about their histories and identities (White). When outsiders confirm a client's identity as he or she presents it, it allows the person to become more self-conscious of that identity and aware of himself or herself in the process of presenting it. This reflexive posture can, in turn, further strengthen the identity as real. Reflecting teams serve as groups of concerned outsiders who perform such functions.

## Supervision

How can a transparent approach be provided to clients when the current institutional context goes against it? Typically, case conferences are held to discuss problematic cases. They take place among professionals without the presence of the clients who are being discussed. Clients' views of their situations are translated, if at all, through the language of the presenting professional. Case conferences tend to be focused on problems, with brainstorming about solutions occurring at the end of the presentation. Many schools of social work have this format in either a practicum seminar or a practice class.

One way to approximate a narrative orientation in a case conference is to have someone in the group role-play the observing client and be interviewed for his or her reactions at the end of the presentation in front of the other seminar or class members (Paquin, 2006). Madsen (2007), who has described a narrative approach to case conferencing in great detail, argues that incorporating narrative principles makes case conferences more accountable to the very clients such conferences were designed to help. For this approach to work, case conference participants need to give permission to change the usual process so that clients' voices are heard.

The process Madsen (2007) employs, which is more extensive than that typically used in social work classes, involves a member of the case conference volunteering to be the client. This person, who does not participate in the case discussion until the end, is asked to experience the role as if he or she were the actual client under discussion. The person who is role-playing the client is asked to focus on his or her experience as an outsider who is being talked about and to refrain from analyzing any solutions that might be proposed. The client's clinician presents the client to the rest of the group and responds to questions of clarification posed by group members. The group then reflects on the material presented, after which the clinician provides his or her reflections on the discussion. The person role-playing the client is then interviewed by the group about the experience. Finally, the group debriefs about the process.

Examples of questions that might be directed to the client include: What was the process like for you? What reactions did you have to it? Were there parts of the discussion that seemed helpful? That did not seem helpful? What could have been done differently? How could we have had the discussion in a way that raised difficult issues and yet felt respectful?

As more people take on "the role of the client, the voice" of clients becomes more fully experienced by the participants (Madsen, 2007, p. 339). To be of value, participants must "fully agree to participate and authorize the use of the client voice to give them candid feedback" (p. 339). Although the use of the client voice can be quite valuable, there are times when it might be less helpful, such as when the focus of the conference is on the therapist's personal reactions to a client and the discussion is more focused on the worker than on the client.

A narrative approach to case consultation can be a powerful learning experience. However, unless there is proper preparation and setup, this approach may simply be treated as a ritual or a novelty, without any learning taking place. In addition to stimulating learning, this approach can reduce the egotistical benefits of showing off one's expertise, which makes case conferences lively but often unproductive..

Supervision in social work field placements usually occurs through case discussions or, less frequently, by process recordings, by video/audio recordings, or by supervisors sitting in or watching from behind one-way mirrors. The discussion of the treatment session typically takes place outside the client's knowledge and is strictly for the benefit (or criticism) of the student.

Madigan (1993) has used a different method of supervision. He outlines a process in which the supervisor sits in the room with the worker during the interview and then in the client's presence interviews the worker about the questions asked during the session. Because, Madigan argues, all questions as speech acts have cultural biases, what is asked can influence the treatment without being visible to the practitioner. These biases, which can be based on theoretical orientation or on gender, race, or class differences, result in some questions being asked and others not. Thus, in Madigan's approach, the supervisor listens for what is and is not asked and then questions the worker about the worker's choices in front of the client. After the discussion, the worker turns back to the client and asks about his or her experience of witnessing the conversation between worker and supervisor.

Examples of questions a supervisor might ask are as follows:

> I observed that you asked Mum a question regarding who reacts most when Johnny "acts up." Were there other questions that came to mind at this juncture that you could have asked but didn't?
>
> How is it that this was the direction you decided to go as opposed to the others you also considered?
>
> If you had asked these other questions, how might you see the family differently?
>
> How do you think they might see you differently?
>
> What does this tell you about yourself that is important for us to know?
>
> What has this family taught you about yourself that you might find helpful in your work with other families?
>
> At this point in the interview what would you consider your most important question and why? (Madigan, 1993, p. 225)

The benefits of this approach are that clients are let in on the thinking of the worker and supervisor and can give feedback on the supervision. They are treated with respect, and one way this respect is expressed is by opening up to them a conversation that otherwise would take place behind their backs, yet would affect their treatment. As with the first example of making clients' voices a presence in the case conference, the end result of this type of supervision is a tendency toward handling difficult topics in a more sensitive way, reducing unnecessary pathologizing, and developing a more client-centered viewpoint.

## Ending With Pomp and Appreciation

Endings in a narrative approach are different from those in traditional social work practice. In the general social work literature, the relationship between the social worker and the client is seen as the instrument of change, and it is through that relationship that the client learns how to interact differently with others. That discourse makes termination very important to successful treatment.

In most traditional approaches, successful termination involves reviewing the results of the therapy and the emotions surrounding the loss of the relationship with the worker. The review allows the client to experience ending a relationship in a more positive fashion than he or she likely has experienced previously. With the worker's support, the client faces up to the experience of leaving and to possible feelings of abandonment.

In fact, many treatment endings are premature or unilaterally undertaken by clients, at least from the worker's point of view. Garfield (1994), in a review of the research, reports that a substantial proportion of clients fail to return after the intake interview and many more do not return after the first few sessions. Hoper (1999) found 30%–60% of terminations in family therapy cases to be premature. Interestingly, studies of those who prematurely terminated treatment report that most respondents say they received at least some assistance from the sessions (Talmon, 1990). Yet, despite possible benefits from even prematurely terminated treatment, some studies have made unilateral termination the measure of ineffectiveness (Kazdin, Mazurick, & Bass, 1993; Prinz & Miller, 1994; Santisteban et al., 1996).

Hoper (1999) conducted a small qualitative study of people who dropped out of narrative family therapy. In Hoper's sample, which consisted of lower income, single-parent, minority individuals, the rate of unilateral termination was similar to that reported for other approaches. Some of those who unilaterally terminated described themselves as frustrated because they wanted advice on what to do with their children and some said the workers' neutrality did not give them the leverage with their children that they expected to get. Although the agency studied was a center for narrative training, the clients could not recall experiences of externalizing their problems or of discussing letters. Clients' examples of questions they were asked appeared to differ little from those that might be used in a traditional family therapy session, raising questions about the extent to which the narrative approach was incorporated into treatment practices.

In narrative work the therapeutic relationship per se is not seen as an element of change but as the vehicle by which the client makes his or her own changes. Thus, the therapeutic relationship is viewed as "facilitative" rather than "mutative" (Richert, 2003, p. 189). Focusing on interpreting the treatment relationship requires the worker's expert knowledge and diminishes the power of the client in the relationship. Discussions of transference or other relationship dynamics are not present in the narrative treatment literature.

One attempt to combine a narrative perspective with a humanistic-existential approach proposes that the therapeutic relationship itself be seen as a story that can be inspected, deconstructed, and reconstructed (Richert, 2003). The story is the tale of the worker-client relationship and it envelopes and affects the client stories brought forth within it. Accordingly, the client is seen as the expert on his or her problem, and the worker is considered the expert on the story of the treatment relationship. Because the worker is accorded the status of treatment relationship expert, this approach has the potential to reinforce power disparities between the worker and the client. As a result, it could set up a dynamic in which there is a confrontation between the worker and the client and it therefore should be considered with caution.

## When to End

A narrative approach to clinical social work puts the client, to the extent possible, in the position of decision maker vis-à-vis the termination of treatment. Whether there is a subsequent session is negotiated at each session's end, thereby affirming the client's power to decide when to terminate his or her treatment. The social worker asks the client to evaluate the session before it ends. For example, a worker might ask a client to describe what struck him or her as significant during the session and whether he or she wished to return.

At some point clients are likely to decide that they can do just fine without the worker. However, instead of a formal termination, they may wish to leave the door open to return in the future (Freedman & Combs, 1996). In agency settings, of course, this can be complicated given that the paperwork and billing systems are set up for intake forms and closing summaries; thus, a new intake form will often need to be completed when a client returns. If there is a formalized intake procedure that restricts the worker's ability in this situation, the client should be informed of the likely hurdles. The conversation might go like this:

> **Worker:** So, we have talked about a lot of things today. What has been most useful for you today?
>
> **Client:** *I found that all the ways I have been pushing anxiety around—you know, getting calm by picturing myself being at my favorite campsite; taking deep breaths when I start to feel uneasy; talking to salespeople I don't know, even when I don't want to, and asking them for help when I need it; you know, those kinds of things—and understanding I really can push back at anxiety has let me take back more and more of my life. I feel like I've come far. I'm feel-*

*ing like these two meetings have been good for me; I don't feel nearly as anxious as I was before I came.*

**Worker:** You really seem to have made a dedicated stand against anxiety. What percentage of the time was anxiety bugging you when you decided to come in?

**Client:** *It must have been between 70 and 80% of the time.*

**Worker:** What percentage of the time is anxiety bugging you now?

**Client:** *Now I'd say it's only maybe 30–40% of the time.*

**Worker:** Does that seem like a big or little change?

**Client:** *Oh, big, very big.*

**Worker:** I would say so. You have really put anxiety in its place by using the ways you just mentioned.

**Client:** *Yes, I feel I can keep it more under control.*

**Worker:** Are you feeling like you want to return for another session or end for now?

**Client:** *I think I would like to meet one more time in about a month, just to check in on how things have been going.*

When a client has been seen for a longer period of time or the termination date has been planned, the worker can recognize the conclusion of treatment by issuing a certificate and/or having a celebration to mark and certify the client's new status.

## Using Certificates, Awards, and the Like

Social work files usually contain information on the deficits or tragedies in people's lives. Files rarely emphasize a person's accomplishments. Yet successful change in a person's life can be a remarkable accomplishment. White and Epston (1990) describe a variety of counter documents that can be used to celebrate a client's achievements, to provide a view of the person different from that contained in the file, and to announce a client's preferred description to his or her community.

Termination of treatment provides an opportunity to memorialize the knowledge and skills clients have used to change their relationship to the problem. With children, in particular, certificates and awards can be an effective way to document progress, and they provide a physical reminder of the accomplishments achieved, which can be especially useful after treatment is completed. With some patience, appropriate certificates can be developed using most word-processing programs; however, specialized software is relatively inexpensive and provides a higher quality document suitable for framing. Children enjoy receiving diplomas or awards for putting the problem in its place. These certificates can have titles such as "Night Monsters and Fear-Buster's Club" or "Night Wetting Reduction Specialist" or "No More Tantrums Diploma."

According to White and Epston (1990, p. 192), some clients find value in drafting a "Declaration of Independence" from their problem. For example, the U.S. Declaration of Independence could be adapted to a specific problem as follows:

> Declaration of Independence From Fear
>
> When in the course of human events it becomes necessary to dissolve those bonds that have connected [Client's Name] with Fear, and to ensure among the powers of the earth the separate and equal station to which the laws of nature and of nature's God entitle [Client's Name] to a good life free of Fear and of having to continually be on the watch for it . . .

A document such as this, which takes a strong and poetic stance against a problem, helps to validate and affirm the client's ability to stand up to the problem. The client could be awarded a certificate, an award, or a diploma during a session or as part of a ceremony before his or her community of concern.

## Celebrations and Ceremonies

Epston et al. (1995) talk about how the metaphor of loss has been used in most therapeutic discussions, particularly those emanating from a psychodynamic orientation, to conceptualize treatment termination. Because the therapeutic relationship is so highly privileged by these treatment approaches, termination is seen as an important step in the client's "going it alone" and can give rise to feelings of abandonment. But just as termination is conceived of as a loss, these orientations also view the self as separate from its cultural contexts; not surprisingly, these therapeutic approaches have been characterized as "therapies of isolation" (p. 279).

By contrast, from a narrative viewpoint, the termination phase is seen as a rite of passage. van Gennep (1960), a cultural anthropologist, suggests that rites of passage involve a series of stages whose specific attributes are determined by the cultural context. Accordingly, a person undergoing a status transformation will experience three stages: separation, liminality, and reincorporation. Briefly, the person must leave his or her taken-for-granted ways of life (separation), enter a period of confusion and disorganization (liminality), and then finally reenter his or her world in a different status (reincorporation).

The process begins when people start to separate themselves from old identities that no longer fit them (Adams-Westcott & Isenbart, 1995). In narrative treatment, separation can be thought of as occurring when the person has externalized the problem. Liminality takes place when the person begins exploring different alternative stories about himself or herself and is "between" identities. Reincorporation occurs when the alternative stories are made available to an audience and the worker is taken out of the person's life. It is this process of rediscovery and support from others that leads to a transformative treatment experience. Therefore, because the end of treatment implies the achievement of a new, better status, it is seen as a "cause for celebration with the persons who have sought therapy rather than commiseration" (Epston et al., 1995, p. 282).

All members of the client's club of life can be invited to celebrate the ending of treatment. At the celebration, the client can receive a certificate and be encouraged to give a speech. People who have witnessed the individual's transformation can be encouraged to speak to the group and tell stories of hope and success about the client. Freeman et al. (1997, pp. 141–142) discuss the use of "honesty parties" in which children who have a reputation for stealing are recognized for getting back their good reputations after successfully completing an extended period of being tested. Professionals involved with the child because of his or her stealing, such as probation officers, judges, and other workers, can be invited to these celebrations. Copies of awards can be placed in the child's case file to counter negative information.

## Consulting the Consultants

People emerge from the client role when they come to be seen as a consultant who can help others with the knowledge they have acquired from their experiences with a problem. The transition from being a client to a consultant allows individuals to feel more in control of and more of an authority on their own lives. Others in their environment become aware of and can affirm these individuals' expertise about the problem. Thus, the gift of treatment is balanced by the gift of consultancy.

This consultancy can occur in a last interview that is designed to document the process by which the person has come into his or her own and found the knowledge and skill to combat the problem. Of particular interest is eliciting the client's understanding of how he or she made this knowledge work for himself or herself, especially how he or she put it into practice. What transpires, with the client's consent, is a session in which the person's historical struggle with the problem is documented either through audio recording, writing, or videotaping, with the purpose of informing others who are confronting the same type of problem. The person is asked to provide a chronological description of how he or she moved from a "problemed" to "nonproblemed" status. The questions asked during the interview focus on the client's agency—the part he or she played—in making things happen in his or her life.

The client's story is his or her property, and its use can be restricted. The client needs to understand that he or she can disguise the information as much as desired. Because the client is only lending the material, the social worker needs to agree that he or she will return it at the client's request. This loaned material is logged into the worker's archive (or collection) to be used with other clients. The client also can access the material if the problem attempts to return and he or she needs to confirm his or her success in standing up to it.

Epston and others have used these materials, with their clients' consent, in workshops and classes. Participants are encouraged to write about their reactions to the information and how it affected them, and they are asked to address their comments to the client. The teacher or workshop leader often passes on these written remarks to the client, who can use them to further strengthen his or her position.

Freedman and Combs (1996) provide a similar opportunity for readers of their popular book *Narrative Therapy: The Social Construction of Preferred Realities*. After discussing work they have done with a client named Julie, Freedman and Combs invite readers to write to her to share their comments and reactions. They ask readers to consider responding to some or all of the following questions in their letter to Julie:

> Besides your general responses, are there things that you wonder?
>
> Have you had experiences, personally or with other people, with extreme forms of self-doubt and self-hate?
>
> What did you or other people that you know find helpful in getting through such experiences?

Might some of the people who consult with you want to form an "anti-self-hatred, pro-connection-with-people league" . . . with Julie? (Freedman & Combs, 1996, p. 218)

Julie's story has come to be widely circulated, and this wide-reaching community has sent her much supportive information. According to Freedman and Combs, Julie is considering starting a league for her own sake and to assist others dealing with the same problem.

# Exercises

## Exercise 1: Finding Your Supports—Your Community of Concern

Getting through a graduate program can be very challenging. MSW students report they are inundated with work and are exposed to many new ideas whose usefulness they may question. They experience the pressure of working with clients at their field placement and often feel they should be getting paid for seeing clients, not paying for the privilege. If the student has a family to worry about and also has a job, the challenge can become a survival ordeal. It is actually the rare student I have met who is delighted with his or her MSW program, which is reasonable given the stresses involved. Few students have not had moments when they felt that they could not do it all or that continuing in the program was not worth the effort. At those times it might be useful to recognize one's own quiet heroism.

This exercise asks you to look at your community of concern. Take a moment to think about who might be a valuable support to you in your effort to obtain your MSW by asking yourself the following questions:

Who sees your ability to succeed in this endeavor?

Who has seen your ambition and determination in the past?

Who sees or has seen you as a caring person?

What do they see about you that you cannot see right now?

Make a list of these people. Then draft a letter to them in the following format:

1. Reintroduce yourself and your reason for writing.
2. Briefly lay out your current dilemma.
3. Explain that you would find it very helpful at this time to receive a letter from them.

4. Ask them to talk about the following in their letter:

   What value your relationship has had to them

   Any specific incidents they remember in which they saw the qualities of ambition, determination, and/or caring in you

   What they hope for you in the future and for their relationship with you in the future

5. Thank them for considering doing this for you, and end the letter with an appropriate closing (e.g., Sincerely).

Decide whether you would like to send these letters as a way to find out how such a campaign works and also to garner support for your getting through your MSW program.

If you decide not to mail the letters, think carefully about the reasoning behind your reluctance, because clients to whom you offer this option may also be reluctant. What is the basis of your reluctance or fear about sending the letters? What might reduce those barriers? How can you use this information in your discussions of letter-writing campaigns with clients?

If you do decide to mail the letters, think about what the experience was like and how getting letters has affected you.

## Exercise 2: Portraying a Reflecting Team

The best way to learn about reflecting teams is to be part of one (Madsen, 2004). Because students are usually in a field placement when in advanced practice classes, they can use a case consultation as a forum for reflection.

Five students need to volunteer to be reflecting team members. The instructor then selects a volunteer who would like to discuss a case. Next, the instructor asks for someone to volunteer to be the client whose case is being discussed. The student playing the client is to try to assume the client's point of view and maintain that perspective while listening to the conversation. The client is interviewed at the end of the exercise about what was said that seemed to be more helpful and what was less helpful.

The students participating in this exercise position themselves as follows: The five reflecting team members take their chairs and form a horseshoe at the front of the classroom. The case presenter moves his or her chair to just in front of the horseshoe. To avoid being distracted, the case presenter positions his or her chair so that, when seated, he or she faces the front of the room. The client moves his or her chair to just outside the horseshoe. The instructor, who will be the interviewer, sits in front of the case presenter, facing him or her, the five reflecting team members, and the rest of the students.

The instructor begins by reminding everyone of the importance of confidentiality and by requesting that the presenter disguise any identifiable information. The first questions should be about the context of the agency and a little about the client as a person. The case presenter describes the demographics of the client, such as age, race, gender, sexual orientation, and income level, all the while being aware of the need to mask the client's identity.

The interview then proceeds to the problem story, and the case presenter describes his or her concerns. The instructor asks questions of the case presenter to try to deconstruct his or her use of any pejorative labels or views about the client or the client's situation. What thinking and assumptions are behind such ideas? Is this the presenter's preferred way of looking at people or would he or she prefer another point of view? What gets in the way of seeing a person from a less negative viewpoint?

To begin to develop an alternative story, the instructor asks if the case presenter has had any success with the client. The instructor questions the presenter about specific incidents and how the presenter was able to do what he or she did. The instructor then asks whether there are other people who see the presenter's skills and abilities and what it would mean if the presenter could continue to build those strengths. This part of the interview is allotted 15 minutes.

Next, the instructor asks the case presenter to move his or her chair to outside the horseshoe. The instructor poses the following questions to the reflecting team members:

> Was anything said that drew your attention?
>
> Can you share what it was about the comment that drew your attention? Any incident in your work or life that would have predicted your interest?
>
> Now that you have considered the comment and your response to it, what impact might this have on your own work or life?
>
> Are there any questions you would have been curious to ask the presenter?

Ten minutes are allotted for this part of the interview. The instructor then interviews the person playing the role of the client:

> What was the process like for you?

> What reactions did you have to it?
>
> Did it feel respectful and empowering or otherwise?
>
> Were there new things you learned about yourself in the process?
>
> Were there parts of the discussion that did not feel helpful?

Five minutes are allotted for this part of the interview.

Finally, the instructor asks the case presenter to return to being in front of the reflecting team and questions him or her about what, if anything, in the process was helpful and why.

> Has the team experience changed your thinking about the client in any way? About the worker-client relationship?
>
> Do you wish to respond to any of the questions raised by the reflecting team members?
>
> What effect, if any, do you think this process will have on your work in the field of social work?

Five to 10 minutes are allotted for this part of the interview.

## Exercise 3: Planning a Class Party as an Ending Ceremony

Students can plan a party such as a potluck for the last day of class to honor each other and review the course. Two weeks before the end of the course, students can give the instructor a synopsis of the notes they have been taking on their fellow students' abilities, knowledge, skills, and experience that predict a good future in social work. If the instructor has time, he or she can summarize the student synopses as a certificate that lists these qualities and that can be given to each student. The certificates can be presented during the party, and students can give short speeches about what they have learned and what they want to do with that knowledge.

CHAPTER 10

# Narrative and Conflict: Advocacy and Mediation

Social workers, even in clinical settings, do not function solely as therapists, and social work training encompasses more than this one role. Social workers have an expertise in the interaction of people and environments, and their job, therefore, encompasses clients' context and situation, as well as the clients themselves. Helping clients to get necessary resources from the environment and to resolve their conflicts are two important social work functions.

Social work educator Dennis Saleebey (1994) notes that a criticism of the narrative approach is that it merely reframes people's lives, focusing simply on stories and restorying and removing people from the reality of the institutions and conditions under which they live. However, Saleebey suggests that when narrative workers construct alternative stories with clients, they do not "blithely reframe individual and family miseries and real pain into more positive and 'moving' language" (p. 357). The alternative stories developed must come from clients' actual experiences and not deny the reality of the problem story. Both problem and alternative stories are linked to context. It is workers' stories (or theories) about what is "really" going on in clients' lives that separate problems from their environments.

Narrative practitioners' belief in both collaboration and clients' expertise in their own lives complements the strong advocacy tone of this approach to clinical practice. Deconstruction looks in many ways like liberation educator Paulo Freire's concept of "conscientization," or bringing into awareness the oppressive effects of the dominant culture's discourses and institutions (as cited in Lee, 2001, p. 37).

For example, narrative practitioners' attempts to instigate leagues of those oppressed by similar problems exemplify empowerment practices. Similarly, through the use of counterreferral documents and the inclusion of other professionals in celebrations for clients who have gained back their lives or reputations from problems, the narrative social worker is directly advocating on behalf of the client, making a new, more positive story of the client part of the institution's records. Narrative treatment's focus on social discourses and their effects leads to a strong social justice orientation that encourages policy advocacy and bearing witness to the stories of people made vulnerable to problems through oppression.

The discussion until this point has centered on how a narrative approach to clinical practice attempts to shift power in the practitioner-client relationship by recognizing the knowledge and skills clients bring to the therapeutic encounter. In this chapter, I examine specific ways in which workers' expertise can be exercised for clients' benefit. I begin by looking at how narrative theory is being used in legal scholarship. I then describe how narrative social workers can advocate for their clients, helping them to secure what they need from their environment. I then discuss how, with clients' agreement, social workers can act as mediators, assisting in the resolution of conflicts. I conclude the chapter by examining in detail the process of narrative mediation.

## When the Social Worker's Expertise May Be of Value to Clients

Social workers have information about resources and systems that can be of value to clients. Providing clients with this information offers them options for acquiring resources to make a stand against a problem. For example, a single father involved in conflict with his 8-year-old son is too exhausted from multiple roles to change his relationship with his child and has no nearby support to help him get breathing space. To change his position toward conflict in his relationship with his child, advocating for access to respite care and other child care resources is appropriate.

Ideally, clients should be encouraged to advocate for themselves. However, there may be times when clients are unable to structure their stories in ways acceptable to the particular forum from which they are seeking resources, exceptions, or a vindication of rights. There are some occasions when an agency possessing resources will not "hear" clients but will respond to a social worker because of his or her "superior status." Although long-term efforts should be focused on changing these situations, given the immediate reality of scarce resources and pressing needs, advocacy efforts by workers can be advantageous to their clients and may be vital in emergency situations.

Narrative workers focus on de-emphasizing their expertise in favor of the clients'. Advocacy requires social workers to take clients' stories and adjust them to be persuasive to those who determine access to concrete resources or who enforce certain rights. Workers must be very careful not to usurp clients' power and to work collaboratively in assisting them.

Advocacy requires flexibility to be effective, and not every decision in negotiations can be discussed in detail with clients before it is made. This puts workers in the position of sometimes arguing on behalf of their clients, without having clients' specific prior approval. The final result of the advocacy in such a situation, if it involves a negotiated resolution, cannot be approved without first discussing it with the client. Yet even with discussion, this type of situation presents the trap of changing the power in the relationship back to workers being in charge and doing what they think is in their clients' best interests, with clients taking a backseat. This leap in worker responsibility becomes obvious when workers find themselves trying to persuade their clients of the benefits of the tentative agreement they have reached with the authorities.

Transparency is achieved only by having clients present during the negotiations. However, as attorneys know, the presence of clients can diminish workers' negotiating ability because negotiators commonly develop mutual trust through using their own "rational approach" to the situation, which allows them to distance themselves from their clients' "irrational approaches."

One way to look at how a narrative perspective can be helpful in advocating for clients is to consider how narrative is instrumental to legal advocacy.

## Narrative in the Law

In law, stating the facts of the case sets the foundation for the legal arguments to follow. Yet facts have no unique meaning in and of themselves until people give them meaning. A decision maker will be influenced by how the facts are presented and whether they form a coherent story with which he or she can identify (Chayes et al., n.d.).

Narrative advocacy occurs whenever an attorney states the facts of the case to his or her client's advantage. A good attorney must be able to look at the same fact situation from multiple points of view, choose the most compelling story given the client's interests, and present it through well-crafted storytelling. This ability to construct a good story sets the stage for developing legal arguments and showing how they apply to the case at hand. The story not only must be interesting but also must be constructed in such a way that it follows a rational legal argument.

As is true for attorneys, being able to see a situation flexibly, to construct the strongest possible story from it, and to present the story in a compelling fashion are skills that assist social workers in advocating for their clients. Good lawyers and, by analogy, good social workers should be good storytellers.

The law has a rich tradition of appreciating the importance of stories and narratives in determining justice. Legal institutions and norms exist through the narratives that locate them in the culture and give them meaning (Mitchell, 1999). Stories can aid in problem solving by providing causal explanations of events and offering a perspective on how an event fits into a broader scheme. They can help people define who they are relative to their lived experiences. Stories can be important therapeutic tools.

Narrative legal scholarship puts forth a number of propositions (Mitchell, 1999). First, communication occurs through storytelling, and the language of our stories forms the template for making sense of our everyday experience. For example, if a stranger walking on a city street pushes you, you might assume that the person is in a hurry and that he or she is not paying attention. If the person does not apologize, you might interpret the shove as an act of negligence or even aggression. You imagine this person to be quite rude or intrusive. You might even attack him or her in return. The shove takes on considerable meaning, and you might experience anger or anxiety for the rest of the day. The legal system appreciates this distinction, developing criminal penalties for intentional acts against another and assessing monetary damages for unreasonable acts that were not intended to cause harm.

Second, although stories give meaning to experience, experience is ambiguous. Thus, different viewpoints allow different narratives to arise from a given experience. In a dispute, each party may have a firm sense of entitlement that is based on the narrative he or she is operating from and that allows the person to act upon his or her desires. A landlord may perceive a tenant's withholding rent because repairs were not made as the tenant taking advantage of him or her. By contrast, the renter may feel that the landlord has not held up his or her end of the bargain when he or she did not provide basic upkeep to the building. Both feel entitled to relief in their favor.

Third, not everyone's story is given equal say. Stories of people from the dominant culture supersede stories of those from disfavored subcultures. Narrative structures shape the form in which legal arguments are heard and legitimized. Stories that do not fit the parameters of older legal stories are discarded or seen as irrelevant. One party will find his or her story is accepted and granted the status of truth, whereas another will find his or her story rejected and seen as untrue (Scheppele, 1989). For example, arguments by a father seeking sole custody of his child would not likely be heard if they were based on claims that it was unfair of his wife to leave him for a lover or that his efforts to provide for his family kept him away so much of the time. These arguments do not coincide with the criteria courts use to make such decisions and, thus, are not seen as relevant.

Fourth, there are no such things as neutral, objective values. As a result, when judges and legislators assume the nonsituated voice of the omniscient storyteller (one who claims universality in his or her edicts), the voices of others are silenced or marginalized. As noted by scholars known as critical legal theorists, those others have included females, racial and ethnic minorities, and gays and lesbians.

Critical legal scholars' work has highlighted the importance of including subjugated and marginalized voices in the legal conversation. Telling the stories of those subjugated is important for at least two reasons. First, having the oppressed tell their stories is healing because it reverses the impact of internalized negative evaluations from the dominant culture and lets people know they are not alone in their struggles (Witty, 2002). This healing can be best seen in the work of South Africa's Truth and Reconciliation Commission, which was headed by Bishop Desmond Tutu after the fall of apartheid. The tortured and the torturers were given the opportunity to have their stories aired in public to heal the traumatized nation (Abels & Abels, 2001). Second, having the oppressed tell their stories allows those stories to circulate, and stories of oppression can influence the oppressors. Most privilege is exercised without the privileged realizing they are doing so. Stories are a way to point out privilege without aggression and to diminish the sense of alienation between the oppressed and the oppressor (Delgado, 1989).

It is perhaps not surprising that the richer the narrative, the more favorable is its depiction of outsiders (i.e., those without privilege in society). For example, legal scholar Kim Lane Scheppele (1989) looks at the facts of a rape case that occurred in the 1970s. The victim in the case stated she was choked by the alleged rapist and was unable to resist, whereas the alleged rapist said his arm around the woman's neck was an affectionate gesture that was misinterpreted. Although legal stories often begin with the "facts" surrounding the event over which trouble occurred, they can be expanded and refined as new facts are brought into play. In the instance described by Scheppele, the case's story was expanded and developed when a judge involved in the matter noted the broader picture of increasing sexual assaults; evidence suggesting that most victims try to resist verbally, not physically; and recommendations by law enforcement officials that women not physically resist and risk further injury.

When the broader picture is developed, sympathy for the victim's position increases and it becomes clearer who the law is really protecting. A legal requirement of physical resistance to show lack of consent to sex favors strong, aggressive, and threatening male rapists over women. In the same way that "sticking to the symptoms" can turn nearly every problem into a medical one, "sticking to the immediate facts" can turn just about every problem into an interpersonal legal one. Both myopic views can hide oppressive social, economic, and cultural factors influencing the problem.

## Use of Narrative in Advocacy

When social workers are in the role of advocates it is incumbent on them to work with clients in developing coherent narratives that will be persuasive. In some forums, a social worker's primary asset as an advocate is based on his or her standing as a middle-class professional communicating with another middle-class professional. The worker's task becomes one of encapsulating the client's rich narrative into a form that will be compelling to the person who is the target of the advocacy without compromising the "logical order" necessary for the argument to be persuasive.

For example, a single mother has been sanctioned by the local Temporary Assistance to Needy Families (TANF) agency for receiving $20 a month extra for the last 6 months because of a clerical error by the agency. When her monthly benefit is docked $120, in a panic she calls a school social worker who is seeing her daughter. She does not know how she will pay the family's basic living expenses for the month. She has attempted to contact her caseworker, who just had a number of her clients similarly sanctioned and is now receiving a barrage of calls of complaint. The caseworker told the woman nothing could be done, and her story was not heard. The woman tells the school social worker that longer-term clients of the substance abuse treatment program she is attending as part of her TANF self-sufficiency contract told her that if she attended all her treatment sessions she would receive a bonus in her welfare check. With her consent, the school social worker contacts her substance abuse worker to confirm her story and follows through with the following letter to the caseworker, which the school social worker has the woman read and approve before sending:

Ms. Jasmine Jones, Caseworker
Department for Employment Opportunity and Financial Assistance
Re. Ms. Tamara Wilkins

*Dear Ms. Jones:*

*My name is Tara Tingle and I am a school social worker at Charlie Chaplin Elementary, where I have been seeing 8-year-old Jenny Wilkins for the past 3 months. Jenny's mother, Tamara Wilkins, whose family is your TANF client, called me upset about her TANF check being docked $120, without notice. She understands that this was because she apparently received overpayments for the last 6 months. However, she is worried about losing her new apartment because of her inability to pay her rent.*

*I have been seeing Jenny and her family because Jenny's schooling is being affected by her night terrors. Jenny has been experiencing panic and has been unable to sleep at night, and she often falls asleep in school from exhaustion. She has been making a stand against these fears with the help of her mother, who reads to her every night to strengthen her against the fear. Ms. Wilkins has consistently tried to help her daughter.*

*The block on which the family had lived was very noisy and had a good deal of drugs and crime. After 2 months of searching, Ms. Wilkins was finally able to move her family to a new apartment in a quieter part of the neighborhood. The landlord was hesitant to rent to a TANF client, and her living situation may be in jeopardy given the large income reduction she has just experienced.*

*Ms. Wilkins started the Chance to Change drug treatment program 8 months ago, as required by her TANF self-sufficiency plan; this is her first treatment experience. Several senior clients, whom she respects, have told her on multiple occasions that she could expect a TANF bonus if she attended the program consistently. I spoke with Ms. Cookie Blurr, Ms. Wilkins's substance abuse counselor at Chance to Change, who confirmed that, on occasion, those rumors had circulated among the clients. According to Ms. Blurr, Ms. Wilkins's participation in the program has been exemplary.*

*The current problem is due to a clerical error by your agency and has been compounded by rumors originating at the treatment program. Ms. Wilkins appears to be doing well in fulfilling her TANF contract and is on the road to successful self-sufficiency. The current dramatic reduction in the financial benefit could jeopardize Mrs. Wilkins's progress, and the progress made by her young daughter at school, should a move be necessary. Although disappointed, Ms. Wilkins realizes that the overpayment must be returned, but she would like to do so over time to avoid further disrupting her and her daughter's progress.*

*I will be calling you in the next 2 days to discuss this further and see if we can come up with a solution. Thank you for your attention to this matter.*

*Sincerely,*

*Tara Tingle, MSW*
*School Social Worker*

This letter attempts to accomplish several things. First, it identifies the advocate as a middle-class professional worthy of consideration. It conveys the professional nature of the communication through its use of formal letterhead and identification of the writer's position and credentials. Second, the letter structures the client's story and notes her achievements in a coherent fashion. Important to that story is the relationship of the advocate to the client. The advocate can draw on the relationship to bolster her assertions that the client is not trying to get away with anything but has a legitimate reason for not previously reporting the discrepancy. Finally, the letter attempts to establish a foundation for problem solving as well as for the problem's urgency by stating that the problem is the result of a clerical error and that the financial loss could undermine both Ms. Wilkins's and her daughter's progress. In the end, the credibility of letters such as this depends in part on the social worker following through by telephoning the other professional.

## Narrative and Mediation

When clients are in conflict with others with whom they will have continued contact, the social worker can sometimes assist by acting as a mediator between the parties. Mediation is the use of a neutral third party to facilitate an agreement that resolves a conflict between two or more parties. The mediation literature describes the process as collaborative problem solving to resolve a dispute (Paquin & Harvey, 2002).

Narrative mediation is an attempt to address mediation's potential for an emotionally unsatisfying result based simply on conflict avoidance or coercion. It was developed as a way for disputing parties to hear the voices of subjugated others. This occurs as the mediator assists the parties to deconstruct the beliefs embedded in the dispute (Winslade & Monk, 2000).

A social worker mediating a dispute from a narrative orientation has the benefit of using externalization and deconstruction to defuse the conflict.

A narrative approach focuses on the dispute as being just one view of the disputants' relationship, one that may well be alien to the relationship in general. Conflict or distrust can be externalized as separate from the disputants' relationship and the assumptions underlying their positions examined. Because some level of trust is needed to establish a satisfactory settlement, a narrative social worker who is serving as a mediator will attempt to open up the possibility of the disputants finding an alternative story about their relationship.

Narrative mediators assume that many cultural stories become internalized, with blame being placed on the self or on others (i.e., women who are abused "ask for it" and men who control their spouses through abuse must be "sick"; Winslade & Cotter, 1997). Yet individualized blame is not the best position from which to make changes ("I am bad and must become good"), which is what makes distinguishing problems from the people who are experiencing them such a powerful technique. Externalizing problems can correct this bias toward internalizing cultural definitions. In mediation, the narrative practice of externalizing problems has led to an approach where "the trouble" or "the conflict" that had been entering the relationship is cast as the problem, rather than the irrational, despicable other or the weak, trampled self.

Deconstruction can reveal additional options for the parties to consider by encouraging them to evaluate the assumptions behind their beliefs and feelings of entitlement. For example, a man determines that he will make his child support payments on time to his ex-wife only if he can be sure that they are being used solely for the care of his children as he defines that. To begin to explore this area of entitlement, the man could be asked, Do you believe husbands have the responsibility to decide how money is spent in a family, and if so, where did you learn that? Further questions could look at the potential costs of this commitment to himself and his children, and whether he thinks an impoverished caretaker can take adequate care of her children: Do you think your position will decrease or increase the level of conflict in the divorce? What effect do you think this will have on your relationship with your children? How will your ex-wife be able to provide for the children? These types of questions could open up discussion of the paternalistic discourse underlying his demand and the costs associated with living up to its standards.

Contrary to the widely held view of their neutrality, mediators are not truly neutral, nor can they leave their own stories at the door. Mediators' cultural biases come into the room with them and are evident in the questions they ask and the information they privilege, which will have an impact on the stories the parties feel free to discuss. It is important, therefore, for mediators to examine their own values and beliefs, and to share these perspectives with clients in order to increase the transparency of the work.

A narrative approach critiques the assumption that the mediator is able to separate the process of the mediation from the content of the communications offered by the parties. The literature talks about the parties to the dispute being responsible for the content of the mediation, or what is discussed. Mediators, by contrast, are seen as being responsible for the process of the mediation, including how the participants act and the steps they go through in discussing their issues (Paquin & Harvey, 2002). Yet an indication of how important the process of mediation is to its content comes from evidence suggesting that who goes first in the mediation frames the issues under dispute, which, in turn, affects the agreements made (Garcia, Vice, & Whitaker, 2002).

Mediation is supposed to allow disputants to tell their stories and describe their feelings of injustice. However, this basic premise is violated when problem-focused mediators attempt to prune stories down to only those portions related to settlement. In addition, feminist critics argue that the cultural messages about how women should act and the inherent power difference in male-female communication are not adequately attended to in the way mediation is generally conducted (Minnow, 1993).

Narrative mediators see cultural discourses on conflict as growing out of a number of assumptions. In the United States, conflict is based on an individual model that comes into play when the satisfaction of people's needs is frustrated. Parties are primarily moved by their internally generated needs, which are expressed in mediation as interests. A personal deficit or a need not met is assumed to be the underlying cause of the conflict.

From a social constructionist point of view, people's needs are not so much determined by internal motivations as they are developed through conversations that are circumscribed by the environment. For example, discourses that say that mothers, rather than fathers, should raise children because it is in their nature to do so, or that mothers who do not raise their own children must be defective and/or bad, arise from patriarchal assumptions and add intense emotions to custody disputes. If disputes can be seen as problem stories, then at least two different stories are possible in each conflict situation, because there are at least two parties in a conflict and each will have a different story about the dispute. Some stories will convey a sense of injustice by citing broader cultural stories that indicate what is fair and expected (i.e., what people are entitled to); other stories will demonize the other participant(s) in the dispute. Conflict, therefore, creates a platform for examining different meanings of the same sequence of events. A mother's negative reaction to an incident in which the children did not use seat belts when the father drove them to an ice cream shop can be seen as based on protection and fear by her and experienced as an attack on his parenting ability for a onetime mistake by him.

Stories organize our reality, yet we do not capture all our life experiences in our stories. There are elements of our experience that do not fit the stories in our head and are therefore treated as irrelevant or are ignored. If stories express the problem and only part of the person's life is explained by the stories, then examining the person's stories and the elements that fall outside of them can open up opportunities for resolving conflict through greater understanding and more alternative solutions. Examples of small kindnesses, even in tense situations, may not be noticed or may be ignored either because such behaviors seem insignificant in the face of the conflict or because such familiar relational behaviors do not fit with the conflict story. Social workers can discreetly point out these examples in individual sessions or note to the parties when small behaviors, such as offering the other a pen or showing any understanding of the other's position, occur in joint sessions. Through questioning, which expands and develops stories, narrative mediators facilitate parties developing their own stories.

By looking at the impact of the conflict story (what harm and benefit the conflict itself has caused the self and others) and at the times when the problem did not have an impact on them (when they were not 100% seduced into the conflict), the disputants may become more receptive to considering what a preferred outcome might be that would be different from the current situation. With the conflict, rather than the parties, seen as the problem, a preferred outcome can be developed that encompasses both emotional and material arrangements.

## The Process of Narrative Mediation

The process of narrative mediation involves engaging the parties, deconstructing the dominant story, and constructing alternative stories (Winslade & Monk, 2000). To begin the process of engaging the parties and deconstructing the dominant story, the narrative mediator initially meets separately with each party to explore his or her conflict story in a more relaxed situation. It is worth noting that experts typically counsel against beginning the mediation by meeting individually with each of the parties for fear that the mediator will be caught in an emotional triangle with one party against the other. Narrative mediators, however, do tend to meet individually with each party; hence, the narrative worker should be especially mindful not to use what was said in one party's individual session to check on stories told by the other.

In the initial session the narrative mediator asks questions that expand and enrich the stories, providing a respectful, empathic audience to each party. The goal is to have the parties hear their own story more fully than they have heard it before. Narrative mediators believe that each telling shapes the meaning of a story; during the process of exploring the conflict story, the worker can externalize, deconstruct, and begin looking for clues to alternative stories through curious questioning.

For example, a client, Peter, comes to a first appointment with a social worker asking for services because of anxiety symptoms. Conflict with his brother, Paul, who lives in the same farmhouse, seems to be the source of tension. According to Peter, Paul, who is the younger son, convinced their father to give him his inheritance about 8 years ago so he could go out and make his way in the world. Peter stayed home and ran the 3,000-acre farm. Not surprising to Peter, Paul threw away all his money on wine, women, and song. A great famine hit the area where Paul was living and he was forced to seek work on a pig farm to survive, living on slop himself.

According to Peter, Paul became weak, ill, and despondent and returned to their father's house repentant. Despite Peter's objections, their father held a big feast for his returning son and treated him as if nothing had happened, because, as the father said, "Once he was lost, and now he is found." Paul stayed on working the farm with Peter.

The father died about 6 months ago, never having changed his original will to reflect Paul's receipt of his share of the inheritance. The will grants each of the brothers a one-half interest in all the property as co-owners. The matter is now in the courts. In the meantime both refuse to leave the family farmhouse, and there is continual tension, along with threats of violence. Peter thinks his brother is selfish and immature and does not feel the need to pay for that stupidity.

The social worker broaches the topic of mediation, stating that he or she would need to meet with Peter and his brother individually first to hear each of their stories, but hopefully by working together they might find a way to reduce the tension in the household and reduce the influence of anxiety over Peter's life. Peter believes that until this issue is handled in the courts things will only get worse at home, so he gives the worker permission to mention to Paul that he has been having trouble sleeping and eating lately, which is why he came to see the worker initially.

The social worker contacts Paul, who states that his brother is a thick-headed lug with the intelligence of a date fruit. Paul says he is also suffering from the tension generated by the conflict and would consider seeing the worker alone. Paul agrees to leave Peter a note that says Paul will see the social worker after discussing such a meeting with his attorney. At the worker's request, Paul agrees to suggest in the note that Peter also consult an attorney.

The parties are asked to place the problem in the context of their full relationship (Paquin & Harvey, 1998) and to use their own words to name the conflict as a way to begin the process of externalizing it. The narrative mediator tries to help the parties speak of the problem as external to themselves rather than as either party's internal characteristics. Externalizing language is used in discussing the problem or conflict to keep it separate from the people involved, thus minimizing blame and reducing the likelihood of differences being internalized as personal weaknesses. To this end, the mediator initiates the dialogue by asking about "the conflict" or "the problem" as the issue at hand, as in the following example:

> **Worker:** As you know from our phone call, your brother, Peter, came to see me and was upset about the conflict going on right now. I was wondering how you saw this problem.
>
> **Paul:** Well, I'm sure Peter told you about my mistake of taking money from my father and being stupid about it. I had never been out of our town, and I just went crazy in Jerusalem. All my money was gone before I even had a chance to invest it. I figured Peter was going to get the farm because he had worked on it and seemed to be in control, and I really hadn't cared about the farm. I was going to invest in wine stock, buying and selling wine for a profit, but I ended up drinking all the profits instead.
>
> **Worker:** You seem pretty honest to me and embarrassed about how things went. How do you think this has affected you since you've returned?
>
> **Paul:** Well, after all the money was gone, I was forced to work on a pig farm, eating and sleeping with them. I returned home expecting to just be a common laborer for my father, if he would have me. My life depended on it because I was so sick. I never expected the reception I got, the feast and all. I really didn't expect to still be in the will; I hope what we are saying is confidential, because I sure don't want Peter to know this. Anyway, Peter got furious at me, like it was my fault our father took me back and treated me the way he did. Peter got real sullen toward me after I returned. He just seemed to

*hate me and brushed me off whenever I tried to talk to him. Like I said, I had never had much interest in the farm, but after my return, I threw myself into it, working just as hard as Peter. I felt I owed my father that for what he had done. Peter just got angrier and angrier, thinking I was trying to outdo him. When our father died of a heart attack, Peter tried to throw me out of the house, but when we saw the will, he couldn't do it.*

**Worker:** What was your relationship with Peter like before you left? Is talking about this something that might be useful? *(Seeking permission to talk about the nonproblematic aspects of the conflicted relationship)*

**Paul:** *I think so. We were always a little distant; he was the big brother ordering me around all the time. I looked up to him until I got to be a teenager. He seemed pretty sluggish to me then; he never talked much anyway, and the only thing he could talk about was the farm. I guess I began disrespecting him then, but I was young and stupid. But dinners were cordial and he did teach me how to do things. He just never had any ability or interest in book learning. I think he will have trouble with the farm because of that. We did work together and enjoyed a glass of wine occasionally. But that all seems to be gone.*

**Worker:** How do you think your experience of going away may have affected your brother? *(Clarifying the impact of the beginning of the problem on the parties)*

**Paul:** *Peter thought I would fail and I didn't let him down that way! But mostly I was just terrified of having nothing. I don't really want half of the farm or to co-own the whole thing. But he won't hear anything from me; he needs to get everything and wants me to get nothing. I had nothing and almost died, and I will fight him to the death if he tries to do that to me.*

**Worker:** So this situation where he thinks you are trying to take what is his and you think he is trying to leave you to die, what would you call this?

**Paul:** *Hell! But I guess I would call it "distrust between us" if I didn't think he was such an unreasonable, greedy idiot.*

**Worker:** So, though you see him as acting unreasonable, it's this distrust that has come and poisoned your relationship? *(Externalizing distrust)*

Once the conflict is externalized, the mediator can begin to question what the conflict's impact has been on the lives of the parties and those around them. In the process of this discussion the mediator can inquire about how each party has coped with the conflict and whether there have been times when the parties were able to maintain some relationship, either before or since the conflict.

Our example continues:

**Worker:** When Peter explained the tension at home, it seemed to me that you might also be under pressure and that talking a bit about it here might be a way to consider ways to handle this with your brother. How has distrust affected you? Your brother mentioned that it had made him anxious, edgy, and unable to sleep.

**Paul:** *Pretty much the same with me. I don't know what to do. I try to make sure I am always on the other side of the farm, away from him. That isn't easy because he won't talk to me and I often don't know what his plans are for the day. I don't eat with him; I have the servants bring my food to my room.*

**Worker:** So you have to worry about being around him and you eat your meals in your room. Anything else?

**Paul:** *I get pretty anxious at night and don't sleep very well. I'm afraid he might come and kill me. I just don't know what he is thinking. I feel like killing him sometimes just so I can live in peace.*

**Worker:** So you also are not sleeping and you're living in fear of what he or you will do if things keep building. Anything else about your health affected by distrust? *(Continuing to question for influence of problem)*

**Paul:** *Well, yes, I guess so. Even though I still work as hard as always, I haven't felt like eating much, so I have been losing weight.*

**Worker:** Is avoiding your brother, eating in your room, not sleeping, and losing weight the way you want your life to go? *(Questioning preferences)*

**Paul:** *Of course not. I want to live a calm life and not feel on edge. I'm miserable, but I have no place to go and can't leave. I won't go out and eat pig slop again.* (Client evaluating the influences of the problem and beginning to discuss preferred outcome)

**Worker:** Given that the results of distrust seem so upsetting and that you have in the past had a calm relationship with Peter, would you be interested in the three of us meeting to discuss the situation?

Language is very important in this approach to mediation. The language and the types of stories available to the parties to understand the conflict are constricted by dominant stories in the culture, such as a "wronged" party must always seek revenge on the person who caused the harm. Another discourse frequently seen is that a parent who is going through a divorce has a grave duty to his or her children to oppose the other parent if that person's parenting style differs from his or hers, even if it is not clearly dangerous to the child. In the example of the prodigal son, discourses about the rights of eldest children to their father's property (primogeniture), the importance of following a father's last wishes as evidenced in a written will, and a family's duties to provide for members' basic needs are at issue.

The mediator attempts to deconstruct these culturally dominant stories in the mediation by asking people where they got these ideas from, if they are interfering in the relationship, and how these ideas seem to be operating in their lives. Seeing that some options are constricted by the dominant stories gives parties the opportunity to consider new and unique alternatives. By directly considering the impact of culture on the conflict, as well as focusing on the relationship between the parties, narrative mediation expands the options available in handling a dispute (Winslade & Monk, 2000).

Once the mediator has met individually with each person, he or she will have a joint meeting with the parties. Both parties need to agree upon ground rules for the joint session. At the meeting, the mediator can pose a variety of questions to the disputants, such as: Would you prefer to have a discussion in which you show a respectful attitude toward each other, or would you prefer a discussion in which you can interrupt each other and use abusive language? Would you like a rule that allows each the ability to call a time-out from the mediation whenever one of you wishes?

One purpose of the joint session is to have each party present his or her story while the other listens. The mediator's function is to slow down the process, to review step-by-step what gave rise to the conflict from each person's point of view. The mediator can then choose to reexplore the impact the conflict has had on each party in the presence of the other.

Next, the mediator helps the parties construct an alternative story. If there were nonconflictual, or even slightly less conflictual, parts of the relationship, the mediator could ask questions to build on those relational aspects. He or she could help the parties explore what it meant to them that they were able to have that type of relationship. These sparkling moments could be just that—moments.

The alternative story is constructed by having each party hypothesize about what type of relationship he or she would prefer to have under the current circumstances and how the problem could be kept from interfering with that relationship. This alternative story is built upon the realities of the current relationship. If one party wishes to continue an intimate relationship and the other party does not, then the story that includes this new, nonintimate reality needs to be discussed. Once an alternative story about what a new relationship would look like is explored, the mediator would ask the parties to examine their understanding further, to see if this expands the possibilities for resolving the current conflict. The worker is trying to open up some emotional space for the parties to take a different view of the conflict and to consider different options for resolution.

An important technique used by narrative therapists and carried over into narrative mediation is the writing of letters by the mediator to the parties after each session. Letters serve several purposes in the context of mediation: to summarize what happened during the session in the parties' own words, to extend the ideas and stories about the conflict that were started in the session, to provide a way for people not in the session to know what occurred, and to lay out the terms of any agreements reached to that point.

A letter is not simply a legal recording; it is a therapeutic technique, too. Letters that use the parties' own words to describe their views of the conflict help to externalize the conflict by letting each party see the other's viewpoint as one story of what occurred. To continue externalizing the conflict, the mediator can pose questions that ask the parties to consider what efforts they can make to defeat the conflict. Lawyers and family members (or others not in the sessions) can be given access to the process if the parties wish to share their letters with them. Letters also provide opportunities for the mediator to pose questions that raise matters not considered during the heat of the mediation session.

## Exercises

### Exercise 1: Negotiating and Presenting the Narrative Advocacy Argument

Read the following scenario:

You are a social worker in a full-service domestic violence agency. This agency not only provides crisis, advocacy, emergency shelter, and counseling services but also finds transitional housing through a contract with another agency that works with the homeless. The application for transitional housing is decided by a panel made up of representatives of both agencies; the panel has made a strict policy of not admitting to the housing program anyone who has had contact with the abuser in a nonlegal setting since entering the emergency shelter. The application for transitional housing is presented to the panel by a shelter resident's primary domestic violence worker. As a matter of policy, the panel does not let an applicant approach it directly.

You have been working with a 20-year-old woman who has been in the shelter with her children for more than 6 weeks. Her former boyfriend had beaten her before she entered the shelter. Her bruises have healed, as has a fracture in her jaw. She has few work skills and little experience. She quit school at age 17 when she became pregnant with her first child. She also has a 1-year-old. Her abusive former boyfriend fathered both children. He has always been careful not to beat her in front of the children and has never been violent with them. Her family abandoned her and her boyfriend kept her away from other people who might have befriended her. Despite these barriers, she has coped with her abuse without striking out at her children and has been fiercely protective of them. She has registered and attended general educational development (GED) classes and is doing well.

However, she has reached the domestic violence shelter's time limit. She seems committed to getting her life back on track. You are optimistic, as is she, that she will be able to work things out for herself if she goes into the transitional living program and is able to get support from the women in it. You think these two elements—the transitional housing and the peer support—will be critical to her being able to maintain herself in the community. Without the transitional living program, she feels she has little option but to go back to her children's father if she is forced to leave the shelter.

When you interview her for the transitional housing application, she tells you that she recently took the children to see their father, her abusive ex-boyfriend, without telling anyone. She says she knows it was a mistake, though he was good with the children and kind to her, as he has been after every other incident of abuse. She says she felt guilty keeping the children stuck in the shelter away from their father. She also tells you that she knows this is just a honeymoon period and that he will turn violent again. She says she would never tell him where she lives and is interested in arranging some kind of third-party visitation, if that is possible. You tell her that because she already knew the rules, you will have to tell the panel members about this contact when they ask you, which you know they will. She begins to cry and you tell her you will do your best to advocate on her behalf.

Here is some further information on the case:

The mission of the domestic violence agency is to reduce the incidence of domestic violence in the community and to protect those who are subjected to violence in their homes. The mission of the domestic violence transitional housing program is to provide the support needed to prevent women who are ready to leave the emergency shelter from having to return to abusive partners. The no-contact policy was put into effect after an incident in which a resident's former spouse who had just had visitation with his children returned to kill the mother in front of the children and the other residents of the program. None of the residents felt safe after this event, and they demanded some type of restrictions be placed on new admissions to the housing program.

Of the women on your caseload, you estimate that this young woman is the one most likely to become independent if she stays in the program. This professional opinion is based on her displaying a commitment to counseling by attending all sessions promptly and being candid; following through on her GED training; demonstrating good parenting skills, which you have seen and have heard about from others in the shelter; and showing the ability to get along with other shelter residents. Shelter staff have told you that she has been a great help to new residents and has shown genuine concern for their troubles. She was doing fine in high school before quitting and needs to make up only 1 year's work before she can take the GED exam. Given the progress she has recently made, she will be able to take the exam within 6 months. She has the realistic future goal of applying for a scholarship to the local community college to study for a medical records degree, a 2-year, part-time program that would provide her with skills in a high-demand field and a livable wage to start. The local children's services agency runs an effective third-party visitation program that your client could use. Of the five panel members, you feel sure you can persuade two members for an exception, but you are unsure about the other three. You only need a majority to get a variance from the rule in this case.

Having familiarized yourself with this scenario, move on to the following role play: Have five students volunteer to be the panel, which consists of the executive director of the domestic violence agency, that agency's clinical director, its senior client advocate, the manager of the transitional housing program, and the director of the housing program that the transitional living program is part of. Have the other students in the class divide into groups of three to six. Instruct the groups to spend 20–30 minutes constructing a coherent argument that in monologue form states the facts most persuasively. Explain that each group is to develop its argument and the way it will be presented so that the panel members will recognize that the argument is based on expertise and will be swayed by it. Tell students to try to predict and prepare for the type of questions they are likely to face from the panel. Select one member from each group to give a 5- to 10-minute presentation of the case to the panel. After each presentation, allow each panel member to ask one question.

## Exercise 2: Initiating Narrative Mediation

Read the following scenario:

A client comes in to see you at the local crisis center stating that she needs medication because of her "nerves." When you ask her how nerves became a problem for her, she tells you about how her new upstairs neighbors, a husband and wife, are continually making noise. The client is a single mother with a 3-year-old girl. She receives TANF and is trying to meet all her TANF requirements. She says the people upstairs are on disability and seem to be having "a grand old time," playing loud music and dancing around up there. She believes they are "dumb as dirt." She says she is trying to better herself by studying for her GED and fulfilling her work hours, but these neighbors are clearly filching the system. She has had several confrontations with them and has called the police. According to the client, things just seem to get worse and worse.

You ask if there was ever a time when she got along with these neighbors. She says there was, when they first moved in. She went up to take them a cake as a welcoming present and found that one of them was on crutches and the other was in a wheelchair. They talked about how they were severely injured in a motorcycle accident and were lucky to have their brains in one piece. They then told her in much detail about the quality of their helmets.

The client says she felt very comfortable with them at first and unloaded to them about her living situation: being on TANF; caring for her daughter; and her on-again, off-again boyfriends. She tells you she took her daughter upstairs so they could meet her and even talked to them about possibly watching her daughter on occasion, as they seemed to get along so well with her. Two weeks later, she did leave her daughter with them. She says they were very "snotty" with her and called her "damn irresponsible" when she returned to pick up her daughter an hour later than she had planned.

She realized that day when she picked up her daughter that the husband was no longer in his wheelchair. This is when, she says, she figured out they were defrauding the Supplemental Security Income people. Shortly afterward the noise started.

You ask her if she would consider having you serve as a mediator to try to work out something with the neighbors. Her response is, "Good luck! They are just too damn stupid to deal with."

Break up into groups of two with one person role-playing the young woman and the other the worker. Pick up the conversation where it ended.

Externalize the conflict, go over its impact on the client (and neighbors), and consider alternative stories of how she would like things to be. Spend 10–15 minutes doing this.

Now switch roles: the former worker will become the person answering the phone at the neighbors' apartment and the former client will become the worker. The worker has agreed to call to see if he or she can avert further conflict between the client and her neighbors. The client has consented to your using any information you wish in the conversation. (A side note is that at least part of the noise has to do with the rehabilitation of the neighbors' injuries; they are an older couple with "strict moral values" and a strong work ethic.) Spend 10–15 minutes in this telephone role play.

CHAPTER 11

# Narrative Approaches in the Area of Children and Families

This and the next two chapters look at three broad areas of social work practice in which narrative approaches are being used: children and families, health and gerontology, and mental health and substance abuse. These chapters are included to provide some appreciation of how narrative methods are being integrated into different areas of social work practice. The narrative approaches employed in these areas are derived from theory, practice, and research. Sometimes they are very exact; other times the practices involved are somewhat vague.

Children and families receive many cultural messages in our society. According to the dominant cultural beliefs in the United States, children should be seen and not heard. Children should accept whatever restrictions the classroom places upon them if they are to find a place in this society. If children "act up," it usually means that caregivers, particularly mothers, are to blame and the state should exercise its powers to correct the deficit. When adolescents are not spending much time with friends, it may be an indication of enmeshment in the family. Yet if they are spending significant amounts of time with friends, it may be a sign of alienation and disengagement within the family. Not surprisingly, children and teens can feel like no one is listening to them, whereas parents, judged incompetent on the basis of their children's behavior, can feel that their children have all the power.

Parents are bombarded with a variety of messages about what they should want; how they should act; and what their obligations should be to each other, to their children, and to other family members. Violence is an all too common part of family life in this country. Even in the absence of violence, tension and stress between adult partners can result in dissension and conflict.

Narrative approaches to working with children and families recognize the impact of social and cultural discourses and their potential to silence people's voices. When we, as social workers, see ourselves as the experts on other people's lives, it becomes easy to think that clients are people who just have not been trained in the right skills; thus, our job is to train them. Although this can be helpful to some clients, it is not the only way to approach working with those who consult us (Monk, 1997).

No single text can cover the subject matter of several books, numerous articles, and many presentations in a comprehensive and in-depth way. Therefore, I present just some broad approaches to working with children, adolescents, and families. I describe some specific techniques that illustrate the remarkable ingenuity of narrative practitioners in making space for clients to develop their own unique skills and knowledge. I illustrate the applicability of narrative methods to a wide range of problems experienced by children and their family members—from children's exposure to neglect and violence; to being labeled with attention-deficit/hyperactivity disorder (ADHD); to problems of enuresis and encropesis; to issues arising in schools; to adolescent "troubles"; to stealing and lying; and, finally, to adult issues of partner violence and couple conflict.

## Methods of Working With Children and Adolescents

Does a language-based form of treatment translate into an appropriate approach for working with children whose language skills may be undeveloped or who may not have yet developed certain skills and understandings? The answer to this question is a resounding *yes*. In fact, narrative practitioners have developed a variety of techniques to meet children's needs.

When problems are separated, or externalized, from children, their imaginations can be engaged with the problem, blame can be lifted from the child and caregivers, and a space can be created for playfulness in the therapeutic work (Freeman et al., 1997). Play is a natural medium for children, and narrative practitioners work with children to use play to develop resistance to the problem.

Sometimes even highly verbal children cannot or will not develop in-depth descriptions of alternative stories. Freedman and Combs (1997) find the use of lists to be helpful in such situations. They employ a format to lay out the benefits of an alternative story, the unique outcomes, the child's achievements, and the names of friends and caring people in the child's life. The list is considered the child's property and he or she receives it at the end of the session. It represents written confirmation of the child's skills, knowledge, and relationships.

Fristad, Gavazzi, and Soldano (1999) describe a somewhat different use of lists. In the technique they discuss, the child's "good" qualities are written on one side of a piece of paper and the problem's bad effects are written on the other. The paper can then be folded in two so that the half containing the problem's effects covers the half where the good qualities are listed. This offers a vivid illustration of how the effects of the problem cover the full person the child is. This technique concretely recognizes the child's abilities and shows how the problem can make people forget them. Thus, for example, acts of kindness and generosity can be hidden by the effects of Temper, which can then be peeled back to reveal the child's positive qualities.

Epston (1997) presents several additional approaches to working with children and their family members. For instance, he suggests that once a unique outcome is discovered, the social worker could speculate about it being a partial solution to the problem and could invite the child and family to acknowledge this as an accomplishment.

For example, a young boy under the influence of Bed-peeing might have tried to get up but did not make it to the bathroom. The family could be asked if this is a step in the right direction. Through curious questioning, the social worker could go into some detail exploring the specifics of this partial solution: How did the boy know it was time to get up? What did he tell himself? What does he think Bed-peeing told him to try to keep him in bed? How did he manage to get up despite that? How was he able to last so long? The worker could then help the boy and his family to identify what significance this event might hold and what it might mean to the problem, to who the child is as a person, and to his relationships with others. Does he think he is beginning to put Bed-peeing in a corner? If he can stand up to Bed-peeing like this, what does that say about him? Is this the direction he wants to take? What will his family think when he continues to stand up to Bed-peeing?

Epston (1997) "invite[s] the attribution of heroic or virtuous properties for discovering these inventions [i.e., the solution practices]; with young people, I suggest the domains of magic, wizardry, 'mental karate,' or the like" (p. 66). For example, the social worker could ask the young boy, "Where did you find the magic to do what you did?" Or, "Do you have a strong spirit that will give Bed-peeing a very hard time?" The social worker could then draw distinctions between these skills and knowledge and the behaviors (e.g., impulsivity, weakness, or aggressiveness) that contributed to the child being seen as part of the problem. When the child has expanded his abilities to take back more of his life from Bed-peeing, he can be recognized as an expert. This recognition increases his confidence in maintaining his gains.

Social workers can ask children to act as consultants to help other children. Young clients can document their knowledge and skills for challenging their problems by writing about or drawing their experiences of standing up to them. For example, a young client's drawings of how he or she put Bedpeeing in its place can be shown to a new client with the same problem, thus bolstering the confidence of the newly arrived client. Among the many benefits of having children act as consultants is that they can see themselves, and are seen by others, as experts on their own lives, understanding and acting in ways worthy of recognition, and as having knowledge important enough to document and share with others (Lobovits & Freeman, 1997).

## Children Exposed to Neglect and Violence

Children who have been sexually abused are a substantial part of any clinical population. It is hard to look at the number of women who report being sexually abused and not see a societal problem. How do some adult males come to believe they are entitled to exploit children's sexuality? A colleague once interviewed a father about his sexual abuse of his adolescent daughter, who had serious cognitive deficits. The father reportedly said, "Well, what else is she good for?" Such a statement, and the behavior it attempted to justify, beg for an exploration of the effect of patriarchal culture on the power relationships in our society. When advertisers use pictures of seminaked waifs who look to be about 12 to sell the newest fashions, what messages are given about sexual desirability?

How do you help children and adolescents challenge abuse-dominated stories and develop different ways of seeing their own competence and expertise? Though victimized by adults, these young people, who have lived experiences of violation and exploitation, can be invited to find ways to see themselves beyond victimhood. Based on their experiences of intense powerlessness and helplessness, they may find their feelings and actions are out of control; yet these young people develop a variety of ways to survive. The experience of being controlled may pass to other parts of their life (running away, fear, anger, etc.) and the sense of regaining a semblance of control may take various forms (substance misuse, eating troubles, and isolation; Adams-Westcott & Dobbins, 1997).

As noted by Adams-Westcott and Dobbins (1997), our culture often confuses intimacy, sex, and violence. The male sexual drive is seen as being intense and compelling; as a result, certain power tactics to satisfy men's sexual needs are legitimized. Historically, rape has been considered a spoil of war when a city was sacked. Today, rape is being used as a weapon of terror in various parts of the world, particularly in those cultures where a raped woman is considered "damaged goods."

Because segments of our society believe "sex is dirty," children and adolescents who have been sexually abused often experience guilt. They may see themselves as responsible for the abuse if they had any pleasure at all during the experience. Or they may feel they somehow should have stopped it. Unfortunately, these stories of sex being dirty rob children of compassion for themselves, and their self-blame makes healing more difficult. Men who are experts in such power tactics know how to exploit these reactions to get their way without consequences.

Narrative workers attempt to help children and adolescents create new ways of experiencing their lives—ways that support stories that lead to preferred outcomes and to identities involving competence and agency. Some workers use expressive arts (painting, drawing, culture, mask and puppet making, sandplay drama, puppet theater, storytelling, music, dance, etc.) to help children express their experiences, separate themselves from problem stories, and perform more preferred stories (Barragar-Dunne, 1997; Freeman et al., 1997; Freeman & Lobovits, 1993).

When first meeting the child, the social worker needs to make a special effort to explore those parts of the child's life that are not entirely dominated by the abuse story to see what the child values in life (Adams-Westcott & Dobbins, 1997). Assuming the child is also involved with state agencies (e.g., protective services, law enforcement), the worker should make it clear that these meetings are not part of the investigative ordeal. Adams-Westcott and Dobbins provide an example for introducing this position:

> Your mother told me that your stepfather touched you in a confusing and hurtful way. I'm really sorry that he hurt you. I understand that you told the police detective, the social worker, and the doctor how he touched you. I'm not going to ask you to tell me what happened. I've talked to a lot of kids who have been touched by adults in confusing and hurtful ways. Even after they get to know me, a lot of kids I work with never talk to me about how they were assaulted. Some of the kids I work with do decide that it's helpful to talk to someone about what happened to them. Those kids may decide to talk to me or to another person they trust. (p. 202)

The message conveyed in this excerpt is that abuse is something that happened in the past, may continue to have effects in the present, but does not have to continue to exert its negative influence in the future. Using creative means, such as collages, the child can explore how the effects of the abuse story are dominating his or her life and consider how things might be different in a future-without-abuse story.

Young people can begin to move beyond the abuse and its damaging consequences with the help of a community that appreciates the child's strengths and abilities. Severely abused children who appear to have difficulty accepting that they can have positive experiences may be particularly well served by engaging with a community of concerned supporters. Support or therapy groups can be a mechanism for developing these types of communities, as can bringing together appreciative others (family, friends, professionals, and so on) from the youngster's life.

Adams-Westcott and Dobbins (1997) discuss how a group of preadolescent girls, who were asked to interview each other for a videotape, came up with the following questions:

> What did you say to yourself to help you overcome secrecy?
>
> How did you decide to listen to yourself and trust yourself?
>
> What does it mean about who you are as a person that you were able to tell someone about the abuse?
>
> Who do you know who would be least surprised to discover that you stood up for yourself in this way? (p. 205)

These questions, generated by young women who had been exploited, suggest how children who have experienced sexual abuse could be approached and what areas they might find valuable to explore.

## Children Labeled With ADHD

Narrative therapists have taken a somewhat antipsychiatry approach to mental health and, as a result, tend to minimize psychopathology. This bias is most apparent with controversial diagnoses such as attention-deficit disorder (ADD) or ADHD. Ian Law (1997), a Canadian therapist, considers ADHD to be affected mainly by societal discourses that interpret and label behavior as pathology, infantilize children, and hold mothers responsible for what takes place in the family. Accordingly, Law argues that the focus of treatment should not be on having the child learn how to "manage" his or her ADHD-related behaviors, but on encouraging the child to "reclaim" the gifts "hijacked" by the problem and to use those gifts to his or her advantage. The narrative treatment approach to working with children labeled

ADD/ADHD begins by helping the children and families to see as special abilities (flexibility, ability to monitor the entire environment, independence, tirelessness) what others consider deficits (e.g., distractibility, short attention span, hyperactivity, impulsivity; Nylund & Corsiglia, 1996).

Carrey (2007), a child psychiatrist, attempts to balance the pressures to diagnose and medicate children with the need to form more collaborative relationships with children and their families. He makes a special attempt to collaborate with children by identifying the meanings the ADHD diagnosis and the medications used for it have for family members and by ensuring that the child's resilience and strengths are acknowledged in the discussions. Thus, in addition to the ADHD label, a child might receive a "diagnosis" of "Too-Darn-Smart-for-His-Own-Good" (p. 90) or "Consummate Multitasker" (p. 91). Simply relabeling behaviors is, of course, not sufficient; turning those talents into ones that will work for the child and will help him or her achieve desired outcomes is the challenge.

Nylund (2002) has developed a five-step narrative process to working with children who exhibit ADHD symptoms. He calls this process the SMART Approach, which essentially is an adaptation of narrative practice for ADHD issues. In what follows, I briefly outline the SMART program and cite questions developed by Nylund to illustrate each step.

The first step is to externalize the problem, that is, to separate the problem of ADHD from the child. This could be broached as follows:

> Families have found it helpful to view the problem as something outside the child. It helps to bring some new ideas on the problem and can pave the way for solutions. Is it OK if we experiment with talking about ADHD in this way? (Nylund, 2002, p. 73)

The second step entails what White and Epston (1990, p. 43) have called *mapping the influence of the problem*, or identifying the problem's effect on the child, on individuals with whom the child has a relationship, and in different areas of the child's life. In this case, the following questions could be used to map the influence of ADHD on the child and family:

> What effect does ADHD have on you at school? . . . What effect has ADHD had on you as his parents? (Nylund, 2002, pp. 90–91)

The third step involves identifying exceptions to the ADHD story. An example of a question that could be used is:

> Are there times when you pay attention, even when the teacher is boring? (Nylund, 2002, p. 109)

During the fourth step, the unique abilities of the child who has the ADHD diagnosis are reclaimed. A question that could be used to draw out this information is:

> What special talents do you think you possess that go unnoticed by your teacher and ADHD? (Nylund, 2002, p. 137)

Finally, the fifth step involves telling and celebrating the new story. An example of a question that could be used is:

> Who needs to be brought up to date with the changes you have been making? (Nylund, 2002, p. 156)

Epston's interactions with a boy who was labeled ADHD nicely illustrate how a narrative approach has been used with this problem (as described in Epston, Lobovits, & Freeman, 1997). Epston employed a wide variety of strategies in his work with this youth and his family members, including meeting with a combative sibling and having the boy and sibling secretly develop a surprise "mother's appreciation day party" (Mother Appreciation section); relabeling the boy as "weirdly abled" (A Burning Question section, para. 1) and misunderstood by those without such weird abilities; writing extensive between-session letters; developing a counterreport that the whole family signed to verify their accomplishments; documenting weird abilities in the extended family as a sign of hope; and, finally, developing an affidavit with the boy to announce his choice to escape his old ADHD lifestyle and to describe what a new lifestyle would look like.

In the process of their work, Epston discovered that the boy's "mind and body seemed to have minds of their own and don't pay you [didn't pay him] any mind" (Epston et al., 1997, Letter to Dave After Fifth Meeting section, para. 5). As a result, self-control meant finding a "weirdly abled way" for the young man to deal with his "mind and body" (Letter to Dave After Fifth Meeting section, para. 5). The case report ends with the youth realizing that although his ability to take on the viewpoints of others will be a lifelong challenge, he was becoming a "New Dave" (Affidavit section, para. 1).

## Problems of "Poop" and "Pee"

Bed-wetting (enuresis) and lack of control over bowel movements (encropesis) are common childhood problems. White (1989, p. 10) worked with one family to help the son get his life back from "Sneaky Poo." When questioned about his influence on the problem, the child talked about times when he did not let Sneaky Poo outsmart him. He said he sometimes stood up to Sneaky Poo by refusing to plaster his feces on the walls or under tables. Though the father was unable to give an example of not being embarrassed by the problem, the mother talked about coping by going upstairs and putting on the stereo. Further conversation with the child indicated that he felt his problem had not yet destroyed all the love in his family. During the two weeks after the first session, the boy fought Sneaky Poo, his mother did not let Sneaky Poo get her down, and his father broke the grip Sneaky Poo had on him by talking about the problem with someone at work. As a result, the family did a remarkable job of reducing the problem's influence on their lives and soon the problem disappeared.

White (2006b, p. 26) illustrates how stuffed animal "colleagues" can be important collaborators when working with children who have problems controlling bladder and bowel functions. These colleagues proved to be particularly valuable assistants for a very young girl who had elimination problems, as well as a history of abuse and trauma that led to her living with foster parents. At their first session, White had the child pick a stuffed animal to serve as a helper; he then interviewed the toy and the girl responded in that persona. The stuffed animal, which the child was allowed to take home, became her consultant, allowing her to begin externalizing the problem and articulating a plan of response. The relationship between the child and the stuffed animal changed over the course of her treatment. From having the toy serving as her consultant, she began to act as the stuffed animal's consultant, helping it with its problems, which were essentially those she experienced. Subsequently, she became the stuffed animal's teacher as her knowledge of and confidence in her own self-regulation strategies increased. With the support of her foster parents, foster brother, and child protection worker, who together served as her audience, she taught the stuffed animal how to recognize cues indicating the need to go to the bathroom.

With elimination problems, alternative stories of success can be hard to come by and families are often stumped for examples. In these instances, the social worker can focus on issues of general identity to find alternative stories. The worker can ask about the child's activities, looking for areas of competence that argue against the problem's definition of the child as weak or incompetent.

For instance, with a 7-year-old boy who continually went to the toilet because of a fear of wetting himself, Epston (1997) looked at the child's sources of strength, including his various activities (e.g., bike riding, swimming) and other possible sources (e.g., strength food [remember Popeye?], special stuffed animals). Epston talks about harnessing all this scattered power to get the better of the problem.

Instead of a narrative letter, Epston (1997) audiotapes stories for children to reiterate what has gone on in the sessions. He then asks the family to play the taped stories for the child at bedtime. Always creative and zealous, he sometimes has gone to a child's house the first night to record the story at the child's bedside. Epston feels that the storytelling element is important because children may not have the reading skills for letters. A bedtime story offers an attractive alternative because children are likely to be familiar with this form of storytelling. The taped stories can quickly become the child's, and he or she can modify and listen to them as often as desired.

One reason these stories appear to work is that children seem willing to attend for longer periods of time at bedtime. If a tape player is unavailable to the family, the worker, after checking on whether the caregiver can read well enough, can write a story to be read at night. The closer in tone a written or taped story is to a bedtime story, the better. For example:

> There once was a little bear who was brave and strong. He was a good swimmer and could catch all the fish he needed to eat. He would go to the side of the lake and bravely jump in, then paddle around to his heart's content. When he saw a fish, he just swam over, dove down, and picked it up for dinner. He was good at games, too, often winning. He could hit a baseball far for his age and could run like lightning. He had all this as well as a loving mommy and friends who cared about him. But he rarely realized how lucky he was.
>
> He had a problem that always got in the way. It told him he was a bad little bear and tried to separate him from those who loved him.
>
> What do you think this problem could be?
>
> The problem would tell him he was a weak little bear, even though he was strong. It used all kinds of tricks to stay in his life. The problem told him that it was the most important thing in his life. The bear never remembered his courage in jumping into the water and his ability to play games.
>
> One day he was getting more and more upset about how the problem was getting between him and the things he wanted to do. He remembered all the brave things he had done and gathered them all into a big ball of strength that glowed.
>
> How bright do you think that ball of strength was? Did it glow like a little flashlight? A nightlight? A bright lightbulb? Or like the whole sun?

When the problem would tell him to forget about what his body was telling him or when it told him to wait just a little longer, he would take that ball of strength, and you know what he would do? He would throw it right in the face of the problem saying, "You can't fool me anymore! I know what you are up to!"

After a while the little bear found that the problem was scared of him, instead of the other way around. He knew he could use his ball of strength to stun the problem and weaken it. Pretty soon the little bear was doing the things he wanted to do and the problem couldn't prevent him.

I like how the bear realized how powerful he was. What do you think?

## When School Is a Problem

Schools provide a particularly interesting arena in which to look at the clash of different discourses. There is an overarching conflict in our country about the purpose of education, and nested within that conflict are other conflicts about such issues as how schools should be structured and whether they are achieving their purpose. Berndt, Dickerson, and Zimmerman (1997) propose several different metaphors for the school system. In each, schools are viewed as serving different functions and, consequently, as operating with different expectations and behavioral standards. These variations, in turn, can exacerbate students' troubles.

One view of school is as a factory whose product is youngsters who are ready for the outside world. Families are seen as distant and ancillary to this mission, as not relevant to creating the educational system's true product, which is the productive student who meets certain requirements for economic competence. The current emphasis on standardized testing and improved test scores as a way of judging the effectiveness of education arises from this discourse. The argument is that students in other countries do better than children in the United States on standardized tests; therefore, this country will be unable to compete globally in the future unless our children's test scores are increased.

A second discourse identifies the school as the surrogate parents of its students. In response to changes in the traditional family and the family's perceived loss of moral authority, it is the school's job to provide character-building experiences to prepare children to live independently as adults. As a result, the school is expected to provide moral education, teach appropriate social skills, and use activities such as sports to develop students' character.

A third discourse says that in a democratic society where merit determines success, the school is the great equalizer. Class differences will become less pronounced in a society built on the merit of each individual's abilities. Students are to be sorted and fitted into slots that show their talents, and this will facilitate their eventual integration into society, where there will be places waiting for them. This discourse ignores the disparate resources, financial and otherwise, between school districts and the way merit is measured in ways defined by class (and race and gender).

A fourth discourse portrays the school as the last bastion of civilization; therefore, it is up to the school to hold the line and preserve what is important in the society. The values and traditional stories of society, particularly in such a culturally diverse nation as ours, should be inculcated and told in a universal setting, namely, the school. High school graduates, for example, should learn the Pythagorean theorem; be exposed to Shakespeare; and receive at least a cursory introduction to how government works and what role they, as citizens, play in it. Where modernity has assaulted the traditions that make us who we are, the school provides an antidote to the overwhelming influence of popular media. Where television portrays children as scantily dressed and belligerent toward adults, the school requires certain standards and specific conduct.

A fifth discourse conceives of the school as a bank. Adults make deposits of knowledge in students, who can then withdraw those deposits later in their lives. In this view, the deposits we make via the school are investments in the society's future. This discourse requires passivity on the part of students who are to learn the truth in its entirety; it rests on the presumption that adults know what students will need to know ten or more years from now. In school, I learned how to balance a checkbook and why it was important to do that, yet I know few people who actually do this now on a regular basis. Where a school's function is seen as depositing knowledge into its students, disruptions to the process are not tolerated. Students who misbehave deprive others of necessary knowledge; thus, disruptive students must face punishment or be placed in another setting.

A final discourse, in sharp contrast to the last, is that the school is a safe arena for exploring and experimenting. Youth's interests and opinions are valuable. Helping them develop their natural curiosity and critical thinking skills will assist them in becoming thoughtful citizens and engaged participants in society. Packaged information is of less value than information experienced in some way.

These different discourses and the demands they incur can leave children, parents, and teachers all feeling manipulated by the system. Conflicts between these discourses become areas of tension in the schools, as exemplified by disputes that have occurred across the country between communities and their school boards, school boards and their administrators, administrators and teachers, and teachers and students or parents. The discourses that are dominant in a community's schools and classrooms can have a significant impact on a child's behavior in school and the school's reaction to it. One school may handle disruptive behavior through detention; another may attempt expulsion to set an example.

A not infrequently cited community discourse is that problems at school are usually the product of poor teachers and bad administrators. In many states, if students are not showing gains in standardized test scores, the school board or state can take over the school, fire all the administrators and teachers, and rehire an entirely new staff. The message is clear: If children do not learn, it is the teachers' and administrators' fault.

All of these discourses place great pressure on teachers and can strain the relationship between the social worker and the teacher. Given the responsibility placed on teachers, it should not be surprising that when a social worker goes into a classroom, removes a child, and attempts to "change" that child, the teacher's reaction may not be positive. Kecskemeti and Epston (1995) discuss several problems that commonly arise when helping professionals and teachers interact. They note that when helping professionals offer consultations to teachers on "problem" students, teachers frequently refuse to make any changes in their own behavior or revert to their prior behavior after an initial period of change, do not acknowledge any changes in the child, and blame the child or the parents for all of the child's problems.

It is easy for teachers to be pulled down by problems in the classroom and to lose sight of their mission and original reasons for teaching. During consultations, social workers can slip into using expert power to tell teachers what they are doing wrong and take away their voice, just as clients can be stripped of their voice in other practice contexts. Teachers can experience social workers as being critical of them, emphasizing their incompetence and leaving them feeling unvalued. It is incumbent on workers, therefore, to find questions that respect teachers' ways of handling problems to bring up alternative stories. Kecskemeti and Epston (1995) give examples of such questions, which were developed during a year-long workshop and consultation process with teachers and school-based helping professionals:

> What respectful practices of your past teachers can you remember that have inspired your decision to take up teaching? What are they?

If you are using those practices, which ones are you finding most useful in overcoming Problems/keeping Problems out of your classroom?

What anti-Problem practices of your own have you developed during your career? Would you be willing to share a few of them? (Remembering Respectful and Helpful Practices section, para. 7–9)

Which one out of all your practices do you think has supported Malcolm the most in putting the Problem out of the classroom?

Would it be helpful to keep this practice alive for the future in case other children might bring the same Problem into your classroom?

What do you think Malcolm is going to remember about you when he is thirty and he remembers his favorite teachers?

How strong do you think Caleb's control over the problem would be without your input? (Teachers as Agents of Change section, para. 3–6)

These questions draw out and appreciate the knowledge and skills of teachers instead of diminishing them, as can happen in a typical consultation. Narrative practitioners also can work with students to write letters to their teachers to show appreciation and to ask for the specific kinds of help they think teachers could provide to assist them in keeping their problems at bay. In this way, the teacher is appreciated, while the student is consulted, listened to, and supported.

## Adolescents in Trouble

In Western cultures, adolescence is seen as a period of turmoil for youth and their families. Although adolescent turbulence is a societal expectation, it is seen as an individual experience of the youth and his or her family, who are all trying to find ways to adjust to the teen's transition into adulthood. For example, traditional approaches to treating depression in adolescent girls tend to ignore the societal discourses (Pipher, 1994) that leave them vulnerable to depression (Nylund & Ceske, 1997). More generally, adolescents in treatment are often seen by themselves, without family members.

In addition to broad cultural discourses about adolescence, modern psychological discourse emphasizes individuation over community, casting adolescents as being essentially alone in fighting the problems they encounter. The individuation discourse can force adolescents to feel they not only have to find their true identity but must do so without those adult relationships that might be important to them (Nylund & Ceske, 1997). (Some time ago, Scottish singer/songwriter Dougie McClean noted during a performance that he had spent much of his life traveling around the world to "find himself" when it turned out all he really had to do was ask his father.) Workers may see parents who are not recruited into this discourse of individuation, and who instead emphasize family closeness, as encouraging enmeshment and infantilizing the teenager.

There is added pressure on teenage girls to be attractive to males if they are to be considered worthy of adulthood. Young women are often asked to compromise their own beliefs and sense of self. According to one teenage girl, "There is pressure to have sex if you have a boyfriend. . . . If you don't have sex, you might not have a boyfriend or be popular" (Nylund & Ceske, 1997, p. 374). Nylund and Ceske argue that "this double bind often invites depression by making a girl feel dirty or inadequate, regardless of her choice" (p. 374). Girls and especially young women feel pressured to adopt behaviors defined as pleasing to others.

Adolescents often believe their delinquent or mainstream-rejecting behaviors contribute to their sense of well-being, despite professional opinions to the contrary (Ungar & Teram, 2000). Narrative approaches, because they are context sensitive (exploring the underlying cultural assumptions behind problems), empowering (giving the client a voice), and focused less on hierarchy in the treatment relationship (diminishing conflict because the worker does not need to be right), provide a particularly good platform for working with troubled adolescents. The more adolescents are engaged in their own empowerment by having their voices heard, the less they seem to need to exercise power over others.

Michael Ungar (2001), a Canadian social work academic/practitioner, looks at ways to use narrative treatment to help adolescents identified as having mental health or delinquency problems. He works with teens to reconstruct their identity based on resilience rather than risk. Ungar employs a three-stage process: reflecting, challenging, and defining.

In the reflecting stage, the worker asks questions about developmental events and stages and whose voice is defining the youth. Included in this exploration can be events the teen does not have direct knowledge of, but whose meaning was constructed and told to him or her by someone else. Stories about conception, birth, and preschool years can be part of this relevant history. For example, when a teen is repeatedly told he or she was a difficult and rebellious baby or is like his or her father's drunken, worthless relatives, a story is constructed about who the teen is that affects his or her expectations of self as well as what the family sees and reacts to in the teen's behavior.

Ungar (2001) reports asking his young clients: "'Who told you about this?' 'How is it you remember what happened?' 'Do you remember it any differently than you have been told?' and 'Did anyone else tell you something different about what happened?'" (pp. 66–67). Through these sorts of questions, the social worker can identify the dominant voices that have had an impact on the youth's identity. These questions also explore what messages may be strengthening or weakening the problem.

The social worker then begins the process of externalizing the problem and further develops the problem's history. Ungar (2001) discusses using a flip chart to record what strengthens and weakens the problem as well as the rules the problem has created. For example, some problems, such as cutting, have rules about secrecy, whereas others, such as fighting, might have rules about how and with whom it should be discussed.

In the confronting stage, the social worker goes over the same territory again only this time looking for indications of stories of resilience. Once a story of resilience is developed through questions, the methods the young person used can be explored: How did you live on the street? Handle such abuse? Find ways to protect yourself? Often these methods are seen as deviant (i.e., fighting and stealing for status, cutting to let the pain out or feel alive), although the intentions and needs underlying them differ little from those experienced by any adolescent.

Through curious questioning, the worker tries to open up a discussion of the methods used by the youth. Questions about who gets hurt, how effective the strategy is, and how it relates to power and responsibility encourage the youth to reflect on his or her behavior, while crediting his or her talents. Ungar (2001) contrasts the stories that tell adolescents of their violent delinquency or insanity with those that speak to their "struggling," "resisting," "functioning," and "surviving" (p. 69). In this way, the teen is recognized and supported for his or her efforts to stand up to the problem, but the stories about who the young person is and how he or she handles the problem remain open to challenge.

In the defining stage, the youth takes this new story of resilience and shares it with those in his or her environment. The great challenge becomes having this new story accepted:

> "Who accepts this new way you see yourself?" "Who does not?" . . . "Who do you need in your life now to help you be more healthy and resilient?" "How are you now different from the people who saw you as vulnerable in your family, among your friends, and in

your community?" . . . "How will you continue to show people how healthy you are?" (Ungar, 2001, pp. 69–70)

These questions look to the future and sensitize the teen to how tricky problems can be (the discourses will not have changed in the society, so the pressure will still be there) and how tiring and sometimes lonely changing can be.

For example, when all of a youth's friends do drugs and he or she is trying to stay clean, trying to find new, clean friends can be a difficult and lonely process. Alcoholics Anonymous and Narcotics Anonymous meetings, though providing sponsors, often do not encourage group activities among younger members, leaving them isolated in a culture saturated with drugs and alcohol. Developing a "clean community" and a commitment to "clean" activities are priorities for youth who are taking their lives back from substance misuse. Remaining clean during the oftentimes trying process of establishing a new, clean community can be a daunting trial for a teen who has just stood up to substance misuse.

## Children Who Have Stealing and Lying Reputations

Persistent childhood stealing is a vexing problem. Children who steal tend to deny they steal when confronted, and some caregivers find the lying about stealing even more upsetting than the stealing itself. Caretakers' interrogations of children about stealing are rarely effective, leaving adults with doubts about punishment and children with the incentive to lie. Because most children who steal do so at a low rate of frequency, it is difficult to set up traditional behavior management programs to address this problem.

David Epston (as cited in Seymour & Epston, 1989) has pioneered work that employs some clear-cut procedures arising from a narrative perspective to help children and caregivers stand against this childhood problem. Epston's initial model for working with childhood stealing took a somewhat punitive approach, with set punishments in place (as cited in Seymour & Epston), whereas his later work focuses more on how community opinion can be used to effect change (as cited in Morkel, 2002). The goal of the treatment is not to "prove" whether a child is stealing or to "change" a child's stealing behavior per se, but to allow the child to reclaim his or her honest reputation. Seymour and Epston report an 81% success rate when Epston's five-part model is employed. The model consists of engaging the entire family, including directly engaging the child, and eliciting the family's understanding of the problem; identifying new information that points to a context for change; defining stealing; developing and implementing responses to stealing incidents; and regarding the child as an honest person with a good reputation.

To draw out how the family understands the problem, the social worker questions all the family members about what has led them to seek treatment at that point, although the worker recognizes, of course, that the child is always coerced. The worker makes clear that "borrowing" and not returning is stealing; he or she uses the terms *stealing* or *robbing* in the conversation to encourage the behavior to be discussed openly without minimizing it. Therefore, caretakers are asked how they account for the child's stealing.

The child is directly engaged in the interview. Change is fostered by looking at those times when the child could have stolen but did not (the alternative story). The family members are asked to confirm times when the child showed honesty instead of dishonesty. The child is asked if he or she would prefer to have a career of crime or one of honesty. All family members are invited to discuss what the impact of each career would be. In this way, stealing and honesty are externalized.

Stealing is a slippery term, because children often have excuses for their behavior. Stealing in Epston's program is defined as possessing something that cannot be completely accounted for, something that is missing based on the accusation of a responsible person or on the caregiver's strong opinion that stealing has occurred. With this definition, the child is not in the position of having to lie about his or her behavior or defend his or her honesty; confrontation is no longer an issue. The focus shifts to the child regaining his or her reputation, not the act of stealing itself. When a person has a reputation as a thief, people will tend to blame him or her whenever anything is missing. Therefore, the child must remain above reproach and actively discourage the appearance of theft.

The caregiver agrees to respond to stealing incidents by enforcing work or other requirements. The child is given a brief period to provide actual evidence that he or she did not steal. If the child cannot do so, he or she is assigned an hour of extra housework, for example. The social worker will require some exacting work in this part of the treatment to ensure that the caregivers are in agreement with the contract and will follow through.

Finally, the child's reputation as an honest person must be won back. Typically this occurs over a three- to six-month period (the exact duration is determined by the family) during which the child is given honesty tests. These tests might include leaving money, or something else the child has stolen in the past, in plain view. These tests are more like pop quizzes, because the child is not informed that he or she is being tested until afterward. Although the child does not know when a test will occur, the child does know that his or her reputation as an honest person will be tested periodically. For example, I might leave money on a table where my daughter can see it and have easy access to it. Later, if the money is gone, I would tell her that she has failed the test, that she is being punished, and that the six-month period to prove her honesty begins again. If she does not steal the money, I would tell her that she has been tested and succeeded, and I would let her know I was very proud of her. If she is young, I might reward her with an ice cream cone or some other treat.

When the child has made it through the designated time period having passed all the honesty tests, he or she would be declared a person who has brought honesty back into his or her life. This achievement could be celebrated with a party to which everyone, including prior victims, with an interest in the child becoming honest again is invited. These individuals could provide the child with a supportive community and could circulate stories about the child's reclaimed reputation to others.

Today, narrative practice in this area has come to focus even more extensively on community involvement through the use of such techniques as honesty parties and has moved further away from using punishments (Freeman et al., 1997; Morkel, 2002). For example, Morkel encourages the use of honesty meetings, which are held after the stories of the child's stealing and honesty are discussed at the initial family interview. Morkel notes that few families have been resistant when she has asked if she could stand alongside them to redeem their child's reputation, if that is what the child wishes to do, and restore honor to the family name by showing that the family has raised an honest child.

The approach described by Morkel (2002) proceeds as follows: At an initial family meeting, the social worker explores in great detail the problem's effect on the family. For instance, the worker could ask the child: What have you been accused of? Has this bad name resulted in your being accused of things that you are innocent of? What do people believe you steal? The parents might be asked: Are you worried that your child is beginning a career of crime? What do people think of you as parents when your child has a reputation of being a thief? Then the worker makes a list of all the people who have an interest in whether the child has a reputation for thievery or honesty, including alleged victims. The worker next asks the child if he or she is willing to make things right with the victims and to make a commitment to the kind of reputation he or she wants: a thief or an honest person.

The worker proposes the idea of an honesty meeting and discusses this possibility with the child and family. The worker explains that the child will be asked to commit to demonstrating his or her honesty through a series of tests whose timing and content will not be revealed to the child beforehand. The worker also indicates the importance of having the child's successes and failures seen for what they are by those who care. The worker then asks the child if he or she is willing to make public his or her commitment to honesty and to undergo the challenge of testing. The child must agree to engage in the tests if the work is to proceed.

Once the child has agreed to demonstrate his or her honesty through the tests, the child, with the worker's assistance, can prepare invitations to the honesty meeting. All the people listed as having an interest in the child's reputation are asked to attend. Here is an example invitation:

*Dear Aunt Jane,*

*I'm sure my mother has told you she thinks I have been stealing money from her and stuff from one of the local stores. She worries that I will become a professional thief and go to jail. I don't want to do that and I am tired of people accusing me of taking things. I want to let everyone know that I will not take things and that I am a good person. The social worker we are seeing, Jill Jones, has told me that I could try to pass some honesty tests over the next four months to get my reputation back. She wants to have a meeting with all the people we thought would care about me and about how I did on these tests, so I am writing to you.*

*Would you please come to a meeting that Jill Jones is having in the conference room at her office on January 10 at 6:00 p.m.? This meeting will start my work of getting my honesty back. I would really like to have you there. RSVP to 999-999-9999.*

*Your nephew,*

*Johnny Jiminey*

At the honesty meeting, the worker asks everyone to sit in a circle. The worker sits in the middle of the circle with the child and interviews each person in turn: "What have you thought about [child's name] reputation for stealing? What has it meant to you? What would it mean if he [she] redeemed his [her] reputation and brought back honor rather than dishonor?"

Afterward, the child is questioned about why he or she wants his or her reputation back and what he or she would lose by continuing to be seen as a thief. The child is asked to consider the commitment to testing carefully because it will involve being closely watched. The child is also told that if he or she is suspected of acting in a stealing way during the testing period, the people who care about him or her will all be informed and the testing period will start anew. After giving the child some time to consider what is being asked of him or her, the worker asks the child in front of the audience if he or she is willing to formally test his or her honesty for an agreed-upon time period. Prior victims are asked if they would like the child to make up the loss to them in any special way.

The child is then sent out of the room and the specifics of the testing are discussed. The tests, like the one described earlier, consist of traps, such as leaving money, or whatever it was the child had been taking, in plain sight. The meeting attendees, or audience, discuss ways they can be sure of the "bait" left out and certain that others are not taking it. The social worker tells them that when the child passes a test, the "tester" is to congratulate and immediately inform the child of the success.

The worker then explains that successes and failures are to be conveyed to the others in the group through notes or e-mails, or via a phone tree. If the child is successful, the whole network is encouraged to praise him or her. Once the challenges set out during the required time period are successfully met, the child will invite all of the members of his or her audience to an honesty party. At the celebration, the child will be awarded back his or her honest reputation, usually with a certificate, and the child can give an acceptance speech.

A narrative approach to working on childhood stealing has the advantage of externalizing stealing as a reputation, which avoids blaming or defensive interactions with the child and/or the caretakers and recognizes the very real impact a reputation can have on a child's life. The approach also looks to the power of community to effect change, involving all those interested in the child and his or her reputation. It leaves the matter of how to avoid stealing to the child's creativity, exemplifying the approach's respect for and trust in people's own knowledge and skills.

## Men Who Have Used Violence to Control Their Partners

Narrative ideas are being used to inform social work practice with forensic clients, which on its face may seem an unusual application given the approach's emphasis on story over truth. Narratives about men's entitlement to use violence as a way to delineate masculinity proliferate in the culture, as any evening spent watching television will confirm. A cultural obligation for men to "take matters into their own hands" when confronted with conflict encourages the use of force to solve problems. But despite this dominant story, other stories about what it means to be a man exist (Nylund, 2004).

Nylund (2004) finds the following types of questions helpful in exploring the cultural context of domestic violence:

- If a man wanted to control and dominate his wife, what attitudes would he need to believe in to justify his behavior and make it OK?
- To what degree have you been influenced into these attitudes?
- What effect have these ideas had on you? On your wife? Your children?
- Where did you learn these attitudes (media, family, school, etc.)? (p. 188)

Unless the sense of entitlement to use violence is explored and found wanting, men will refrain from violence solely because of fear of punishment, not because it is the right choice.

The dominant story is not the only story, and most men, in fact, desire to have loving relationships, as well as control. From a narrative standpoint, if social workers are to understand men's full experience, including how abuse may be one part of it, they need to listen to men's stories. And they need to listen without allowing stories of irresponsibility to multiply. Listening to stories of men's own oppression outside of the relationship and of their desires other than to control and hold power over their partners allows social workers to examine the discrepancy between what men want and what their behavior is getting them (Augusta-Scott, 2003).

The dominant narrative in work with men who physically or sexually abuse their partners is that men want power and control and use violence and threats to get their way. They continue using violence because it works. This discourse does not consider that men may also experience injustice and powerlessness, feel ashamed of their actions, and be isolated, feeling, therefore, tremendous dependency on their partners (Augusta-Scott, 2003). These stories are avoided in treatment because they are thought to deflect responsibility from the offender for his actions. However, these stories can be used as a tool to genuinely engage men in making changes in their lives, if it is recognized that stories of power and control and of powerlessness, shame, and dependence can take place simultaneously. Listening to one need not negate listening to the other.

A client once told me he did not feel bad for his child victims because at least they were getting help now, whereas he received none after his long history of rape by his father. The question became: Did he think that his experience of terrible pain enlightened him to the exquisite harm his behavior had done to others or had it callused him, making all others' pain seem insignificant relative to what he felt? His affirmation of the latter led to a discussion of the help and the harm this "callusing over" had accomplished, as well as of whether it clarified or distorted his vision of others' suffering.

Alan Jenkins (1990), an Australian clinical psychologist, began writing about his work with spouse abusers shortly after narrative approaches started to be discussed. Most who work in this area refer to Jenkins and his current work with adolescent sex abusers (Jenkins, 1998). Jenkins argues that offenders need to develop an alternative story of their identity and they should begin this process in individual work before entering groups.

Jenkins (1990) is clear that the story of nonviolence given by men who have abused their partners is not truth in the sense that it is not necessarily an indication of readiness to stop using violence. However, he sees it as an expressed goal against which to measure future behavior. For example, a social worker might say, "You said previously that you would give up a lifestyle of pushing others around. Do you think your angry warning to your wife to leave you alone fits into the nonpushing-around lifestyle you want to have or into a lifestyle of pushing others around?"

Jenkins (1998) suggests three intervention principles that should guide work with men who have abused women: holding those who are abusive responsible for their behavior; making the intervention accountable to those who have the least power, such as victims; and ensuring that the intervention demonstrates respect, including being respectful to those who have abused others. Often men who abuse have themselves been abused, oppressed, and neglected. If these stories are not listened to first, the client is likely to feel it is unjust to expose himself to full responsibility for his actions when his own experience of injustice has not been understood. Giving the client the space to talk about his own subjective experience of maltreatment is not an invitation to irresponsibility, to allowing him to minimize or rationalize away his actions; rather, acknowledging the harm the client has experienced may open up the possibility for him to take responsibility for the harm he has caused others.

Jenkins (1998), in talking with a young man who was accused of sexually abusing his younger half sister, said:

> I don't want to push anything on to you. I don't want to tell you to do anything. That would be unfair and I guess you've probably had enough unfair things pushed on to you already. . . . I don't even want

to talk about what you did to Amy until I understand what you think is important. (p. 173)

Jenkins (1998) reports the young man responded hostilely to this statement. Yet Jenkins's remark affirmed for the young man both that he, the client, would have some control over the sessions and that eventually the work would have to focus on his abusive behavior.

Speaking out about past hurts is identified as an act of courage, while recognizing that prior abuse never entitles one to abuse others. The client's stands against injustice are identified and explored to reduce feelings of helplessness and blame. His own pain is recognized: "How fair would it be to expect you to face up to what you had done to Amy and try to understand what you might have put her through, if nobody understands or has thought about what you have been through?" (Jenkins, 1998, p. 179). By sensitively focusing on the client's ability to suffer through and cope with oppression in his own life, the stage is set to begin looking at whether the current abuse situation matches up to the client's preferred views of himself.

Jenkins (1998) talks about the engagement process as consisting of invitation, declination, and acknowledgment. Invitation involves asking questions that are geared toward "providing opportunities for the young man to consider respectful and responsible positions in relation to his abusive behavior that accord with his stated preferences and values" (p. 179). Declination means that the social worker refuses to be an audience to minimizing and rationalizing the abuse. Rather than confronting the individual or collusively remaining silent, the worker shifts the conversation to a previously agreed-upon fact: "You know what it is like to be let down and hurt yourself"(p. 180). Finally, acknowledgment, which often goes hand in hand with invitation, involves helping the client to recognize responsible and respectful actions and their meanings. "Facing up," for instance, is treated as an accomplishment and explored.

Discussing one's abuse of others is seen as an expectable part of treatment and a natural consequence of the behavior. The client's acknowledgment of his abusive actions and the shame or fear involved in discussing them are treated as indications of self-respect, caring for others, and integrity, rather than weakness. The social worker recognizes the client will likely leave out some details in the first telling because most people panic about what will happen to them and what others will think, as well as because of their own shame. Knowing this, the worker encourages repeated retellings of the story, which are likely to expand and get closer over time to the full details of the event. In this way, clients gradually take a more detailed and firmer stance regarding their abuse of others.

## Families

Families are collections of individuals with bonds and rules for interaction developed over time and with declared commitments to the future. The family itself can be the focus of change, as when certain patterns are identified as the intruding problem. The family also can be the audience for a member's stand against a problem and development of a new identity.

Family relationship patterns can be sources of distress. These patterns can be externalized as problems in themselves. Family therapist William Madsen (2007), drawing on psychiatrist Karl Tomm's work, looks at patterns that develop over time and repeat themselves in families and can be externalized. In what follows, I have summarized the five common patterns Madsen (see also Zimmerman & Dickerson, 1996) identifies:

- Being overresponsible/underresponsible, where one member denies or minimizes the problem, while the other intensely focuses on it;
- Minimizing/maximizing concerns, where one member overly emphasizes a positive or optimistic view of the situation, while the other assumes a negative or pessimistic perspective;
- Emotionally pursuing/withdrawing, where one member seems to desperately need to be close, while the other feels smothered and wants more distance or wishes to run away altogether;
- Demanding disclosure/secrecy and withholding, where one member demands information, while the other meets such demands with even greater secrecy;
- Engaging in correction and control/protest and rebellion, where one member imposes ever more rules, while the other continually tries to find additional ways to circumvent or break the new requirements.

When members of a family identify these constellations of behavior, the pattern can be named and externalized. For example, a couple might describe how their fights have been increasing in intensity and frequency as follows:

**Jill:** *Sometimes I just get so lonely, and I need Amy to talk to me about what is on her mind, what is going on with her, how she feels about me.*

**Worker:** So tell me what you do when you have these feelings.

**Jill:** *I just ask her how her day was and she says, "Fine." So I get kind of frustrated and ask her what was so fine about it, and she says that she's too tired to talk and goes off to watch TV. So I start to get angry because if she cared for me, she could at least be civil, so I go over and tell her I just really need to talk with her.*

**Worker:** Sort of pursuing her for an answer or some sense of connection?

**Jill:** *Right. Then all hell breaks loose. She goes into the bedroom swearing and slams the door.*

**Worker:** So you feel lonely and ask Amy about her day and she says she is too tired to talk, and when she leaves, you continue to pursue her for connection.

**Jill:** *Yeah.*

**Worker:** So, Amy, what is your experience of Jill's attempts to connect with you when you get home from work?

**Amy:** *Pretty overwhelming. I mean I'm exhausted. The last thing I need is lots of questions coming at me when I get home.*

**Worker:** So how do you experience Jill's attempts to be close?

**Amy:** *Like I can't breathe, like I just need a break. When she comes after me I feel like I need to get away.*

**Worker:** So you find yourself trying to put distance in some way between yourself and Jill?

**Amy:** *I guess I do but I haven't thought of it that way. It makes sense!*

**Worker:** So maybe what happens is something like pursuing and distancing going on. Is this one way you can consider these arguments? Does it fit what you've been experiencing?

**Jill:** *Yes, it seems to.*

**Amy:** *Makes sense to me.*

**Worker:** Let's talk about what pursuing/distancing is doing to your relationship, if that's okay.

Lobovits and Freeman (1997) note:

> If the problem of Fighting, for example, has taken over family life to such an extent that it is the primary mode of interaction between family members, initial and validating steps would be identifying the

Fighting interactions and acknowledging the deep pain, distrust, and destruction that accompany them. However, this is not a place to dwell indefinitely—nor is merely understanding the roots or workings of the Fighting and waiting until the problem works itself out. Instead, family members can be invited into a conversation that clarifies the family's preferences for communication—spotting and highlighting Fighting-free interactions, while contrasting their effects with the Fighting-dominated ones. (p. 176)

Each small accomplishment should be explored and expanded. Lobovits and Freeman (1997) report that families can often be skeptical of any change noticed. They give the following example:

"Well it's easy to have a good time at the zoo, but what about on a school morning?" This challenge creates an opening to explore similar questions: What would be the impact on the family and its members if Peace stood up to the rigors of getting off to work and school? If this occurred, would it prove that Peace not only had broken out for a moment at the zoo, but had found a place in the day-to-day life of the family? (p. 178)

Again the emphasis is on building an alternative story despite the family's feeling of hopelessness. It would be rare if at least one family member did not initially see the situation as repairable.

## Problems That Grow Between Couples

Couple counseling is an important clinical social work function. However, some students are uncomfortable with this work because it can evoke a high level of conflict and intense animosity.

Neal et al. (1999) describe narrative couple work as involving a series of phases: establishing transparency; engaging with how the couple experiences the problem; rediscovering preferred experiences; disentangling oneself from gender practices in favor of preferred re-remembered experiences; exploring previous, current, and future possibilities for performing one's preferred identity and preferred relationship; and reauthoring practices.

When the social worker situates himself or herself as a person in relation to his or her work with the couple, the worker models an ethic of transparency. This practice entails the worker offering to answer questions the partners may have so that they can understand where the worker is coming from. For example, a worker might note, "If you are unclear about why I am asking a particular question, please let me know and I will tell you my thinking behind it." This type of statement is a way to reduce some of the power differential between the worker and the clients by allowing greater transparency of the worker's thinking process.

The next phase involves the social worker engaging in the couple's experiences of the problem by looking at the problem's effects on the individuals and their relationship. The worker explores with the couple the effect of the problem on each person's view of himself or herself, the partner, and the relationship. The social worker asks questions that continually draw out each person's perception of himself or herself in the relationship and a description of his or her experiences of the relationship. Eliciting each partner's story permits the worker and the clients to see where the stories coincide and where they contradict each other.

From a social constructionist perspective, self-identity is fluid and constructed in communication with others. How a person's partner experiences the person can influence how a person experiences himself or herself. Whereas partners often focus on the other as the source of the problem, looking at one's "relational identity" (e.g., Who can I be with this person?) focuses on each individual's own responsibility in the relationship (Freedman & Combs, 2004, p. 29).

Freedman and Combs (2004) discuss the importance of helping people witness the perspective of the other without defensiveness to bring hope for the future back into the relationship. Care needs to be taken to set up the proper circumstances for this to happen. The social worker needs to explain to the couple that while one partner talks with the worker, the other will listen without interrupting; each will have a chance to be the "talker" and the "listener." In one example, Freedman and Combs skillfully ask the observing partner, "Would you be willing, as I talk with Vernon, to listen as you would to a friend? With friends, sometimes you can suspend your own point of view and listen just to understand. Would that be all right?"(p. 37).

Sometimes, as in cases of infidelity, partners will need to apologize and possibly seek forgiveness from the other before they can develop the necessary trust to continue their relationship (Segal, 2004). Partners need to be helped to place their behavior in the context of their values, commitments, and preferences:

- "Has any of your own behaviour taken you away from your own values or beliefs and undermined your sense of personal integrity?

- What would it take to bring your own values and behaviours closer together? . . .
- What do you imagine the impact of your behaviour has been on your partner?" (Segal, p. 109).

A partner who has been greatly hurt by the other should expect more caring behaviors in return for forgiveness.

In the process of exploring the problem, the social worker collects dissonant experiences—those times or events where the problem has not captured the couple. This moves the process into Neal et al.'s (1999) third phase: finding and exploring preferred experiences of self and of the relationship that are separate from the influence of the problem. Exceptions to the problem story always exist. No couple is the same 24 hours a day, 7 days a week since the first day the pair met, and it can be difficult for a couple in conflict to remember this when tension is high. The social worker seeks out and notes periods of time when the couple is not or has not been under the influence of the problem and when the couple's intentions, experiences, or behaviors do not show or have not shown the effects of the problem.

The fourth phase involves separating the influence of gender practices, or gendered role expectations in the case of same-sex couples, in favor of preferred re-remembered experiences of self and the relationship. Separating the identities of the clients from the problem is only part of the externalizing process. Gender messages, which can have a negative impact on the kind of relationship the couple desires, need to be examined and deconstructed, too. For example: What does it mean to be a man or woman in this society? How do those meanings affect the couple as a unit? Does playing a particular gender-based role increase or decrease a partner's satisfaction? When one's partner has had a difficult day, does doing the dishes despite a schedule indicating it is the partner's turn lead to feeling that the partner is abdicating responsibility or that appreciation is being expressed for the partner through the act of doing the dishes? The answers to these sorts of questions provide the basis for examining the assumptions behind gender roles in families.

When the couple can see themselves, each other, and the relationship somewhat differently, then the fifth phase of Neal et al.'s (1999) model begins. The partners are encouraged to explore their past, present, and future performance of preferred identities and a preferred relationship by coconstructing a coherent narrative. The definition of the problem is shifted from the troublesome personality of the other to the influence of a cultural discourse by looking at issues of gender. The blame for the relationship problem is taken off the partners, and they now have choices about how to develop their relationship based on their preferred images, which may or may not coincide with cultural expectations. Clients can gain greater agency in their lives as they consider which experiences with their partners they wish to continue and what they believe the relationship is capable of allowing them to become. This phase is a foundation for the next step, which is the development of an anchored alternative story.

Finally, during phase six, reauthoring practices help partners relate preferred experiences to preferred narratives. Through questioning, the couple explores those times when they were able to have their preferred relationship, when the conflict or the problem was absent and something they desired was present instead. By stringing these incidents together across time, the couple is helped to remember

> their shared history as a couple. . . . things that were important about themselves, each other and the relationship. . . . The reauthoring process reconnects persons to historical moments in order to place preferred experiences . . . into a meaningful (alternative) story about themselves, each other, and the relationship. (Neal et al., 1999, pp. 392, 395)

The more each partner can get inside those experiences, the more he or she can retrieve the strong parts of the relationship. The social worker can help the couple do this by questioning in detail the specifics of each historical moment that formed an exception to the conflict, developing those events into a story, and projecting the story's meaning into the future.

Typically partners come in and say the other person is the problem in the relationship. This puts social workers in the position of judge, a role with which they rightfully feel uncomfortable. White (1993a) suggests that this discourse about couple relationships, in which each partner sees the other as being at fault and the partners' anger and bitterness permeate the relationship, seems common in the Western world. White asks:

> Have you ever had the suspicion that these adversarial interactions are common enough to be represented as institutionalized practices of relationship? . . . Have you ever observed that partners who are locked into such interactions are in pursuit of an individuality that denies relationship? . . . Have you sensed that the version of individuality . . . performed . . . is one that distances and isolates partners from each other? (pp. 191–192)

He goes on to state that alternative forms of individuality do not have to deny collaboration between people; rather, they can acknowledge aspects of the other's preferred identity—of the partner's desires, purposes, goals, and so on. Individuality in relationships does not have to diminish empathy for the other. Without some sense of empathy it is hard to imagine any success in rescuing relationships.

Epston (1993, p. 183) developed a style of interviewing known as *internalized other questioning* to break people out of the patterns of argument and reproach that often occur in couple therapy. Epston begins by telling the couple that they have probably been asking each other and themselves a good many questions before coming to see someone to help them with their relationship. He informs them that he does not wish to repeat those same questions because they have not been helpful. Instead, he says, he would like to ask different kinds of questions, kinds that may take them by surprise and may require them to take a few minutes before responding. Epston states:

> I need to warn you of their [i.e., the questions'] difficulties and to seek your permission to pursue a course that may cause you discomfort. You might not have quick or ready answers. . . . So I apologize to you now for their difficulty. You may be stretched in ways you have never been stretched before. Do I have your permission to go ahead with this questioning process? (p. 186)

As can be imagined, this type of preamble is likely to get most couples' attention if delivered sincerely. For example:

> Who would like to go first? . . . Jill, what do you think Jack would say if I asked him the following question: "Jack, how do you account for the deterioration in your relationship over the past 10 years?" . . . Jill is invited by the question to render Jack's complaints about her. . . . Even if Jill's answer is self-condemning (e.g., "Jill isn't giving me enough love."), I then ask a further question of Jill: "Jack, what effect has this 'lovelessness' had on your relationship?" . . . "Do you think a loveless direction is good or bad (healthy or unhealthy, adds to or takes way from, increases or decreases) the . . . value of your relationship?" . . . "Jack, you have come up with three theories for the shape your relationship is in. There must be more than that! Are there any little reasons you think are too small to mention out of embarrassment or any big reasons you think are so big you are reluctant to mention them out of fear?"

The answers are then cross-referenced. "Jack, Jill thought that you would explain the downfall of your relationship by way of an 'I'm all right and you're all wrong' patterning. How close is her representation of your experience to your actual experience of how your relationship is declining?" (Epston, 1993, pp. 186–187)

These types of questions require partners to listen to each other and consider the other's perspective. These questions also help the partners to begin to externalize the relationship problem, to see it as separate from themselves as individuals and as a couple. The narrative practitioner uses these sorts of questions to get the couple to work on the problem instead of each other.

Several pilot studies have found the narrative practice of using a reflecting team to be helpful in working with couples. In Griffith et al.'s (1992) study, family members were more likely to demonstrate positive interactions after a reflecting team session than before one. According to Sells et al. (1994), couples reported that the distance provided by being unable to interrupt the team members' discussion required them to give the comments more thought. The couples also said they were less embarrassed because the comments were not made to them face-to-face. In addition, they indicated that their comfort with the experience was increased by having a mixed-gender reflecting team. The couples' therapists, however, did not see these points as important to the session (Sells et al.).

## Exercises

### Exercise 1: Practicing Couple Counseling

You are the social worker who has been asked to work with Jake and Millie. Put yourself in this role, keeping in mind whatever your actual characteristics are (e.g., age, gender, race/ethnicity, sexual orientation, marital/relationship status). Following is the information you received from Millie when she called to make the initial appointment.

Jake and Millie are a biracial couple who have been having difficulties. Jake is a 32-year-old African American who works as an accountant at a small firm in town. Millie is a 30-year-old Italian American who works part-time as a nurse at the local hospital and cares for their 8-year-old son, Sam, and 4-year-old daughter, Angel. Lately, the couple is averaging three arguments a week over Jake's late nights out and his "not following through on promises" to Millie and the children. When Jake came home at 2:00 a.m. last Friday night, he and Millie had a big argument. When he woke up the next morning, Jake found his clothes packed in boxes on the porch. Rather than get into another fight, he loaded up his clothes and drove to his brother's house, where he stayed over the weekend. Millie told him he could move back if he would go with her to see a counselor about their marriage, to which he agreed.

In the following transcript several multiple choice responses are inserted. Select the one that would best fit a narrative format. As in real life, no answer will be perfect.

**Worker:** Okay, at this point I have only talked to Millie on the telephone. She said there has been friction between her and you, Jake, over what she sees as your late-night hours. This came to a head in an incident on Friday night, when you came home later than Millie could tolerate, and ended with your moving out of the house. Millie made seeing a counselor to talk about this problem a condition of getting back together. Is that what you told me, Millie?

**Millie:** *Yeah, he never comes home when he says he will and he never keeps his promises to me and the kids.*

**Worker:** You're saying that Jake has never kept his word to you, or maybe you have some specific concerns.

**Millie:** *Yeah, I think he's lying to me and going out on me and this is what I have to live with. He is never there for me and the children. All he ever thinks about is himself.*

**Jake:** *See, this is why I don't want to go to counseling. This is what I go through day in and day out. She wants to strangle me; everything is my fault. She thinks I lie if I don't do what she tells me to. She can always find something to bitch about.*

1. Possible worker responses:

    (a) Don't you think you are being a bit harsh here, denying her experience?

    (b) I don't think that name-calling will be helpful because it doesn't work at home.

    (c) Jake, I wonder if you would tell Millie why you think she is so difficult.

    (d) So far I have heard that Millie feels betrayed and upset over your staying out and that you, Jake, feel distrusted and belittled by Millie's complaints about you to me. Is that accurate so far or did I miss something?

**Worker:** Has the problem always been like this or has it gotten worse lately?

**Jake:** *Worse—she never lets up. All the time; it never stops.*

**Worker:** So things feel worse right now. Has this distrust completely taken over your relationship or are there ever times when things feel a little more like normal?

**Jake:** *Like I said, she never lets up. Don't you get it! I would think this is obvious!*

2. Possible worker responses:
    (a) I think I get it, but I just want to be sure it is as bad as you say.
    (b) You seem to be very angry at me, as if I'm to blame here.
    (c) I'm wondering if maybe I made a mistake and led you to think I didn't believe you.
    (d) I'm just trying to find a way so you can talk to each other, so each can hear the other.

**Millie:** *It has gotten tougher lately. It seems since Angel turned two and needed more watching things have gotten tougher. I feel like I need him more and he's not there. He just gives me more trouble.*

**Jake:** *Again, me giving her trouble. You have no idea what it's like living with this woman!*

3. Possible worker responses:
    (a) How could I?
    (b) You seem to think that this problem is all her fault.
    (c) So, what is good about living with her?
    (d) This is the second time you mentioned that I can't understand how difficult life is for you right now. Perhaps you can give me a specific example to help me understand how you are feeling.

**Worker:** Are either of you happy with the way things are going? I mean, do you want things to stay the same?

**Millie:** No!

**Jake:** *No! I'm tired of this. If this keeps up we won't be together.*

**Millie:** *Right, just leave the kids; what difference do they make!*

**Worker:** Whoa! Neither of you is happy with this situation, nor was it always this bad. If I can, let me change the subject a bit. Who supports your being a couple?

**Millie:** *What do you mean?*

**Worker:** Well, who wants to see you stay together?

**Millie:** *Maybe we do, at least sometimes. That's why we're here.*

**Worker:** I was just wondering if the fact that you being Black, Jake, and, Millie, you being White has made things tougher or easier.

**Millie:** *That don't mean anything.*

**Worker:** So you feel accepted all the time and supported as people who should be together?

**Jake:** *People give us looks sometimes. I used to just hold her tighter when that happened, to let them know they could just shove it.*

4. Possible worker responses:
   (a) How do you cope with this?
   (b) Do you think you could be misreading people's intentions?
   (c) What meaning do these looks have for you?
   (d) You sound like a very protective man.

**Worker:** I was just wondering, actually, how you tell when someone disapproves.

**Jake:** *Oh, they either turn away or get a goofy smile on their face. Pisses me off.*

**Millie:** *I think he sees it more than I do. I don't let it bother me; he is my husband and it's none of their business.*

**Worker:** Does it ever get wearing? I mean feeling like people don't support you for who you are.

**Jake:** *Sometimes I just want to punch out some of these clowns who check us out. I feel like I have to protect her and me sometimes.*

**Millie:** *I just ignore it and don't let it bother me. I figure, if they're assholes then it's their problem.*

5. Possible worker responses:
   (a) What other coping strategies do you have?
   (b) Do you see a way to talk to each other about this?
   (c) Do you think there are messages in our society that encourage people to act that way?
   (d) What have you done to take care of this problem?

**Worker:** So despite the pressure on you, you have stayed married for how many years?

**Millie:** *Nine.*

**Worker:** Nine years! Who can you turn to when it feels like it's overwhelming? Who supports your being a couple?

**Millie:** *Not many people. We have a couple of close friends and they seem okay with it, but this shouldn't be a problem anymore—hell, we're married.*

**Worker:** So who specifically does support you? Who are they?

**Millie:** *Jill and Gene, friends of ours. We try to get together at least once every two weeks. She's Black and he's White.*

**Jake:** *My older brother, Sam; he's always there for us.*

**Millie:** *That's true.*

6. Possible worker responses:
    (a) What do they do that is supportive?
    (b) Do you really talk to them about what is important?
    (c) How often do you see your brother?
    (d) Let's imagine something for a minute, and play along with me if you can. Jake, let's imagine you're not Jake in this room but Sam. Would that be okay? Sam, what do you see in Jake and Millie's marriage that is worthy of saving that they may not be able to see right now?

**Worker:** Do your kids face any problems in your neighborhood because they are biracial?

**Millie:** *No, they seem pretty protected and accepted.*

**Jake:** *You have to worry some. I know they're different; wait until dating and that stuff comes around—then we'll see what's really going on.*

**Worker:** Despite the pressure, it seems you have done well until lately with this. Do you want to handle this issue differently between you or are you satisfied with the way it's going?

**Millie:** *I'm not sure how it's connected.*

**Jake:** *No, this worker's right. The hassles add up over time, and we can't ignore that it makes me edgy.*

**Millie:** *Maybe that's something we need to talk about, but what does that have to do with his being irresponsible?*

**Worker:** That's true. How does this conversation meet your needs? Did the conversation we just had strike you as irresponsible?

**Millie:** *No, he sounded responsible here, but that anger gets us nowhere.*

**Worker:** Actually, I was trying to think of what you would call this problem that comes in and sits in the middle of your lives taking away your joy. You both sound pretty unhappy with it.

**Millie:** *Well, it's his irresponsibility.*

**Worker:** Okay, perhaps I haven't allowed you the time to talk about where you stand on this. I wonder, though, if maybe we could set up some ground rules that would make this a different experience than you have at home.

7. Next possible worker comment:

   (a) During the rest of our session I would like you to listen to each other's story of your lives as if you were good friends. We usually cut our friends some slack and hear them out before jumping to conclusions, whereas spouses tend not to listen to each other and are quick to judge.

   (b) During the rest of the session I would like to try practicing a different kind of listening. After one person speaks, I would like the other person to say what you think you heard, then decide if that was what was meant before responding.

   (c) Before you speak I would like you to think about what you are telling yourself about what is being said that is making you so angry.

Here are possible responses to the multiple choice items in this exercise and an explanation of each:

1. (d) Provides a simple summary and checkout
2. (c) Assumes a more equal status between client and worker by admitting a possible mistake
3. (d) Responds to a client's answer that the client's problem story has not been listened to
4. (c) Uses a landscape of meaning question that begins discussion of discourses
5. (c) Begins discussion of societal discourses that may be affecting couple's commitment
6. (d) Uses an internalized other question to bring outside party into the room and provide some distance in the discussion

7. (a) Invokes the concept of friendship to create some distance for the listening party, while giving the talking party the space to discuss his or her story without interruption

## Exercise 2: Presenting the "Colleagues"

Sometimes those things that seem to be the easiest to do are difficult when you first try them. For this role-play exercise, you will need stuffed animals. However, if none are available, you can do the exercise with imaginary animals.

Break into pairs. One of you will role-play a child and the other a social worker. The child is under the influence of bed-wetting, bowel movements in the wrong place, temper tantrums, or some other problem over which he or she does not seem to have control. For the person playing the social worker, begin by explaining to the child what colleagues, or helpers, are and introduce the child to the stuffed animal colleagues that are available for consultation. Ask the child to choose a helper. Once the child has picked a stuffed animal colleague, tell the child about the unique problem his or her helper confronts, which is the same problem the child is experiencing. Ask the child to do what he or she can to teach the helper to deal with the problem. The focus is on helping the child use his or her own knowledge and skills to teach the animal helper, not telling the child what to do.

Make the role-play more interesting by having the person playing the child ask questions such as "Why do I have to do this?"; "How do I teach her not to have tantrums?"; and "What if I lose him?" Role-play for no more than 10 minutes, and then switch roles. What seemed to work? What seemed less effective?

## Exercise 3: Interviewing Around Reputation

Interviewing adolescents to secure accurate information can be challenging. This chapter described the technique of using reputation as an alternative to asking about behaviors. Reputation requires no judgment of truth. Therefore, inquiry about it can be made without prying. Adolescents are usually concerned about their reputation with others and can suffer long-term personal, relational, and system consequences from a bad reputation. Actual patterns of behavior are not necessary; the simple appearance of engaging in troubling behaviors is enough to create and/or maintain a "bad" reputation. In this exercise, you will work on laying the foundation for reputation as an area of focus in the conversation.

Break into pairs. You will be engaging in a 20-minute interview, after which you will switch roles and start the exercise all over again.

One student will role-play a social worker in a juvenile court diversion program who has just met a new client. The other student will be the client, who is a 12-year-old child, either a girl or boy, recently arrested for shoplifting a CD at the local department store. The youngster has no other delinquency record. However, the social worker learns in a phone call from the mother that the child has been stealing change from the family for the last year to play video games at the local arcade. In addition, change has turned up missing at the homes of extended family members after the child has visited, although family members have not confronted the child about this. The mother says her child is hanging out with the wrong crowd, and she thinks they might have put the youngster up to stealing the CD. The parents could not make this first session but plan to come to the second.

For the person playing the social worker, begin the interview by introducing yourself. Then explain that you are interested in what the child enjoys and is proud of, as well as what troubles he or she has. Describe what a court diversion program is supposed to do (avoid a child's having further contact with the court), and make sure the child understands that as an arm of the court you have to tell the court about criminal behavior (as well as take action if abuse, neglect, or danger to self or others is suspected).

Discuss the troubling behavior that has brought the child to you by reminding the child why he or she is being seen. Ask the child how his or her behavior might affect his or her reputation as an honest or a dishonest person. Ask the child whether this is entirely positive or entirely negative (realizing that it may be positive in the eyes of his or her peer group). Ask him or her why it is positive or negative. Go into specifics.

For example:

**Worker:** So you say having a dishonest reputation is bad. What makes it bad?

**Client:** *It's just bad, that's all.*

**Worker:** I'm just curious, because in some places being seen as a thief is not something bad. What specifically about a dishonest reputation makes it bad?

**Client:** *People don't trust you, I guess.*

**Worker:** So what's so bad about not being trusted?

**Client:** *They won't talk to you about stuff or they are always watching their things or they are always blaming you for stuff, hassling you.*

**Worker:** How would you like people to treat you instead?

**Client:** *I want to be the kind of person people can talk to, not have to watch out for. I don't want to get blamed for stuff I haven't done.*

Next, ask the child how his or her reputation has affected family, friends, and school, as well as his or her feelings about himself or herself. Finally, ask the child what kind of reputation he or she would like to have and what it would be called.

After each student has played both roles, work together on the following questions:

Did anything in the exercise interest you? What part?

What would be the biggest encouragements for using reputation in your client interviews at your placement or work? What are the greatest barriers?

If you currently have a client for whom focusing on reputation might be a helpful way to proceed, tell your partner how you might go about integrating it into your work with that person.

CHAPTER 12

# Narrative Approaches in Health and Gerontology

Health and aging are sensitive subjects in a culture that emphasizes growth and productivity. Those confronted by illness or old age are seen as "stalled," and our society continually finds ways to indicate their need to progress against their illness or despite their aging. Octogenarians are praised when they run marathons, but not when they care for their grandchildren. In the same fashion, those who "triumph over" an illness are lauded for not "succumbing" to it, as if these were wholly individual choices. And death, whether from illness or age, is something to be "resolved" as quickly as possible.

Health and aging are also places where tensions between discourses about individual versus community responsibilities play out. Does society have any responsibility to provide wellness and preventive medical services? Or, are individuals responsible for their diseases? Have people done everything they could to prevent disease or injury or to minimize its impact? Have they exercised enough, eaten the right kind of foods, and reduced stress in their lives? If you are diagnosed with cancer and yet have not made radical changes in your lifestyle, are you then responsible if you come out of remission? These are the subtle questions of an individualistic discourse that ill people must struggle with every day in addition to the suffering and uncertainty they endure.

Similarly, in the United States, if people are entitled to the often stigmatized label of "disabled," they are allowed minimal living expenses. As other income subsidy programs are being dismantled, programs for the disabled encounter intense scrutiny, and questions about who is disabled by injury or physical or mental illness are resolved in the decisions made by examiners and hearing officers. Individuals with disabilities, an already marginalized population given our society's emphasis on fitness and ability, become a suspect group as debate swirls around the question of who is "truly" disabled.

And although we all age, the need to deny that fact runs deep in our culture. Just as the ill are held responsible for their sicknesses, older adults are seen as responsible for growing older and for experiencing the physical and cognitive changes that aging can bring. Who should provide the assistance elders may need? Who determines what type of help is provided? Who has a say in where the assistance is provided? Does aging strip people of their voices? Of their dreams and hopes and preferences?

I begin this chapter by looking at the importance of illness stories and the various forms such stories can take. Next, I talk about how change and growth can emerge from trauma. Then I discuss a form of narrative medicine that is being developed to increase empathy and collaboration in the doctor-patient relationship. I next describe how narrative approaches can provide new ways to assist the aging and the dying to claim their dignity. Finally, I look at how narrative practice can be especially well suited to working with issues of grief and loss, allowing those who remain to "keep a place at the table" for those who have died by keeping their stories alive.

## Illness Narratives

Through stories people make sense not only of their lives but of their illnesses, too. There are many narratives that arise from illness that despite their individual differences typically start with an experienced sensation (pain, itching, dizziness) leading to contact with a health professional who turns the sensation into a symptom of a deeper problem (Kierans & Maynooth, 2001). The problem then takes on a life of its own as a disease or an injury for which there are treatments. From the health care professional's point of view, the condition has a likely trajectory, a course of progression and/or regression termed a *prognosis*. In a desire to improve, the person often adopts the medical version of the illness, even though this may require the individual to deny or revise his or her actual illness experiences. "Good" patients get better; resistant, stubborn ones do not.

Illness and suffering become the ground for many stories, and these stories touch upon the core of existence and help alleviate the aloneness of pain. As Frank (1995) notes:

> One of our most difficult duties as human beings is to listen to the voices of those who suffer. The voices of the ill are easy to ignore, because these voices are often faltering in tone and mixed in message.... These voices bespeak conditions of embodiment that most of us would rather forget our own vulnerability to. Listening is hard, but it is also

a fundamental moral act; to realize the best potential in postmodern times requires an ethics of listening. (p. 25)

If illness narratives are difficult for the listener, they are even more so for the teller. Illness requires people to stand up to our culture's discourses of fitness, accomplishment, success, individualism, and progress, as illness means people cannot perform to their maximum ability at all times. They are "less than" and therefore diminished according to these standards (Weingarten, 2005). These cultural discourses are part of the identity of the person standing up to them, having been inculcated in childhood and continually reinforced as he or she matured. The dependency on others that disease, illness, and aging incur can become the focus of conflict, and then the unrealistic societal messages about who is productive or worthy escape with little scrutiny or challenge.

Frank (1995) hypothesizes three forms of illness narratives: restitution, chaos, and quest. He developed this classification to make illness narratives easier to hear, not because he thought these categories embodied the truth.

The restitution story is the medical story of health, illness, and ultimately health regained: "I have a physical problem; it is not a mystery, but a series of small problems that can be dealt with one at a time, and once these problems are dealt with, I will get better." This is a convenient story and television advertisements for medications readily capture its essence: "I'm sick and can't enjoy life. I take the magic pill and then I can enjoy life and even become a more active participant with my family than before or have an improved sex life." This is a comforting story for patients, though it is the story of the medical profession's offerings and often not of the patient's experience of the illness.

The restitution story constructs illness not as a narrative in and of itself, but as simply the life story of a person placed on hold (Kierans & Maynooth, 2001). The "hold" will be lifted once the illness is dealt with, and the person's life story then will pick up where it left off and continue as if there had been no interruption. However, in some cases, people die or the illness worsens. Spending all their time focusing on the multiple treatments in cases of chronic or terminal illness can push people to never confront their mortality. For example, "This new chemotherapy is just the thing to kill this tumor, even if it has only a 50% success rate. I won't think about what comes next while we are trying this out." There are comforts and there are denials in the restitution story.

The chaos story is one of disjointed emotion and terror of life not improving or returning to what it once had been. It is the often unspoken story behind the illness, the one that people do not wish to talk about for fear of seeming crazy. When it does come out, the chaos story is often squashed by other stories. Shame and rage can overwhelm the person. Kaethe Weingarten (2005), a family therapist and cancer challenger, notes, "I am a ghost. My purpose and my meaning have been surreptitiously removed. I know I look like a person, but I am not" (sect. II. Restitution, Chaos and Quest Narratives, para. 10). She characterizes her experience as being out in the middle of the ocean hanging on to a Styrofoam coffee cup.

The chaos story is one of experience and can be impossible to set into a coherent narrative when the person is in the experience. It is frequently a difficult story for social workers to listen to. Giving people the space to state their experience without trying to change it is very challenging initially because workers often find the experience too raw and painful and it comes too close to the chaos and hopelessness that everyone feels at times (Weingarten, 2005). As Frank (1995) notes, "Chaos stories show how quickly the props that other stories depend on can be kicked away" (p. 114).

Listeners intuitively want to inject hope so that the chaos story can begin to look like a restitution narrative. As social workers, we often feel we can best serve people if we reduce their anxiety or depressive symptoms. But when we focus on alleviating these symptoms, do we take the experience away from our clients? Do we tell them we cannot listen to their emotion-driven story? Here, perhaps, is the place for feeling our own suffering as well.

Because of the sense of panic, of being out of control that chronic and terminal illnesses can cause, people may question their own sanity. A social worker's ability to listen, to question the idea that craziness is unreasonable in such circumstances, and to convey the belief that the feeling will not always be so intense can let clients know that they are not alone in their struggles. Not being alone seems important for people to get beyond this story, at least for a while.

Chronic or terminal illnesses can involve a variety of new experiences that along the way can push a person into a chaos story. Every test, treatment, or weigh-in can trigger panic. Unfortunately, hospitals, in particular, separate patients from the community of people who love them, and, as a result, patients often face these anxieties alone or only in the care of professionals. Illness remains a problem of the individual who has it and who has now been detached from his or her community. The burdens and joys of caring for the person are not distributed to the community that cared for him or her before the illness. Instead, caring is assigned to experts with specialized knowledge and skills.

Sometimes, the chaos story leads to a different type of story, one that Frank (1995) calls a quest or journey narrative. This narrative involves trying to make sense out of the illness experience. The central idea is that suffering is transformative in some way. It is a narrative that comes from the voice of the sufferer but is usually framed by the dominant discourse of hero stories: a person is drawn in, usually unwittingly, to suffer challenges and returns with some sort of benefit. The benefit may seem elusive, and the journey itself may be the only benefit—the experience of being with suffering.

As a faculty member who has survived cancer so far, I have been approached by students when they or their family members are struggling with cancer or other life-threatening illnesses. I do not think I am a particularly sensitive or even empathic person, but by virtue of my confronting the limits of my mortality and experiencing the terror of death by cancer, I am sought out. I am on a journey that I have experienced some portions of. Students just want to know that there can be another side to suffering. I have remarkably little to offer in terms of any solace, other than just to say I am sorry for their pain and the panic will not last forever but will likely return on occasion. I believe my subjective experience with suffering and with confronting my more limited life expectancy allows me to hear these stories without judging them. For this reason I am sought out.

A videotape (Andrews, 1996) of Jill Freedman, a well-known narrative therapist, author, and trainer, shows her conducting a session with a couple in which the husband had acquired a strange and apparently terminal illness. Added to the disruption of the family's life caused by the husband's illness is the strain created by the medical profession's inability to offer much in the way of treatment.

The interview shows the couple struggling to name what they are going through and what they envision for the future. The restitution story is clearly not applicable. Given the unpredictability of the husband's disease, the couple might easily find themselves in chaos for long periods of time. However, they finally come up with a journey metaphor. The conversation, which students often do not see as therapy, leads to the couple thinking about how they will face each new unpredictable event in this "journey to nowhere." They are realistic about the ending of this journey but see meaning in the journey itself.

As this videotaped session illustrates, the object of narrative treatment is not to get people to move into a quest narrative form just for the sake of doing so. Rather, by being open to their experience of chaos and accepting the chaos for what it is, individuals may enter a more reflective stance, if they are capable of doing so. Should they arrive at a quest narrative, a transformation of meaning may occur that influences their self-identity and their relationship to others.

## Posttraumatic Growth in the Face of Serious Illness

Some people find new sources of strength in the process of struggling against trauma. Some writers hypothesize that individuals' meaning structures are devastated by trauma, and, as a result, some people find new structures to hold their world together. This transformation can happen while they also are experiencing considerable distress. This "posttraumatic growth" can take place in five domains: "greater appreciation of life and changed sense of priorities; warmer, more intimate relationships with others; a greater sense of personal strength; recognition of new possibilities or paths for one's life; and spiritual development" (Tedeschi & Calhoun, 2004, p. 6).

This predominantly cognitive perspective on the transformation of trauma experiences disguises the impact of interpersonal and societal influences (Neimeyer, 2004). The cognitive view also minimizes the strong role played by culture in interpreting trauma and recovery (Pals & McAdams, 2004). In cultures focused on appearance, for instance, extensive disfigurement may be less likely to induce growth than cancer or heart disease. Nor does the cognitive perspective account for those consequences that occur not by cognitive restructuring but simply by virtue of acquiring a more vulnerable and diminished role and experiencing the social environment's reaction to it (McMillen, 2004). For example, in a society that is relatively wealthy and that values individualism, the options to recognize new possibilities or paths for one's life and to experience a changed sense of priorities may be privileges that not only are unavailable but are unimaginable in poorer, communal, or duty-bound cultures.

For example, when an individual's illness results in an outpouring of support from others, the significance of these relationships to the patient may be heightened. It is not uncommon for people to suffer greatly from a trauma yet eventually develop a positive ending to their narrative (i.e., being a better person or discovering others are important). The exact content of the ending and the meaning ascribed to it are likely determined by the culture's dominant narratives (Pals & McAdams, 2004).

The concept of posttraumatic growth itself may well come from a broader cultural discourse about wisdom through suffering. Opening space in conversations for considering these narratives and their impact on people's lives makes available new options for discovering meaning in chronic or terminal illnesses (Petersen, Bull, Propst, Dettinger, & Detwiler, 2005).

## Narrative Medicine

Medicine has been engaged in looking at lives narratively for some time. In stark contrast to concerned detachment, the style typically seen as the professional ideal, some medical educators have come to see a narrative approach as one that would humanize the medical professional and make medicine a more fulfilling and ethical profession. The emphasis in this orientation is not on helping people find the space in which to see different narratives in their lives, but on helping the doctor understand the patient and vice versa. Additionally, with a career seen as a journey, a narrative approach puts the stresses of medical practice in perspective (Charon, 2001).

The goal of a narrative approach to medical education is to develop a doctor's "narrative competence," which requires "a combination of textual skills (identifying a story's structure, adopting its multiple perspectives, recognizing metaphors and allusions), creative skills (imagining many interpretations, building curiosity, inventing multiple endings), and affective skills (tolerating uncertainty as a story unfolds, entering the story's mood)" (Charon, 2004, p. 862). This is important because medicine often lacks an "attunement to patients' individuality, sensitivity to emotional or cultural dimensions of care, ethical commitment to patients despite fragmentation and subspecialization, acknowledgement and then prevention of error" (p. 863).

Medical narratives have become popular literature, as seen by the success of Oliver Sacks (1983, 1985), a neurologist, among others. Such narratives are therapeutic in that they develop empathy in the physician for the patient and allow the physician to use his or her relationship with the patient as a tool for healing through concern. Even brief accounts, such as notes, can be valuable. When a physician shares his or her written notes with a patient, the individual can get a glimpse of the physician's personal reactions to his or her story. This technique has been valuable in helping patients feel understood, valued, and joined in their struggle against disease (Charon, 2001).

When physicians do not have the time to conduct the types of interviews envisioned in a narrative approach, a patient can still feel better understood if other personnel, such as trained volunteers, conduct the interview and write it as a short story for the physician (Heifetz, 2003). By exploring the existence and intensity of symptoms, the trouble is placed in the context of the person's life and the way he or she is experiencing his or her suffering. Obviously confidentiality issues would have to be resolved and the patient would need to have the ability to review the story before it went to the physician. Reading a story is not the same as hearing it from the teller's lips, but it is a good deal quicker and, hence, is more feasible.

## Adults Who Struggle Against Physical Challenges

Johansen (2002) and Nochi (1988) employ a narrative perspective to depict the journey involved in standing up to acquired brain injury. These individuals, who both experienced severe brain injury, had to change their former identity and (re)discover a new identity in order to find the motivation to continue in the long, arduous rehabilitation process.

Hogan (1999) describes the use of a form of narrative treatment to help a male patient who experienced a brain injury that limited his verbal skills and placed him under the influence of aggression. The patient's aggression seemed to arise from his frustration at being unable to communicate. Hogan would write down all that the patient said and then read the notes back to him the next day, giving him a voice to tell his story. Aggression became less a part of the patient's life, and he was able to become more involved in rehabilitative efforts.

Hogan (1999) notes that narrative work with people standing up to severe disabilities can lead to coauthoring stories instructive in "the value for all of us slowing down, recognizing our interdependence, and growing emotionally through accepting loss as a part of life" (p. 24). Earlier, when considering taking-it-back practices, I discussed how clients' stories can impact practitioners' lives. Hogan's work suggests that posttraumatic growth perhaps can occur vicariously, that social workers can be transformed by the struggles of clients who are standing up to the consequences of their particular trauma.

## Narrating and Populating the World of Elders

The social discourse about aging is one in which growing older is seen essentially as a medical condition, a deficiency. Because many older adults are not employed, they are seen as less productive and less valuable. In the United States, elders are seen not as having wisdom to provide, but as being used up, as a potential drain on resources that could be better used for other purposes. When aging is considered a stage of life, the aged compete against other age-defined populations for resources. It is not uncommon to hear this tension posed in the form of a question, such as: Should society invest in adolescents or in the aged? The dominant culture has appropriated an investment metaphor for distributional decisions that are made within a zero-sum framework, thus rationalizing the view that resources are better spent on younger, more productive members.

The medicalization of problems disguises the impact of ageism, poverty, and a shortage of safe, low-income housing. Rather than a social problem, the difficulties facing older adults are interpreted as individual medical ones. Social workers who do hospital discharge planning for the elderly are well aware of the impact that resources and social conditions have on the prevention of disease and the maintenance of health. Discharging a 75-year-old woman with complications from severe diabetes directly from a hospital cardiac unit to an apartment in a neighborhood with a high crime rate where she will have little family contact and only periodic visiting nurse's care is an ethical struggle that hospital social workers frequently face.

Social workers are not immune to these societal discourses about aging. Research conducted in the 1980s by Gantz and Pearson (1988) indicates that helping professionals have their own stereotypes about older adults. They found helping professionals thought older people were less talkative and less amenable to "talk therapies." As a result, much of elders' "aberrant" behavior is attributed to organic causes, and drug therapy becomes the treatment of choice. Despite elders enduring losses of family members, friends, and status, and having to find ways to adjust to those losses, they are commonly portrayed as rigid and unwilling to make changes. This story about elders being "rigid" can lead to their being identified as "reluctant" clients, who, in turn, are provided fewer social work services.

The message that "old is bad" is part of workers' cultural background in the United States. The dominant culture shapes us in the very language we use. Think of how many negative adjectives are associated with aging compared to how few positive ones there are. An attitude that aging is good goes against the dominant culture's messages and requires strong protest.

Work with older adults requires certain skills and understandings. Knowledge of community resources is critical, as is a willingness to engage family members, when they are available. Identification and coordination of services can make an important difference in outcome. Office treatment with elders can be very challenging, especially for those who have physical ailments or memory difficulties. In-home sessions may be the only viable option.

Grimm, Maki, and Morales-Long (1995) note that death, loss, and pain are inevitable issues when working with older adults. They say social workers need to examine their own beliefs in these areas in order to remain open to and curious about elders' ways of coping. These are difficult stories that go to the core of human experience and are often cut off because they are not easy to listen to.

A narrative approach to clinical practice in the field of aging requires social workers to not accept societal biases about elders; it demands that workers be willing to question themselves about what beliefs trigger these biases, how they are learned, and what can be done to protest against them. As part of this, social workers can reacquire optimism, which is not often associated with working with older adults.

Externalization is a little different when working with elders and with those who are chronically or mortally ill. When problems are externalized in order to gain power over them, to fight them, to challenge their influence, and to protest against them, such metaphors may lack meaning against chronic or deteriorating conditions. There are problems elders may need to learn to live with and will not be able to fight and defeat. They have to develop a different sort of relationship to the problem, a relationship where they are living in spite of the problem (Grimm et al., 1995).

Grimm et al. (1995) have developed some questions to illustrate this point:

- "What ideas do you have about your own health care, that the doctors may not know about?" (p. 11). This question brings out the special knowledge a person may have despite feeling disempowered by the medical system.

- "You discussed how you feel overwhelmed with your pain. Are there times or moments when you've gained control over life such that the pain seems secondary to your choices?" (p. 11). This question to sufferers of chronic pain helps people to think about their own techniques of coping with pain and opens up the possibility of their lives moving along despite the pain.

- "Your children have expressed that you're getting older and they want to take care of you, even though you state their choices for you are not pleasing to you and invite depression into your life. You've also said you feel obligated to follow their wishes, rather than explore your own wishes. What ideas do you feel exist in our society that tell someone that just because they are older, they no longer are qualified to make good choices for their lives?" (p. 11). This question attempts to draw out the assumptions behind certain decisions, such as when a placement feels too early to an elder, but the elder feels he or she cannot trust his or her own judgment.

- "I was wondering how life might be different for you if instead of seeing a life of dying, you saw a life which is living with the process of dying" (p. 11). Here the focus is on helping a terminally ill patient begin to get a small degree of distance to reflect after a period of disorganization.

Maintaining or renewing a community can be very difficult for older adults because of the death of relatives, friends, and peers; the mobility of adult children; and possible restrictions on older adults' activities. Letter-writing campaigns, in which a person lets the members of his or her community know what each has meant, can be one way to attempt to re-member one's life (Madigan, 1997). (See the exercise at the end of this chapter regarding the memory box for another way to do this.) Re-membering conversations can be another way to help elders feel less alone when the loss of community is a problem.

Every person's life is constituted by a myriad of interactions with others. These others can include living or deceased friends and family members, people who have been lost from contact, professionals who have taken a special interest in the person, and even former or current pets. This constellation of others constitutes a person's club of life (White, 1997). (I recently saw a decorative pillow that read, "Be the person your dog thinks you are." A high standard indeed!)

Exploring with an elder those others, both living and deceased, who are in his or her club of life can develop what this membership looks like as well as what gaps exist in it. In conversation, people can adjust the status of their club members, elevating those who support a preferred lifestyle and downgrading those who diminish it. In this way, older adults can determine whose voices, or which portions of people's voices, they hear in defining their identity and whose no longer are authorized to speak to them on certain matters.

One person can, in fact, create distinct voices in the life of another. For example, a specific voice from a person can be privileged over another, more negative voice from that person:

**Mrs. J. (an 80-year-old who, according to her doctor, may be depressed):** *Well, my husband, when he was drinking, would just call me all these names, things he really didn't mean. When he died he apologized, but those names—"lazy," "useless," "bitch"—still ring in my head when I am alone.*

**Worker:** So there were times when your husband was drunk that he would call you names, and sometimes his voice sticks with you. That can be painful. Did he call you things other than those angry names? *(Separating different voices of a single club member)*

**Mrs. J.:** *Well, he used to call me sweetheart a lot and honey.*

**Worker:** *Did he mean those words, that you were a sweetheart and a honey to him?* (Exploring the significance of the labels)

**Mrs. J.:** *Yes, he actually did love me. He turned nasty with the drinking.*

**Worker:** *What did he see in you that led him to think of you as a honey or sweetheart?*

**Mrs. J.:** *Well, I think I was a good wife. I was there for him when he wasn't drinking. We went through a lot together.*

**Worker:** *Can you give me a specific example?* (Thickening the alternative story)

**Mrs. J.:** *Well, I remember one time when there was talk of lay-offs at his plant and he was real worried about losing his job. I told him that everything would work out, that I would love him no matter what. I told him I would get a job if need be. I know he didn't want me to do that, but in a funny way I think it made him feel a little better. Anyway, things worked out and he didn't lose his job, but it was a hard spell.*

**Worker:** *Do you think the "honey/sweetheart" or the "lazy/useless/bitch" best represented how he felt in general about you?*

**Mrs. J.:** *His words were hurtful to me, but I think in general the nastiness was from the drinking, so I guess I'd say the honey part.*

**Worker:** *Which group of names better describes who you are?* (Beginning to explore a possible preferred outcome)

**Mrs. J.:** *I'd like to think that honey describes me better than bitch, but we did have our fights.*

**Worker:** *So being a "honey" person is positive to you?*

**Mrs. J.:** *Yes, of course!*

**Worker:** *Just to be clear, what about being a "honey" person makes it positive?*

**Mrs. J.:** *That person would be loving and lovable.*

**Worker:** *Okay. Because your husband is still very important to you in your heart, I wonder how you could stick with your husband's "honey" voice and downgrade his "bitch" voice?*

**Mrs. J.:** *I don't know.*

**Worker:** *Is there anyone who is currently treating you as if you were lazy, useless, or a bitch?* (Exploring if there are other members of her club who degrade her)

**Mrs. J.:** *What do you mean?*

**Worker:** I just wondered if anyone was disrespecting you and making it easier for you to remember your husband's negative voice?

**Mrs. J.:** *No, no one is.*

**Worker:** Okay, are there, or have there ever been, other people in your life who have seen the "honey" in you? *(Wondering who might be a more positive member of her club)*

**Mrs. J.:** *Let me think.*

According to Grimm (2003), "Many older adults have lost opportunities to perform a preferred story to a supportive audience because of deaths of significant people in their lives, poor health, poverty, ageism, and other social factors" (p. 265). It is important that the social worker explore the older adult's current community and social environment to see how they might be affecting the person's current mental state. Other factors that can impinge upon someone's functioning, such as physical abuse, financial exploitation, prescription drug abuse, and the like, should be explored, too. Following the internal story without exploring potential external constraints would place narrative treatment in the category of just one more individualistic psychological approach. As social workers, our profession's aspirations and commitments encompass both the individual and the environment and demand that we, as practitioners, attend to both.

The previous conversation continues:

**Mrs. J.:** *I think the biggest supporter in my life was my mother, but she's been gone for about 40 years now. I really miss her, even now. She could always find the good in me and I could always go to her.*

**Worker:** When you are hearing your husband's drunken voice, do you still ever go to her?

**Mrs. J.:** *What do you mean? She's dead.*

**Worker:** Is she still alive in you the way your husband is?

**Mrs. J.:** *I guess.*

**Worker:** How do you keep her memory alive?

**Mrs. J.:** *Sometimes on Mother's Day I think about her. And on her birthday. And also on the day she died. I will never forget that day.*

**Worker:** Yes, the last day is always there. I wonder, do you ever hear her voice in your memory?

**Mrs. J.:** *Only occasionally.*

**Worker:** If you asked your mother in your mind whether she thought you were, let's see, "lazy, useless, and a bitch," what would she say?

**Mrs. J.:** *I don't think I would ever ask her about that last name; I mean, I never would have said that word to my mother. But she would have said it was just baloney and I shouldn't let words like that get me down.*

**Worker:** What did she see in you that told her you were not all those names?

**Mrs. J.:** *She would say that she saw me as a caring, sensitive, and sometimes naive person.*

**Worker:** Can you think of a time with your mother when she said that or you did something that showed her that that was who you were?

Recalling conversations can reactivate old relationships by reengaging the older adult with others from his or her past. People can reexperience those relationships through conversation even if they cannot physically meet those people again. For the elder, discovering the relationship's "historical truth" is less important than reconnecting with those parts of the relationship that may be of value. Such conversations can act to re-member the elder's life—to repopulate it by having the presence of those lost or missing, either literally or figuratively, felt once again (Madigan, 1997). Re-membering conversations that focus heavily on both the detail and the meaning of each event to the client can help bring his or her experiences of the relationship into the present. Through these mechanisms, re-membering conversations can help elders retain their preferred stories (Grimm, 2003).

## Preparing for the "Final" Journey

The narrative approach has a unique perspective on the dying process. One task of people facing death is to be remembered, to have their stories carried on after they are gone. Here it is again important to consider the concept of membership in a club (Myerhoff, 1982; White, 1997). Recall that the idea of a club of life considers the network of a person's relationships to be a system in which the importance of each voice is defined either by culture or by the person exercising control and making choices that may challenge societal assumptions. Thus, for example, should the strategies that family members sometimes use to emotionally torment each other be given priority over the strategies of supporters? Similarly, parents, partners, and children are supposed to offer caring and trustworthiness; when they do not, should the person subjected to the betrayal be found at fault?

Narrative treatment, reflecting its emphasis on client strengths and empowerment practices, recognizes that club membership is not defined exclusively by kinship. Choosing the members of one's club and establishing a "charter" for the process of membership (White, 1997) provides a story in which the person has a voice and agency in determining his or her social support system. Selecting those individuals who will cherish, not denigrate, a person's stories on his or her death is an important task.

Membership in someone's club of life can be downgraded or eliminated as well as upgraded. When a club member is not available, the importance and repetition of his or her voice in the life of the person can be increased or diminished. This is a natural process of life that occurs all the time. In divorcing couples, it is not uncommon for the "left" spouse to have better continued relations than the "leaver" does with the leaver's extended family. Membership for the spouse who was left has stayed the same, but membership for the spouse who left is downgraded. In the same way, those confronting their mortality may reconfigure membership in their clubs of life as they face this final stage of life.

This view of membership allows the dying person to exercise control in his or her life. The experience of the AIDS crisis in the United States has shown how important this kind of choice can be. When the families of those dying of AIDS abandon them or are otherwise unavailable, these individuals with AIDS would die in conditions of scorn and self-regret if biology were the sole determinant of membership in their clubs of life. However, many find caring from partners, friends, and other caregivers, and it is these individuals who are the members of the dying person's club of life and who carry on his or her stories.

The common tasks said to face the dying, such as saying good-bye to family and friends, look solely at the impending loss rather than at what will live on. Focusing on which memories an individual wishes to have passed on and by whom is a very useful way to consider the dying process. Who keeps a person in memory and which stories are passed on are important decisions that the dying person faces (Hedtke & Winslade, 2004). Dying is a sad affair for most, partially because the sense of loss, of "seeing the future occur," is so poignant. This sadness often closes off people from having talks about death, although many, especially those who are dying, see such discussions as important. Considering what will live on is a way to broach the sadness, not run away from it. It provides an opportunity for the treasured parts of a person's life and acquired knowledge to be looked at; it allows the sadness to be experienced without the parties being so caught up in the loss that they withdraw from the conversation, because of either one's own or the other's distress.

Recognition of the person's continued relationship is comforting for all involved and can be an antidote to guilt over not seeking forgiveness, hearing someone's last words, or being with someone at the moment of death. It is lore among hospice workers of dying people's ability to "pass on" when those closest to them are out of the room. If possible, many would wish to spare their loved ones their death rattle. Those moments are just part of much bigger stories about how someone is remembered.

People can think over and then describe to loved ones, either in writing or, better, verbally, what about their life they would like to leave: What stories about who you are as a person would you like your family members to know? What wisdom or advice would you pass on? What have you found important in your life? A general life review can be undertaken with the purpose of creating a legacy for those who are living as well as for yet-to-be-born future generations (Garland, 1994). In addition, questions can be posed about the dying process itself, putting it into the relationship context.

Hedtke and Winslade (2004) offer the following questions:

> "What do you want your loved ones to say about how you approached death?"
>
> "What aspects of the way you have handled your illness will you want your loved ones to be proud of?"
>
> "How do you want the last part of your life to be recalled?"
>
> "How do you hope that the story of your death might help your loved ones when it is their turn to die? What lessons might there be for them here?"
>
> "How might you want your story told to the generations yet to come?" (p. 70)

These questions are future oriented and give the dying person the opportunity to consider such issues as legacy and connections with his or her present club as well as with members across the generations. Because this approach is language based, it becomes a problem when the person is unable to talk coherently or is in a coma. Here it is up to the club to come together and discuss stories of the person's life, hopefully in the dying individual's presence, as a way to pull together his or her legacy. As Hedtke and Winslade (2004) note in relation to persons experiencing loss of memory:

> If we assume that remembering is not an individual psychological process but one that happens in relationship, then we can take up the

task of remembering on behalf of someone who is struggling to do so, just as we help push others in wheelchairs when they cannot be completely in charge of their own locomotion. Remembering conversations can serve as the function of reincorporating a person's thoughts, feelings, stories, and presence into their communities, even when they are struggling to achieve this on their own behalf. (p. 114)

Hedtke (2002) provides a nice example of this sort of work. She met with a man who had struggled with depression all his life, a story that in and of itself would not likely be of much value to his estranged son. Hedtke reports:

I asked him what was the story that his son did not know about him that would help guide his son when he too faced challenges. How had the father been courageous in facing these times when depression had tried to get the best of him? How might he hope that his son would describe his father as he faced what lay ahead with his illness? (p. 291)

The focus of Hedtke's questions was on agency and strength. The depression-influenced stories were real, but so, too, were other stories that might be of help to and cherished by his son. Yet, without probing, these other stories were not visible under depression's veil.

## Keeping a Place at the Table

Modern grief theory focuses on the idea of closure, of getting beyond the loss of a loved one, of coping better. This is a problem because it implies a specific period of time that grief can be allowed, although this view may complement well the often limited bereavement leave available from employers. The implied time period for grieving (be it 2 months or 6 months) can cause people whose grief extends beyond that point to be labeled as having "complicated grief reactions." But delimiting time in this fashion is arbitrary, an artifact of our culture.

I was brought up in the Portuguese American culture. When I was growing up, widows generally wore black until they either remarried or died themselves. Grieving was a lifelong process.

Seeing the dead, talking to them, consulting them on important decisions, as well as leaving a place setting for them at the table or celebrating their birthdays, are acts of remembering. These acts, however, are looked down upon and are not discussed for fear of appearing irrational, given this country's dominant cultural definitions. Taking the stories of the past and incorporating the wisdom of the dead into current relationships is not an easy thing to do and often is seen as a quaint, anachronistic practice when it is done, rather than as an act of remembrance.

Workers can encourage such remembering by recognizing that these practices are common (though not usually publicly discussed) and play an important part in allowing the living to remember the person who died. Social workers can sensitively inquire about how the dead person continues in someone's life and how the deceased would want to be remembered. Sorting out which stories would be most helpful in keeping the person's memory alive and whom they should be told to can be important, although often overlooked, aspects of grief therapy.

Not all deaths are heroic in the eyes of society and not all relationships benefit the living by remembering. Survivors can experience a range of emotions in situations in which the death was a true relief or was not "acceptable" (e.g., due to suicide or to a disease or condition that has been stigmatized, such as AIDS or drug abuse), the relationship was one of unmitigated abuse, or the survivor feels (or is) responsible for the death.

Where remembrance of a "should-be loved" one brings up only memories of abuse, part of a person's task is to forgive himself or herself for hating the person and, if possible, to look at what was gained in the relationship. For example, how has the abuse made the survivor more sensitive to protecting himself or herself? Harder and tougher against life's struggles? Willing to rely on himself or herself? How have all these things benefited as well as weakened the person? What worldview has the dead person left and where does the survivor stand in relationship to that perspective? Were there also times when the deceased was not abusive? How does the person who is left make sense of this and what did he or she learn from it?

When a person dies under "tainted" circumstances, the challenge is to see the suicide, drunk-driving death, or overdose, for example, as only one part of the individual's story. What other stories about the person are available and worth extending? How can the suicide or overdose be seen in the context of the person's whole life?

Another problem is when no one attends a funeral. The assumption is that a person does not amount to much if no one attends the service. However, without progeny and when one has outlived friends and family or when they are all too frail to attend, this assumption would be wrong. The narrative approach allows workers to more easily express their own reactions and what they have learned from clients, and to help the deceased's memory be carried on in this way.

Hedtke and Winslade (2004) give this example:

> One minister told of how he preached a sermon to an audience of one—the deceased's spouse. As he was planning the service, he interviewed her and learned of the strong love that grew in their 60-year marriage. Their only child had been killed many years before and they had outlived most of their friends. Like the minister's father, the deceased man had worked as a carpenter.
>
> During the funeral, the minister read scripture and sang a hymn and then sat with this man's widow. He shared with her what it meant to him to be introduced to her husband. Even though they had only met after this man's death, he was certain that he learned a lot from this man. He recalled special times with his own father. . . . he made the occasion meaningful by affirming the dead man's membership for her and by offering to carry forward his membership in his own life. (p. 122)

Current grief theory is focused on loss and moving the survivor to resolution. Looking at condolence cards is a good way to see society's current discourse on death. Compare the usual condolence card message with this one, which is from a card given to a client of Hedtke's (2002):

> I recall years ago we were all together for a New Year's Eve celebration. Your husband asked you to dance and as he did so he bent over to kiss you. From across the table, I was moved to tears as this moment between you was so love-filled. (p. 289)

This is not a message that says move on, but instead appreciates the relationship between the couple and honors it. The card stirred up a conversation about the client's deceased husband's loving relationship with her and how they might have been a model for others. This is an appreciation message, a message to carry a relationship on in life despite the death of one of the partners.

# Exercises

### Exercise 1: Talking About Those We've Lost

Lorraine Hedtke, an expert on how narrative methods can be applied to issues associated with death and grieving, has developed an exercise to help students experience this different approach. This exercise, which comes from a 2004 workshop conducted by Hedtke and used with her permission, can provide people with a sense of what it means to notice how relationships continue to live on following the death of a person.

Start with students dividing into pairs. Each person will talk about someone he or she knew who has died. Given that this exercise is a teaching tool, a student may not wish to discuss someone for whom he or she still has very raw feelings. The student to go first will discuss the following (for about 15 minutes):

> Introduce him or her (the person who has died) to your partner.
>
> Who was this person to you at the time of his or her death?
>
> How has his or her relationship with you continued? What has it meant to have the person as part of your club of life?
>
> How would you like the person's connection with you and with others in your life to grow in the coming years?

The listener will then respond to the following questions (about 10 minutes):

> Acknowledge your partner's connection to the person who has died.
>
> Share what it has meant to you to hear of this relationship—how have you been touched or moved?
>
> What aspects of the stories link to connections and moments in your life?
>
> How will being introduced to this person affect your life?
>
> How do you hope this way of thinking will affect your work and your life?

The introducer will then discuss the following (about 5 minutes):

> Of the things you discussed about your loved one, what surprises have there been? What has caught your interest?

The students should now switch roles and repeat the exercise.

For more information about Hedtke's approach, see www.remembering-practices.com.

## Exercise 2: Deciding Which Stories to Pass on and Who Should Pass Them On

Few of us in Western culture look forward to dying, despite our religious beliefs. Some worry a lot about the dependency that illness can bring and the burden that it might cause others. Some may feel that they did not accomplish what they had hoped for in life or that they are somehow letting down those who depended on them. One way to assist people in facing their mortality is to help them consider who in their clubs of life they would want to carry on their stories and which stories they would want carried on.

Break into pairs. Decide which of you will go first and have that person answer the following questions (about 15 minutes):

> If you were to face your mortality head-on, what stories about you would you like told? (This would be more than just an obituary with generalities; think about the specific stories you would like told about you and your life as a whole.)
>
> Who would you bequeath these specific stories to? Why?
>
> If you told these stories to the person (people) to whom you want to give them, might this in any way change your relationship with that individual (those people)?

For the next 10 minutes, have the listener respond to the following questions:

> Share what it has meant to you to hear these stories—how have you been touched or moved?
>
> What aspects of the stories link to events or moments in your life?
>
> Now that you have listened to these stories and heard about whom they will be passed on to, how will this affect your life? How you practice as a social worker?
>
> Switch roles and repeat the exercise.

## Exercise 3: The Memory Box

An alternative method of generating stories is through mutual prompts. In pairs, select from the following list one prompt that you both would be willing to discuss:

1. Supper at grandma's house
2. First day at school
3. Your child's first day at school
4. A special birthday
5. A special Halloween
6. The first day of your first job

Spend 15 minutes describing the event. If the teller seems to have exhausted his or her memory of the story, the listener is to ask questions to more fully re-create the event. The listener can ask about who might have been there at the time, what people were wearing, the color and design of the rooms, the level of sound, whose voice was most recognizable, and so on. These types of questions may help the teller become more in tune with the event in his or her memory and may set off further recollections of the event. After the teller has completed his or her description of the event, the listener will then talk about what it has meant for him or her to hear the story.

Reverse roles, so that the former listener is now the teller. He or she will launch into a story of a similar event in his or her life and the listener will ask the kinds of questions previously suggested. At the end of 15 minutes, the listener will tell the teller what it has meant to him or her to listen to the story.

This exercise is called a memory box because it is based on a practice arising from an AIDS project among the poor in South Africa. As originally developed, excerpts of a dying person's stories were written down and placed in a personally decorated box. The person afflicted with AIDS would designate who should receive the box, and after he or she died, the box would be handed down as a legacy to the people chosen to receive it. The person's stories thus become these people's inheritance, something that may be particularly precious because the deceased may have had few, if any, material possessions to leave.

CHAPTER 13

# Narrative Approaches to Mental Health and Substance Abuse

Current discourses in the field of mental health about the advent of new medications, evidence-based treatment technologies, and the efficacy of intensive community-based mental and behavioral health services, for example, suggest we are well on our way to a mentally healthier society. But are we?

I have already discussed postmodern concerns about diagnostic schemes such as the DSM and have noted how a mental illness label (or diagnosis) can act to define the entirety of who a person is. In this chapter, I examine how narrative methods allow social workers not only to respond to the needs of people under the influence of mental health and substance abuse problems, but to do so in an innovative fashion that honors and respects those who seek our assistance.

Many clusters of behaviors are categorized as mental illnesses, and an entire separate book could be written about the topics of mental health, mental illness, and narrative treatment. Here, I explore how a narrative approach is used to help people take a stand against voices (auditory hallucinations), eating disorders, trauma, and substance misuse. I offer general explanations of the narrative methods used to deal with these four specific problems. Although clearly not exhaustive, these descriptions provide beginning social work practitioners with insight into the ways that mental health and substance misuse issues can be approached from a narrative perspective.

## The DSM and Thin Stories

Narrative workers, like family therapists before them, have taken a dim view of diagnostic categories that center mental health or mental illness solely in an individual's psyche or neurobiology. A medical diagnosis, consisting of a cluster of behavioral symptoms identified as a disorder, takes problems out of their social context and makes them a disease of the individual. From a narrative perspective, there are two major objections to the DSM: the implied ownership of the problem by the person, and the potential for "totalizing" descriptions of people once they are fit into a particular category.

In an instance described by Simblett (1997), for example, a young woman who had left a psychiatric hospital against the advice of her doctors depicted herself as a tiger with nine lives. She talked about how various events, including her hospitalization and treatment, each took away a life, leaving her tiger self with few remaining lives. For her, the psychiatric hospitalization was an acute indignity that diminished her.

Perhaps an even more telling example is the story of a man who was diagnosed as having schizophrenia. Earlier in his life, this man had studied art. He recounted the story of an event from his education when one of his art teachers held up a white canvas with a black dot in the center and asked the class to describe what they saw. The students, he said, all replied that they saw a black dot. The instructor then pointed out they had missed the rest of the canvas, the white part. The man described his life experience as being seen as only the black dot—as the schizophrenic. He said he had even come to believe that that was all he was (Stockell & O'Neill, 2001).

A final example: It is commonly known that psychiatric histories are scrutinized carefully before a political party will put forth a candidate. Yet, about 30 years ago, a presidential campaign was nearly scuttled when it was discovered that the vice presidential candidate had an undisclosed history of depression and electroconvulsive therapy. The candidate was forced to leave the campaign, despite his successful career as a respected senator. For many, what this individual once experienced continued to define him years afterward.

In all these cases, the people who were diagnosed received a label that affected how others saw them and, to a greater or lesser extent, how they saw themselves. A richer description of people would include not only the "black dot" of the diagnosis but also the wider canvas of their thoughts, skills, knowledge, values, and commitments that are not encompassed in the diagnosis.

Students preparing for clinical social work devote much time to learning DSM categories and to gaining skills in applying and interpreting the psychiatric diagnoses suggested by those categories. It is important for students to consider the power that diagnosing gives to them and the influence it has on their relationship with their clients. Unlike a broken leg, strep throat, or diabetes, psychiatric diagnoses still carry a social stigma that can harm the person diagnosed. Diagnosing implies that the social worker's knowledge of what is going on is truth, and the client's knowledge is either an expression of confusion or a symptom.

A balance is appropriate here; for some people, the diagnostic label can provide a way to characterize the problem that has been externalized and the diagnosis is not an all-encompassing description of identity (Wetchler, 1999). A person can stand up to depression yet not be a depressive. Whenever possible it is preferable to use the client's words for the problem, especially if they are different from the medical terminology.

An additional caution is warranted here: Where the diagnostic label includes the term *chronic*, it is almost always totalizing. Madigan (1998a) describes an older man who had made two suicide attempts and who spent nearly a year in an institution undergoing not only medication trials but also extensive electroconvulsive shock treatments. The interventions had little positive effect. The man identified his problems as boredom and a sense of having accomplished little since his retirement. These became the named problems, not the chronic depression named by the hospital staff. By allowing him to name the problems he was experiencing, his expertise was given priority over the professionals' view of the problem.

## How Medication Fits Into the Story

On one level, medical science and new research on neurobiology have produced numerous chemical agents that have reduced the symptomatology of hundreds of thousands, if not millions, of people. However, even the new atypical antipsychotic medications have side effects. In one investigation, these side effects were severe enough that 74% of a sample of nearly 1,500 patients discontinued their medication use within the first 18 months (Lieberman et al., 2005). And there is some suggestion that placebos compare favorably with the much-touted selective serotonin reuptake inhibitors (such as the ubiquitous medication Prozac) in the reduction of depressive symptomatology (Taylor & Stein, 2006).

Although not ultimately the answer, medication can reduce many people's suffering. Again, a balance needs to be struck between antidiagnosis/antimedication and prodiagnosis/probiological treatment perspectives. Medication can be a tool, but not the sole answer for people's troubles.

## Living With Voices

One important area of mental health–related problems is "voice hearing," or auditory hallucinations. The experience of hearing voices that apparently come from outside the body can be frightening and disconcerting. However, it is not so for everyone, and there is evidence that the relationship between the voice hearer and the voice is as important as what the voice says (Vaughan & Fowler, 2004). When people feel that the voice is in control, they then suffer distress.

Pioneering clinical work in this area comes from the United Kingdom and the Netherlands. Professionals in these two countries are developing nontraditional ways of working with people who have auditory hallucinations. Rather than viewing them as just a serious symptom of a psychiatric disorder, these professionals consider voices as a subjective experience that can be worked with. Information about voice hearers and networks of support for people who hear voices is available online. A good initial source of information is http://www.intervoiceonline.org

Not all people who hear voices are psychotic. Many individuals report hearing their name called by a newly deceased loved one, for example. It even has been suggested that some of the behaviors seen in schizophrenia, such as the inability to make decisions and the isolation, might be coping reactions to the voices, in which case the symptom might cause the illness instead of vice versa (Romme, 1998).

Clients who hear voices identify as important having groups in which they can talk without feeling stigmatized, writing documents that can be reviewed when the voices get strong, and using objects that can remind them of their unity with others when they are standing against ridiculing voices (Sue, Mem, & Veronica, 1999). Keeping clients in control of their treatment appears to help them have the confidence to stand up to the voices. In a group for people with long histories of psychiatric hospitalizations, for example, clients were encouraged to create rules about how the group should operate. Having their expertise recognized and honored seems to have positively influenced the clients' ability to share their knowledge and skills with each other in standing up not only to voices, but also to stigma, a mechanistic public health system, and isolation (Vassallo, 2002).

## Lies That Depression and Anxiety Can Tell People

As is well known in cognitive behavioral research, what people tell themselves can affect or modify their mood. The narrative perspective adds to this assumption and takes it further. Narrative treatment actively supports clients' control of their thinking and opens up space for them to consider broader interpretations of their lives, interpretations that emphasize hopefulness and condone imperfection. Even where medication is used as a response to symptoms, placing the symptoms in the broader context of clients' lives should help them cope better with the problem over the long term.

By looking at cultural discourses that might be influencing the continuation of the problem, the client is helped to see both where these negative messages are reinforced in the present and where there are sources of positive messages in his or her life. Madigan's (1998a) work with the retired man who had made previous suicide attempts, for instance, could lead one to ask: What messages do people who are entering retirement get that would reinforce their feeling a lack of accomplishment? In a similar vein, one could raise the question: What messages do Japanese students get that would encourage them to suicide when they find out that their college entrance exam results were not what they hoped them to be? Or, the question could be posed: What messages do women get that would encourage them to feel responsible for having experienced physical or sexual abuse?

Our society emphasizes individual economic success as a measure of identity and self-worth. Given this societal orientation, if a person is not rich, is it because he or she has a "poor" mentality? If someone is not achieving excellence or has not been more productive, then the fault must, of course, lie with the individual. It should not be surprising that the psychiatric disorders most closely related to societal discourse are eating disorders, which affect primarily young women influenced by Western standards of beauty and success.

## Struggles Against Eating Disorders

Eating disorders, including anorexia nervosa (self-starvation) and bulimia (purging cycles), have been of particular interest to narrative workers. Eating disorders draw strength from cultural standards of attractiveness and desirability; they target and dominate mostly girls and women through isolation, continual self-evaluation, and the promotion of a lack of entitlement (Zimmerman & Dickerson, 1994). The messages women get through media, friends, and sometimes family are that if you are not thin, you do not deserve to be loved, and the thinner you are, the more lovable you are. As an old quip reminds us: You can never be too rich or too thin. (Although men are not immune from eating disorders, the vast majority of people struggling with these problems are women and the majority of the literature discusses female clients. I, too, focus on women's experiences and use feminine pronouns in this discussion.)

Eating disorders require continual attention to detail, which can preoccupy those experiencing the disorder. At the same time, the changes in appearance from anorexia serve to ward off close relationships. The result is isolation. The person does not seek connection with supportive members of her club of life, and these individuals eventually give up trying to offer support in the face of the person's apparently illogical and sometimes suicidal behavior.

An eating disorder requires a woman under its influence to continually compare herself to others and find herself wanting. Self-evaluation captures her thoughts continuously. She sees herself as having little value and finds what value she has in her ability to control her body. A woman under the control of an eating disorder is not entitled to self-respect or a sense of accomplishment. It is particularly important, therefore, that therapeutic practices not replicate the power tactics of the problem.

In a narrative approach the client is helped to see the impact of the eating disorder on different areas of her life and the relationships she has with others; she is also helped to look at what the eating disorder tells her about herself. Externalizing questions can take the focus away from the perceived failures of the client and place it instead on the strength of the problem and its influence on her. These sorts of questions help to put a wedge between the client and the eating disorder. To rephrase Michael White's famous dictum about problems, clients are not the eating disorder; the eating disorder is the eating disorder.

Following are examples of helpful questions:

- How does anorexia convince you that you are not worthy of love?
- How does it manage to slowly kill, all the while telling you that it is your savior?
- What are its tricks?
- What are its allies in taking control of your life?
- How does it hide its true intent from you, its target?
- What about you does it not want you to see?
- How does it hide your true strengths from you and get you to believe you are weak?

It is through the struggle against anorexia that some of narrative workers' most powerful techniques to create community have been developed, such as letter-writing campaigns (Madigan, 1997), leagues (Grieves, 1998), and archives (Archive of Resistance, 2000).

## Lives Ruled by Trauma

People subject to trauma can experience some relief in the telling of their story, though they need to control how, when, where, and with whom this happens. When people are pressured to tell their stories of trauma before they are ready, as is seen in some debriefing programs for emergency first responders, they can experience further pain and their coping abilities can be further compromised. Trauma takes away people's sense of an independent self and leaves them feeling vulnerable to upsets triggered by cues from the surrounding world.

The self that is read in the story of someone who has experienced trauma is one that emphasizes brokenness and in some cases, as with abuse, badness. Stories of victimhood reduce people's sense of agency. Such stories can reinforce people's sense of helplessness in the world, and this sense of helplessness can become hardwired with changes in brain chemistry. Individuals subject to trauma may engage in inner dialogues in which they demean themselves; they can begin to experience others as being more in control of them than they are of themselves. These are the voices of abuse and the abusers.

People exposed to trauma can find themselves living out victim stories and can become involved in interactions that reinforce this view of themselves. The intense emotional and perceptual experiences involved in trauma stories can short-circuit a person's typical narrative. If asked to express his or her experience of self, someone who has experienced trauma might say: "I'm not the person I once was" (Neimeyer & Stewart, 1998, p. 168) or I have lost my "sense of myself" (White, 2006c, p. 26).

From a narrative perspective, trauma and its aftermath can best be reduced through a restorying of the incident to focus on the client's agency as a survivor. The social worker and client can work together to help the client access his or her internal knowledge and skills and external supports to challenge the oppressive story of being completely vulnerable, broken, bad, or guilty. The worker would try to coconstruct with the client a future that has more alternatives than the past. "Disempowering stories are maintained by restraints that prevent people from noticing exceptions to their constrained descriptions of self" (Adams-Westcott, Dafforn, & Sterne, 1993, p. 262).

Clients experience their own agency as they begin to separate from and reflect on disempowering or disqualifying self-stories, and they can then begin to challenge those destructive self-stories. This, in turn, allows them to reconnect with what they think, rather than what others have told them (Adams-Westcott et al., 1993). They have the opportunity to see how their lives over time became increasingly restricted as the disqualifying beliefs gained more and more influence.

As people begin to escape the grip of the disqualifying stories, they can begin looking at alternative stories of competence (i.e., How have you done so well despite . . . ?). Clients' sense of agency can be further extended by questioning them about how these alternative stories might lead them to change their relationship to themselves (i.e., How will they treat themselves differently given their growing recognition of their competence?). Adams-Westcott and colleagues (1993), for instance, describe asking a woman who experienced trauma as a child to consider what it would have been like if at that earlier time there had been an adult like herself available. To draw out and develop this alternative story, they posed the following questions

- How would her future have been different if, during her latency years, she would have had herself as a parent?
- What would that 7-year-old have appreciated about her as a parent?
- Would the child have trust in her ability to protect her from further abuse? What about her would help the child know this?
- What qualities would that 7-year-old appreciate about her as a person?
- How would her awareness of the experience of this 7-year-old make a difference in how she pictured herself? What difference would it make in how she treated herself? (p. 269)

If a client relapses into panic and fear, then the relapse should be brought into perspective within the context of the individual's entire life story.

I focus in the rest of this section on White's (2006c) work in the area of trauma and describe a case he presents to illustrate his approach. White begins by discussing "double-listening" to trauma stories, which entails a worker attending not only to a client's suffering but also to "what the person has continued to give value to despite all that they have been through" (p. 28). White believes that the continued pain and suffering caused by trauma are evidence that something quite important to the person has been taken away. Without those things people hold dear to them—their beliefs, values, hopes, and dreams—they lose their sense of self. Recovering that story of self, therefore, is an important therapeutic task, one that places clients in a less vulnerable position, allowing them to discuss the trauma without retraumatization. All people in their own way attempt to defend themselves against trauma, and the stories of their response to the trauma are often even more hidden than the trauma stories themselves. Double-listening requires listening for what is "absent but implicit" (White, 2006a, p. 153).

White's concept of "absent but implicit" goes to the heart of what double-listening is. Every experience in life can be described not just by what it is but also by what it is not. Describing yourself as "sad" means you also are describing yourself as "not happy" or "not joyful," as not having happiness or joy in your life at the moment. Feeling "damaged" by trauma means that something has been taken from you, that you are not whole; the more upset you are, the more precious that something is. White (2006a) provides some examples of what those precious things might be:

(a) cherished purposes for one's life;

(b) prized values and beliefs around acceptance, justice and fairness;

(c) treasured aspirations, hopes and dreams;

(d) moral visions about how things might be in the world;

(e) significant pledges, vows and commitments about ways of being in life; etc. (p. 154)

From this perspective, ongoing emotional distress represents a tribute to the person's ability to maintain a relationship with what is held precious but has been violated, and what is held precious shapes the person's response to the trauma (White, 2006a). The pain can also represent a legacy, as people will or cannot forget despite what the environment might be telling them. Having gone through trauma, the pain of it opens individuals up to compassion for others with similar experiences, which, in turn, can lead to connection. Understanding trauma in this way does not lead to denying the existence of great suffering; rather, it identifies it with a noble meaning upon which the self can be reconstituted.

White (2006c) provides an extended story of his trauma work with a woman identified by others as having a "borderline personality disorder"

(p. 31). The woman had a history of abusive relationships and was engaged in self-cutting behavior. At the time of the consultation, she was living once more at the local women's shelter, having again left an abusive relationship.

With the client's permission, White invited two of the shelter workers who knew her best to attend the session to act as "outsider-witnesses" (White, 2006c, p. 33). As such, they listened carefully to the interview and afterward in the client's presence responded to questions from White.

As the woman talked about the array of hardships and traumas she struggled with, she described no sense of agency and talked about herself only as the passive recipient of pain. However, one example she gave led White to wonder if there was something different about it. She mentioned seeing a child run down by a car and described herself as having been paralyzed by what she saw. In contrast to her own response, she said, other bystanders rushed to assist.

White (2006c) returned to this story later in the interview, asking the woman:

> When you were telling the story of the child being injured by a motor car, I sensed an expression of some significant feelings. Was this about relief that there were people present who were able to attend to the child, or was it about shame that you were unable to attend to the child yourself, or were these feelings about something else? (p. 32)

She replied that although she had not considered it before, it was probably shame, which upon further questioning was revealed to be quite severe.

White then proceeded to question her about why that event incurred such shame. She replied, "Can't you see . . . there isn't anything in life that's worth much, but a child's life, that's different" (White, 2006c, p. 32). From that statement began a story of a woman who not only was miserable and beaten down but also cherished the lives of children.

White then used the two workers as a reflecting team and interviewed them in the client's presence. He inquired about the impact of the interview on them as people, not merely professionals. He asked what caught their attention in what the client said; they noted that she treasured children. He then asked how this new information influenced their view of the client or perhaps what she stood for in life, why this new information struck a personal chord or resonated for them as people, and what changes or movement in their own lives might be stimulated by this revelation. White carefully formatted his questions to discourage advice giving, praise, or negative labeling by the observing shelter workers.

White then turned back to the client and asked her these same questions in reaction to what she heard from the observers, thus enriching the story further. The client described the session as "like coming out of hibernation" (White, 2006c, p. 43).

White began the second session by recapping the client's reactions to the workers' observations. He then said, "I became curious about the sorts of stories you might be able to tell me about your life when you were younger that would reflect the high value you give to children's lives" (White, 2006c, p. 60). The client said she could not think of any. White noted that she had a younger brother and sister and wondered what stories they might tell that indicated this value in her.

In response to White's comments and questions, the woman recounted a remarkable story of how as a 9- or 10-year-old she found a hiding place in some nearby woods that she stocked with food, water, and games. When her father became drunk, the precursor to abuse, she would take her younger siblings to the hiding place and bring them back only when she believed her father had passed out. When asked about what meaning her siblings might attach to this behavior, she indicated that they would see her as standing for fairness and against injustice.

With further questioning the client was able to see how she was taking these stands even in the present, by, for example, befriending an isolated woman at the shelter. She also came to realize that these were important values that she continued to try to live by despite her history of trauma. These interviews began with a client in despair and experiencing emptiness; they ended with her beginning to recognize that she had a "self" of value, in contradiction to her history of trauma and abuse and her psychiatric label.

## The Stories Around Substances

The abuse, or more accurately misuse, of legal and illegal substances is a widespread problem in the United States, one that can disguise the impacts of inequalities due to poverty, class, race, and gender (Raven, 1997). Substance use and abuse is associated with being a man in some subcultures, where it is said that real men can hold their liquor and will not shy away from doing drugs with their friends, or risk being viewed with suspicion by their peers if they do not drink or take drugs (Smith & Winslade, 1997). Substance misuse is also reflective of a culture of consumption, where pressure to consume to achieve the "good life" underlies much alcohol or tobacco advertising.

There are many cultural pressures to drink, and in some subcultures to use other substances, perhaps to the point where asking what keeps people from being troubled drinkers is a more appropriate question than asking why people cannot leave alcohol (White, 2004). For many people, their stories of pain and suffering are interwoven with their stories of substance misuse and both need to be externalized (Callahan, 2001).

Narrative workers have displayed both supportive (White, 2004) and dismissive (Sanders, 1998) attitudes toward 12-step recovery programs. Narrative workers appreciate the nonjudgmental character of Alcoholics Anonymous (AA) and Narcotics Anonymous as well as their ability to forge new identities through disclosure narratives. At the same time, some narrative practitioners are concerned about 12-step programs' adherence to a disease model that locates the problem firmly within the individual. Sanders (1997), who works with young people whose sense of themselves has been shaped by their involvement with AA, tries to draw out the stories of these youths' identities by asking the following sorts of questions:

- Who helped you begin to think of yourself as an "alcoholic" and/or "addict?"
- What meaning is there in these words for an understanding of your life?
- Do you imagine this to be hereditary identity, or did some members of your (extended) family refuse this identity?
- Do others in your life know you as an "alcoholic/addict," or as someone else?

...

- Do you have other intentions for the paths your life could take? (p. 405)

Through these questions, Sanders (1997) attempts to give these young people the space to consider identities other than the addiction-based problem one they have had.

Before looking in more depth at the narrative practices employed in this area, I wish to acknowledge a criticism made about using a narrative approach with individuals who misuse substances, which is that by externalizing alcohol or drug misuse, responsibility for irresponsible behaviors may be placed on the externalized problem, rather than assumed by the person who is responsible for those behaviors. This concern is understandable, but misplaced. People always have the responsibility for their relationship with substances and for establishing and extending their resistance against them. Alcohol and drugs may blind people to opportunities to act responsibly, but they do not create people's irresponsibility.

Narrative workers have used a variety of techniques in working with people whose lives are under the influence of substance misuse. These techniques include deconstructing substance-related discourses, externalizing the many supporting allies of alcohol/drugs, predicting periods of misuse through a rite of passage or migration of the identity metaphor, and writing therapeutic letters.

The cultural pressure to take substances needs to be deconstructed as part of the therapeutic process if people are to confront their long-term cravings. For some young men, backing off from substances can create a crisis in their sense of who they are as men. Deconstruction takes the form of asking men to look at their underlying assumptions about manhood and decide which they buy into, which they find helpful, and which allow them to grow and change as people. Narrative workers are curious about how the cultural stories that shape people's lives support a substance-misusing lifestyle.

Smith and Winslade (1997) talk about several themes that are part of the process of working with young men under the influence of an alcoholic lifestyle: deconstructing alcohol's place in one's relationships with others, deconstructing the identity claims of alcohol, renegotiating the place of alcohol in one's life, renegotiating one's relationship with self once free of alcohol's domination, and renegotiating one's relationships with others. These themes are often interwoven and do not develop in any particular order. They occur naturally when the social worker and client explore alcohol's supports and effects as well as the client's possible new ways of being. The main caveat for workers is to maintain a spirit of flexibility.

When discussing the substance's effects on the person, it is important to consider what the positives of the substance use are as well as the negatives. People take, or at least initially took, substances because they wanted to and they became committed to that lifestyle because of some of the substance's benefits, as well as because of the chemical barriers to quitting. Looking at both positives and negatives is also recommended in motivational interviewing as a way to lessen clients' resistance, particularly when people are ambivalent about making a change (Miller & Rollnick, 2002).

Substance misuse does not occur in a vacuum. Often it allies with other problems. Sometimes these other problems mask the substance abuse, and sometimes the substance abuse masks these other problems. Examples of other externalized problems that have been described as allies with alcohol and drug misuse are pain, alcoholic lifestyle, cravings, grief, depression, and always pleasing others versus caring and kindness toward oneself.

It is not uncommon to hear those under the influence of substance misuse described as "being in denial" about the problem's influence on them. However, what looks like denial at times may actually be a unique outcome. Smith and Winslade (1997) discuss a situation in which a person who drank every day and had a history of multiple counts of driving under the influence stated that he did not have a problem with drinking but that drinking and driving was something he needed to stop. This was seen as a unique outcome because his desire to stop drinking and driving was not a commitment he had made after his prior offenses. This commitment developed into what became a major turn in the person's drinking lifestyle.

As Prochaska, DiClemente, and Norcross (1992) note, relapse is a natural part of the recovery process. People attempting to quit alcohol have on average six spells of treatment before it "takes." The reality is that people intent on leaving an alcoholic or drug-using lifestyle are likely to go back to it on several occasions. Unfortunately, the shame and guilt that accompany these relapses allow alcohol or drugs to convince people of their inability to make a change, and, as a result, individuals end up spending a longer time in a substance-misusing lifestyle.

Prochaska et al.'s (1992) model of change identifies relapse as a normal part of the change cycle, not as a failure. This view of change can be useful for short-circuiting the relapse/shame cycle. Yet although often employed, this cycle metaphor is not well-suited to storytelling because the stages are determined by professional assessment and the cycle may be hard for people to relate to in a narrative sense.

White and others have developed the image of a journey that encompasses both migration of identity and rite of passage metaphors (Man-kwong, 2004; White, 2004). People must be prepared for the long haul when changing from a substance-misusing lifestyle. The migration of identity metaphor acknowledges that the road is rarely straight but is instead filled with ups and downs; that what initially might be exciting and new can become difficult and dreary, testing the person mightily; and that it always takes much longer to adapt to a new environment than imagined.

Man-kwong (2004), in his work with young people who are trying to change their relationship to drug misuse, makes three predictions to clients. First, if people lapse into drug use again, they may experience a sense of total failure and forget all the successful experiences they have had. Second, if they do experience a relapse, they may feel too ashamed to tell the worker, which, according to Man-kwong, is particularly a problem with individuals from the Chinese culture. Third, if someone has gained control over his or her drug-using lifestyle for a few months, the person may think that the journey is over, but the cravings will last much longer than that.

Thinking about what is involved in making a migration of identity—the anxieties, fears, longings, and misgivings as well as the strength and courage—can evoke the image of a journey—a story with characters, a plot, and a conflict. A migration of identity also represents a rite of passage of sorts where between the separation stage, during which there is excitement about the initiation of the event, and the reincorporation stage, where the person's new identity is integrated and recognized, lies the liminal stage, a period in which the person is "betwixt and between" (White, 2004, A Rite of Passage section, para. 1). The works of anthropologists van Gennep (1960) and Turner (1969) focus on the problem of this betwixt and between stage, where confusion and despair are to be expected. It is only when the liminal stage is surmounted that the person can incorporate the various elements of his or her identity—both old and new—into a new identity. What is learned and survived in this period of confusion and dissociation is crucial for the final product: new identity.

Encouraging people to take this journey while still making them aware of its difficulties requires the development of an active community of concern because such a journey is not successful without support and hope. This realization is important for both the client and the worker, and its exploration can influence the maintenance of change. For example, although AA provides support for a sober lifestyle during meetings and encourages a close relationship with a sponsor outside of meetings, it has no mechanism to encourage people's involvement in nonsubstance-related activities. Young people, in particular, need sober peers from whom they can get support and with whom they can engage in recreational activities. Being sober in an intoxicated adolescent subculture can be very isolating, and loneliness can ally to encourage a relapse.

Letters represent an important tactic in assisting people influenced by substance misuse. Having a concrete representation of the treatment session can make a difference to those clients who are likely to read and reread such letters. Though efforts should be made to assemble a community of concern to assist people with their cravings and despair, a significant letter can be a source of some small comfort when a community is not immediately available. Wixson (2004) discusses the poignant example of a letter he had given to a homeless alcoholic woman he talked with on the street. He notes that for the long-term homeless, items of value are often taken from each other, and a prized item might have several different owners. He found out that his letter (which he replaced for the woman) had been taken several times, passing among those homeless individuals like other valuable property. He saw this circulation of the letter as an indication of its value.

## Exercises

### Exercise 1: Role-Playing a Substance Abuse Interview: Drugs

Substance abuse is a clearly defined entity in this culture and there are many ways to treat it "correctly." Colin Sanders (1998) developed questions for a clinical practice exercise, and with permission I have included these questions as a way to give you experience role-playing a different kind of interview.

Break into pairs, with one student taking the role of someone whose life is being controlled by substance misuse, and the other taking the role of social worker. Engage in an interview for 15 minutes using the following questions as guides:

1A. Mapping the influence of substances in the person's life, or in the life of the family, etc.
- How has cocaine/pot/valium etc. been affecting your life?
- Has cocaine/pot/valium created a wedge between you and persons who care for you?
- Describe the negative effects cocaine/pot/valium etc. has upon your life at school/home/work/etc.
- Describe how activities you used to enjoy have been affected by substance misuse.
- Would you say that a substance-misusing lifestyle is working for you, or against you?
- Does it sometimes appear to you that drugs are ripping you off?
- Could you describe some of the ways in which drugs are doing this to you?
- Are there specific situations or contexts in your life that drugs are more likely to take advantage of?

- Would you agree that valuable time has been stolen from you by cocaine/pot/heroin etc.? Describe some of the plans or dreams you had that drugs interfered with.
- Would you agree that substance misuse created isolation in your life?
- Are there times when drugs seem to be your jailer?

2A. Mapping the influence of the person, or family, etc., in the life of the problem

- Describe a time recently, or in the past, when you talked back to heroin (etc.).
- What was it like to protest against heroin's domination of your life?
- What is it you now know about cocaine/pot/valium/alcohol that can help you in escaping its influence, or standing up to its influence?
- What actions have you taken to reclaim your health/relationship/mind (etc.) from cocaine's grasp (etc.)?
- Who among your friends/family (etc.) is standing alongside you against drugs?
- Now that you have reclaimed your health/relationship/mind (etc.) from cocaine (etc.) what actions are you taking to ensure these changes will be maintained?

3A. Questions for those who have escaped the grasp of drugs for some time

- Having been drug-free for __ days/weeks/months, how has your thinking changed?
- With whom have you been celebrating this victory, and these new developments in your life?
- Do you think drugs are revising their opinion of you as weak and vulnerable?
- With the courage you're showing to practice moderation, or, be drug-free, who in your life is the least surprised? who is the most surprised? (Sanders, 1998, pp. 157–158)

Switch roles without discussion and again engage in a 15-minute interview. Then debrief by asking each other about his or her experience of being the interviewer and the interviewee. What did you find significant in the interview? What did you feel unhelpful? How might you take the helpful part into your work?

### Exercise 2: Role-Playing a Substance Abuse Interview: Alcohol

In this exercise, you will interview someone about his or her addictive thinking in relation to alcohol misuse. Break into pairs; if you have any uncertainty about which role to take, the person with the larger shoe size is the client first. I have included the following questions, which were developed by Trina Crowe (n.d.) and are used with her permission, to help you think about areas to explore in the interview:

> Some externalizing questions in relation to addictive thinking (self)
>> How does addictive thinking get you to use more than you intended to?
>>
>> What are some things that give addictive thinking more space [to influence you]?
>>
>> How does addictive thinking get you to use during times when you don't want to?
>>
>> Does addictive thinking get you to believe that you are not in danger when in fact you are?
>>
>> Does addictive thinking cause you to be dishonest with yourself?
>>
>> What emotions accompany addictive thinking that may lead to using or over-consuming?
>>
>> What does addictive thinking tell you is the reason why you drink?
>>
>> Does addictive thinking get you to lie about the amount you use?
>>
>> Does addictive thinking convince you that you are capable of driving when in fact you are not?
>>
>> What values is addictive thinking capable of separating you from?
>>
>> Are there hopes of ways you prefer to be that addictive thinking will not allow you [to] be?
>
> Some externalizing questions in relation to addictive thinking (relationships)
>> Does addictive thinking separate you from people who really care about you?

Does addictive thinking cause you to be dishonest with others?

Do you find that addictive thinking interferes with your abilities to be the parent that you prefer to be?

How has addictive thinking changed one of your relationships?

Do you find that addictive thinking causes you to associate with others who are also having problems with addictive thinking?

Do you find that addictive thinking causes you to avoid other people who do not have problems with addictive thinking?

Do you find that addictive thinking interferes with your abilities to be the partner that you prefer to be?

Do you find that addictive thinking interferes with your abilities to be the son/daughter that you prefer to be?

Has addictive thinking convinced you that no one understands, in an attempt to isolate you from others?

Does addictive thinking cause you to become angry towards other people?

How has addictive thinking changed the way you see yourself? (Crowe, n.d., first and second sections)

This time, instead of just asking the questions, reflect in the client's words what was said and explore each answer for a specific incident if it seems appropriate. You can add your empathic reaction where appropriate to extend the story. Use evaluation and justification questions. For example:

**Worker:** So, Jean, I wonder if we could talk today about this addictive thinking that you brought up in our last session. Do you think this could prove of some value to you?

**Client:** *I guess.*

**Worker:** The first thing I was curious about was how does addictive thinking get you to use more than you intend to?

**Client:** *Hmm. Well, I guess it tells me it's okay and, what the hell, it doesn't really matter. I mean, once you are a little high why not just keep drinking? It says I can be braver and more at ease if I drink a little more.*

**Worker:** So addictive thinking tells you that it doesn't matter if you are already a little high and that you can be braver and more at ease if you drink a little more. Did I get that right?

**Client:** *Yep!*

**Worker:** I can see where that could be tempting. Can you remember any time recently when that happened?

**Client:** *Last Saturday night. I went to Joe's Grill out on Broad Street and had a beer just to let me relax, and then I saw some people down the bar from me laughing and figured if I had a few more I could maybe be laughing with them.*

**Worker:** What did the addictive thinking tell you?

**Client:** *Well, that I could be laughing, too, if I got a little higher, that I wouldn't care about my problems with work or the bills.*

**Worker:** So it told you that if you drank more you could be happy, laugh, and forget work and the bills.

**Client:** *Yeah, that's it.*

**Worker:** Well, do you think this is a good thing or a bad thing? (*Evaluation question*)

**Client:** *Both, I guess.*

**Worker:** Why do you say both? (*Justification question*)

**Client:** *Because I like the release, but then I spend money and feel lousy the next morning. And I don't think those folks thought I was such good company, one of the guys tried to hit on me in a way I didn't like. Scared me some.*

**Worker:** So you did find some release, which felt good, but you also spent money when you have bills, felt bad in the morning, and felt scared because there was a risk in that situation. Is that right? Or do you see it differently than that?

Spend about 20 minutes going as far as you can in the interview, and then switch roles and again interview for 20 minutes. Finally, ask each other whether you were able to keep an externalizing frame of reference and what your experience as a client was like. How were you able to stay in an externalizing frame? What pulls did you experience to become more causation based and judgmental? How did you stand up to causal and judgmental thinking?

## Exercise 3: Interviewing a "Mental Illness"

Break into pairs. One person will be a "mental illness personified," and the other will be a curious interviewer. Select a category of mental illness that you know something about, through either friends, family, clients, or your own experience. Look at the exercise "Interviewing a Problem" in chapter 4. Use that interview format for this role play, but this time the mental illness as the interviewee.

# Epilogue

A narrative approach to clinical social work offers a value-based, strength-focused way of engaging individuals, families, and groups in helpful conversations. Accepting people as capable experts about their own problems and as creative coconstructors of their own identities frees social workers from the often frustrating role of expert applier of theories of change.

What is most exciting about using narrative methods is that we, as social work professionals, get to see clients as people, not symptom carriers. Of course, narrative is not the only viewpoint that can be taken of people and their troubles, but it is a respectful one. It honors people in a helpful way. It respects people's pain and helps them consider how they have been able to avoid having problems completely take over their lives. It leads one into a complicated and detailed approach to solving problems.

There are a number of centers in the United States that will train social workers in narrative principles. A good way to get information about training opportunities is to visit the following Web sites: http://www.narrativeapproaches.com and http://www.dulwichcentre.com.au.

# References

Abels, P., & Abels, S. L. (2001). *Understanding narrative therapy: A guidebook for the social worker*. New York: Springer.

Abramovitz, M. (1996). *Regulating the lives of women* (Rev. ed.). Boston: South End Press.

Adams-Westcott, J., Dafforn, T. A., & Sterne, P. (1993). Escaping victim life stories and co-constructing personal agency. In S. Gilligan & R. Price (Eds.), *Therapeutic conversations* (pp. 258–271). New York: Norton.

Adams-Westcott, J., & Dobbins, C. (1997). Listening with your "heart ears" and other ways young people can escape the effects of sexual abuse. In C. Smith & D. Nylund (Eds.), *Narrative therapies with children and adolescents* (pp. 195–220). New York: Guilford Press.

Adams-Westcott, J., & Isenbart, C. (1995). A journey of change through connection. In S. Friedman (Ed.), *The reflecting team in action: Collaborative practice in family therapy* (pp. 331–352). New York: Guilford Press.

Akamatsu, N. (2002). Cultural racism—the air we breathe. *International Journal of Narrative Therapy and Community Work, 4*, 48–55.

American Psychiatric Association. (2000). *Diagnostic and statistical manual of mental disorders* (4th ed., Text Revision). Washington, DC: Author.

Andersen, T. (1987). The reflecting team: Dialogue and meta-dialogue in clinical work. *Family Process, 26*, 415–428.

Andersen, T. (1991). *The reflecting team: Dialogue and dialogues about dialogues*. New York: Norton.

Andersen, T. (1995). Reflecting processes: Acts of informing and forming: You can borrow my eyes, but you must not take them away from me. In S. Friedman (Ed.), *The reflecting team in action: Collaborative practice in family therapy* (pp. 11–37). New York: Guilford Press.

Andrews, J. (Producer). (1996). *Partners in strength: A consultation with Jill Freedman & Gene Combs of the Evanston Family Therapy Center* [Videotape]. (Available from Andrews & Clark Explorations, 10650 Kinnard Avenue, Suite 109, Los Angeles, CA 90024)

Archive of Resistance: *Anti-Anorexia/Anti-Bulimia*. (2000). Retrieved August 21, 2006, from http://www.narrativeapproaches.com/antianorexia%20folder/entry_conditions.htm

Arciero, G., & Guidano, V. F. (2000). Experience, explanation, and the quest for coherence. In R. A. Neimeyer & J. D. Raskin (Eds.), *Constructions of disorder: Meaning-making frameworks for psychotherapy* (pp. 91–118). Washington, DC: American Psychological Association.

Association of Social Work Boards. (2006). *Candidate handbook: ASWB licensing examinations, 2006–2007*. Culpeper, VA: Author.

Augusta-Scott, T. (2003). Dichotomies in the power and control story: Exploring multiple stories about men who choose abuse in intimate relationships. In Dulwich Centre Publications (Ed.), *Responding to violence* (pp. 203–224). Adelaide, Australia: Author.

Banks, S. (2003). From oaths to rulebooks: A critical examination of codes of ethics for social professions. *European Journal of Social Work, 6*(2), 133–144.

Barragar-Dunne, P. (1997). "Catch the fish": Therapy utilizing narrative, drama, and dramatic play with young children. In C. Smith & D. Nylund (Eds.), *Narrative therapies with children and adolescents* (pp. 71–110). New York: Guilford Press.

Beauchamp, T. L., & Childress, J. F. (2001). *Principles of biomedical ethics* (5th ed.). New York: Oxford University Press.

Benard, B. (2002). Turnaround people and places: Moving from risk to resilience. In D. Saleebey (Ed.), *The strengths perspective in social work practice* (3rd ed., pp. 213–227). Boston: Allyn & Bacon.

Bennett, J. S., Daugherty, A., Herrington, D., Greenland, P., Roberts, H., & Taubert K. A. (2005). The use of nonsteroidal anti-inflammatory drugs (NSAIDs): A science advisory from the American Heart Association. *Circulation, 111*, 1713–1716. Retrieved June 10, 2005, from http://circ.ahajournals.org/cgi/content/full/111/13/1713

Berndt, L., Dickerson, V. C., & Zimmerman, J. L. (1997). Tales told out of school. In C. Smith & D. Nylund (Eds.), *Narrative therapies with children and adolescents* (pp. 423–454). New York: Guilford Press.

Biever, J. L., & Franklin, C. (1998). Social constructivism in action: Using reflecting teams in family practice. In C. Franklin & P. S. Nurius (Eds.), *Constructivism in practice: Methods and challenges* (pp. 259–276). Milwaukee, WI: Families International.

Brown, C., & Augusta-Scott, T. (2007). Introduction: Postmodernism, reflexivity, and narrative therapy. In C. Brown & T. Augusta-Scott (Eds.), *Narrative therapy: Making meaning, making lives* (pp. ix–xlii). Thousand Oaks, CA: Sage.

Brown, L. S. (2000). Discomforts of the powerless: Feminist constructions of distress. In R. A. Neimeyer & J. D. Raskin (Eds.), *Constructions of disorder: Meaning-making frameworks for psychotherapy* (pp. 287–308). Washington, DC: American Psychological Association.

Bruner, J. (1986). *Actual minds, possible worlds*. Cambridge, MA: Harvard University Press.

Bruner, J. (2002). *Making stories: Law, literature, life*. New York: Farrar, Straus and Giroux.

Callahan, T. (2001). *Alcohol, drugs and suffering*. Retrieved June 10, 2005, from http://www.dulwichcentre.com.au/alcohol.htm

Carlat, D. J. (1999). *The psychiatric interview: A practical guide*. Philadelphia: Lippincott, Williams & Wilkins.

Carlson, T. D. (1998). The virus metaphor and narrative therapy. *Journal of Family Psychotherapy, 9*(3), 63–68.

Carrey, N. (2007). Practicing psychiatry through a narrative lens: Working with children, youth and families. In C. Brown & T. Augusta-Scott (Eds.), *Narrative therapy: Making meaning, making lives* (pp. 77–101). Thousand Oaks, CA: Sage.

Chambon, A. S. (1999). Foucault's approach: Making the familiar visible. In A. S. Chambon, A. Irving, & L. Epstein (Eds.), *Reading Foucault for social work* (pp. 51–81). New York: Columbia University Press.

Charon, R. (1994). Narrative contributions to medical ethics: Recognition, formulation interpretation, and validation in the practice of the ethicist. In E. R. DuBose, R. P. Hamel, & L. J. O'Connell (Eds.), *A matter of principles?: Ferment in U.S. bioethics* (pp. 260–283). Valley Forge, PA: Trinity Press International.

Charon, R. (2001). Narrative medicine: A model for empathy, reflection, profession, and trust. *Journal of the American Medical Association, 286*, 1897–1902.

Charon, R. (2004). Narrative and medicine. *New England Journal of Medicine, 350*, 862–864.

Chayes, A., Fisher, W., Horwitz, M., Michelman, F., Minow, M., Nesson, C., et al. (n.d.). *The bridge: Legal reasoning: Introduction.* Retrieved July 28, 2007, from http://cyber.law.harvard.edu/bridge/r1_intro.htm

Clark, D. C., & Fawcett, J. (1992). A review of empirical risk factors for the evaluation of the suicidal patient. In B. Bongar (Ed.), *Suicide: Guidelines for assessment, management, and treatment* (pp. 16–48). New York: Oxford University Press.

Cohen, B. (1999). Intervention and supervision in strengths-based social work practice. *Families in Society, 80*, 460–466.

Coleman, L. (1984). *The reign of error: Psychiatry, authority, and law.* Boston: Beacon Press.

Combs, G., & Freedman, J. (1994). Narrative intentions. In M. F. Hoyt (Ed.), *Constructive therapies* (pp. 67–91). New York: Guilford Press.

Compton, B. R., Galaway, B., & Cournoyer, B. R. (2005). *Social work processes* (7th ed.). Pacific Grove, CA: Brooks/Cole.

Cooper, M. G., & Lesser, J. G. (2002). *Clinical social work practice: An integrated approach.* Boston: Allyn & Bacon.

Cowger, C. D. (1998). Clientilism and clientification: Impediments to strengths based social work practice. *Journal of Sociology and Social Welfare, 25*(1), 25–37.

Cowger, C. D., & Snively, C. A. (2002). Assessing client strengths: Individual, family, and community empowerment. In D. Saleebey (Ed.), *The strengths perspective in social work practice* (3rd ed., pp. 106–123). Boston: Allyn & Bacon.

Crowe, T. (n.d.). Some externalising questions in relation to addictive thinking (self).
Retrieved October, 20, 2006, from http://www.dulwichcentre.com.au/some_externalising_questions_in.htm

Decker, P., & Buckley, E. (2003). *Workshop materials: From isolation to collaboration: Narrative approaches to children and families in crisis.* Conference on Narrative Therapy, Evanston, IL.

Delgado, R. (1989). Story telling for oppositionists and others: A plea for narrative. *Michigan Law Review, 87*, 2411–2441.

Dickerson, V. C., & Zimmerman, J. L. (1996). Myths, misconceptions, and a word or two about politics. *Journal of Systemic Therapies, 15*(1), 79–88.

Dorfman, R. A. (1996). *Clinical social work: Definition, practice and vision.* New York: Brunner/Mazel.

Drewery, W., & Winslade, J. (1997). The theoretical story of narrative therapy. In G. Monk, J. Winslade, K. Crocket, & D. Epston (Eds.), *Narrative therapy in practice: The archaeology of hope* (pp. 32–52). San Francisco: Jossey-Bass.

Drewery, W., Winslade, J., & Monk, G. (2000). Resisting the dominating story: Toward a deeper understanding of narrative therapy. In R. A. Neimeyer & J. D. Raskin (Eds.), *Constructions of disorder: Meaning-making frameworks for psychotherapy* (pp. 243–263). Washington, DC: American Psychological Association.

Dunst, C. J., Trivette, C. M., & Deal, A. G. (Eds.). (1994). *Supporting and strengthening families: Methods, strategies, and practice* (Vol. 1). Cambridge, MA: Brookline Books.

Ecker, B., & Hulley, L. (2000). The order in clinical "disorders": Symptom coherence in depth-oriented brief therapy. In R. A. Neimeyer & J. D. Raskin (Eds.), *Constructions of disorder: Meaning-making frameworks for psychotherapy* (pp. 63–89). Washington, DC: American Psychological Association.

Epstein, L. (1999). The culture of social work. In A. S. Chambon, A. Irving, & L. Epstein (Eds.), *Reading Foucault for social work* (pp. 3–26). New York: Columbia University Press.

Epston, D. (1989). *Collected papers*. Adelaide, Australia: Dulwich Centre Publications.

Epston, D. (1993). Internalized other questioning with couples: The New Zealand version. In S. Gilligan & R. Price (Eds.), *Therapeutic conversations* (pp. 183–189). New York: Norton.

Epston, D. (1997). "I am a bear": Discovering discoveries. In C. Smith & D. Nylund (Eds.), *Narrative therapies with children and adolescents* (pp. 53–70). New York: Guilford Press.

Epston, D. (1999). Co-research: The making of an alternative knowledge. In Dulwich Centre Publications (Ed.), *Narrative therapy and community work: A conference collection* (pp. 137–157). Adelaide, Australia: Dulwich Centre Publications.

Epston, D., Lobovits, D., & Freeman, J. (with Murphy, S.). (1997). *Annals of the new Dave: Status: Abled, disabled, or weirdly abled*. Retrieved August 20, 2006, from http://www.narrativeapproaches.com/narrative%20papers%20folder/new_dave.htm [Simultaneously published as A chronicle of therapy: Annals of the "new Dave." *Gecko: A Journal of Deconstruction and Narrative Ideas in Therapeutic Practice, 3*, 59–85.]

Epston, D., White, M., & "Ben" (1995). Consulting your consultants: A means to co-construction of alternative knowledges. In S. Friedman (Ed.), *The reflecting team in action: Collaborative practice in family therapy* (pp. 277–313). New York: Guilford Press.

Epston, D. (with Maisel, R.). (2000). *The history of the archives of resistance—anti-anorexia/anti-bulimia*. Retrieved August 15, 2007, from http://www.narrativeapproaches.com/antianorexia%20folder/history.htm

Eron, J. B., & Lund, T. W. (1999). Narrative solutions in brief couple therapy. In J. M. Donovan (Ed.), *Short-term couple therapy* (pp. 291–324). New York: Guilford Press.

Fast, B., & Chapin, R. (2002). The strengths model for older Americans: Critical practice components. In D. Saleebey (Ed.), *The strengths perspective in social work practice* (3rd ed., pp. 143–162). Boston: Allyn & Bacon.

Fisher, D. D. V. (1991). *An introduction to constructivism for social workers.* New York: Praeger.

Flexner, A. (1915). Is social work a profession? In *Proceedings of the National Conference of Charities and Corrections* (pp. 576–590). Chicago: Hindmann.

Focht, L., & Beardslee, W. E. (1996). "Long speech after silence": The use of narrative therapy in a preventive intervention for children of parents with affective disorder. *Family Process, 35,* 407–422.

Foote, C. E., & Frank, A. W. (1999). Foucault and therapy: The disciplining of grief. In A. S. Chambon, A. Irving, & L. Epstein (Eds.), *Reading Foucault for social work* (pp. 157–187). New York: Columbia University Press.

Foucault, M. (1973). *Madness and civilization: A history of insanity in the Age of Reason* (R. Howard, Trans.). New York: Vintage. (Original work published 1965)

Foucault, M. (1975). *The birth of the clinic: An archaeology of medical perception* (A. M. Sheridan Smith, Trans.). New York: Vintage. (Original work published 1973)

Foucault, M. (1979). *Discipline and punish: The birth of the prison* (A. Sheridan, Trans.). New York: Vintage. (Original work published 1977)

Foucault, M. (1988). Technologies of the self. In L. H. Martin, H. Gutman, & P. H. Hutton (Eds.), *Technologies of the self: A seminar with Michel Foucault* (pp. 16–49). Amherst: University of Massachusetts Press.

Frank, A. W. (1995). *The wounded storyteller: Body, illness, and ethics.* Chicago: University of Chicago Press.

Franklin, C. (1998). Distinctions between social constructionism and cognitive constructivism: Practice applications. In C. Franklin & P. S. Nurius (Eds.), *Constructivism in practice: Methods and challenges* (pp. 57–94). Milwaukee, WI: Families International.

Freedman, J., & Combs, G. (1996). *Narrative therapy: The social construction of preferred realities.* New York: Norton.

Freedman, J., & Combs, G. (1997). Lists. In C. Smith & D. Nylund (Eds.), *Narrative therapies with children and adolescents* (pp. 147–161). New York: Guilford Press.

Freedman, J., & Combs, G. (2003). *Questioning marginalization.* Unpublished manuscript.

Freedman, J., & Combs, G. (2004). Relational identity in narrative work with couples. In S. Madigan (Ed.), *Therapeutic conversations 5: Therapy from the outside in* (pp. 29–40). Vancouver, Canada: Yaletown Family Therapy.

Freeman, J., Epston, D., & Lobovits, D. (1997). *Playful approaches to serious problems: Narrative therapy with children and their families.* New York: Norton.

Freeman, J., & Lobovits, D. (1993). The turtle with wings. In S. Friedman (Ed.), *The new language of change: Constructive collaboration in psychotherapy* (pp. 188–225). New York: Guilford Press.

Fristad, M. A., Gavazzi, S. M., & Soldano, K. W. (1999). Naming the enemy: Learning to differentiate mood disorder "symptoms" from the "self" that experiences them. *Journal of Family Psychotherapy, 10*(1), 81–88.

Gantz, M., & Pearson, C. G. (1988). Ageism revised and the provision of psychological services. *American Psychologist, 43,* 184–188.

Garcia, A. C., Vise, K., & Whitaker, S. P. (2002). Disputing neutrality: A case study of a bias complaint during mediation. *Conflict Resolution Quarterly, 20,* 205–230.

Garfield, S. L. (1994). Research on client variables in psychotherapy. In A. E. Bergin & S. L. Garfield (Eds.), *Handbook of psychotherapy and behavior change* (4th ed., pp. 190–228). New York: John Wiley & Sons.

Garland, J. (1994). What splendor, it all coheres: Life-review therapy with older people. In. J. Bornat (Ed.), *Reminiscence reviewed: Perspectives, evaluations, achievements* (pp. 21–31). Buckingham, England: Open University Press.

Gergen, K. J. (1999). *An invitation to social construction.* London: Sage.

Gergen, K. J., & McNamee, S. (2000). From disordering discourse to transformative dialogue. In R. A. Neimeyer & J. D. Raskin (Eds.), *Constructions of disorder: Meaning-making frameworks for psychotherapy* (pp. 333–349). Washington, DC: American Psychological Association.

Germain, C. B., & Gitterman, A. (1996). *The life model of social work practice: Advances in theory and practice.* New York: Columbia University Press.

Goncalves, O. F. (1995). Cognitive narrative psychotherapy: The hermeneutic construction of alternative meanings. In M. J. Mahoney (Ed.), *Cognitive and constructive psychotherapies: Theory, research, and practice* (pp. 139–162). New York: Springer.

Gonzalez, R. C. (1998). A technically eclectic blend of paradigms and epistemologies for multicultural clinical relevance. In C. Franklin & P. S. Nurius (Eds.), *Constructivism in practice: Methods and challenges* (pp. 349–375). Milwaukee, WI: Families International.

Grieves, L. (1998). From beginning to start: The Vancouver Anti-Anorexia/Anti-Bulimia League. In S. Madigan & I. Law (Eds.), *Praxis: Situating discourse, feminism & politics in narrative therapies* (pp. 195–206). Vancouver, Canada: Yaletown Family Therapy.

Griffith, J. L., & Griffith, M. E. (1994). *The body speaks: Therapeutic dialogues for mind-body problems.* New York: Basic Books.

Griffith, J. L., Griffith, M. E., Krejmas, N., McLain, M., Mittal, D., Rains, J., et al. (1992). Reflecting team consultations and their impact upon family therapy for somatic symptoms as coded by Structural Analysis of Social Behavior (SASB). *Family Systems Medicine, 10,* 53–58.

Grimm, R. (2003). Narrative therapy with older adults. In J. L. Ronch & J. A. Goldfield (Eds.), *Mental wellness in aging: Strengths-based approaches* (pp. 237–271). Baltimore: Health Professions Press.

Grimm, R., Maki, B., & Morales-Long, L. (1995). Developing narrative approaches with the elderly. *Journal of Collaborative Therapies, 3,* 4–14.

Guidano, V. F. (1991). *The self in process: Toward a post-rationalist cognitive therapy.* New York: Guilford Press.

Gutierrez, L. M., Parsons, R. J., & Cox, E. O. (1998). A model for empowerment practice. In L. M. Gutierrez, R. J. Parsons, & E. O. Cox (Eds.), *Empowerment in social work practice: A sourcebook* (pp. 3–24). Pacific Grove, CA: Brooks/Cole.

Hacker, H. M. (1976). Women as a minority group. In S. Cox (Ed.), *Female psychology: The emerging self* (pp. 156–170). New York: St. Martin's.

Haley, J. (1976). *Problem-solving therapies: New strategies for effective family therapy*. San Francisco: Jossey-Bass.

Hardy, K. (2004). *Working with low income minority families*. Workshop presentation delivered at the Ackerman Family Institute, New York.

Harper, K. V., & Lantz, J. (1996). *Cross-cultural practice: Social work with diverse populations*. Chicago: Lyceum.

Hartman, A., & Laird, J. (1983). *Family-centered social work practice*. New York: Free Press.

Hedtke, L. (2002). Reconstructing the language of death and grief. *Illness, Crisis & Loss, 10,* 285–293.

Hedtke, L., & Winslade, J. (2004). *Re-membering lives: Conversations with the dying and the bereaved*. Amityville, NY: Baywood.

Heifetz, J. (2003). Why write a patient's life as a short story? *Lilith, 28*(4), 12–13.

Helms, J. E. (1992). *A race is a nice thing to have: A guide to being a white person or understanding the white persons in your life*. Topeka, KA: Content Communications.

Hoffman, L. (1981). *Foundations of family therapy: A conceptual framework for system change*. New York: Basic Books.

Hogan, B. A. (1999). Narrative therapy in rehabilitation after brain injury: A case study. *NeuroRehabilitation, 13,* 21–25.

Hoper, J. H. (1999). *Families who unilaterally discontinue narrative therapy: Their story, a qualitative study*. Dissertation Abstracts International-B (DAI-B), 60(06), 2945. (UMI No. 733663491)

Hugman, R. (2003). Professional values and ethics in social work: Reconsidering postmodernism? *British Journal of Social Work, 33,* 1025–1041.

Irving, A., & Young, T. (2002). Paradigm for pluralism: Mikhail Bakhtin and social work practice. *Social Work, 47,* 19–29.

Jenkins, A. (1990). *Invitations to responsibility: The therapeutic engagement of men who are violent and abuse.* Adelaide, Australia: Dulwich Centre Publications.

Jenkins, A. (1998). Invitations to responsibility: Engaging adolescents and young men who have sexually abused. In W. L. Marshal, Y. M. Fernandez, S. M. Hudson, & T. Ward (Eds.), *Sourcebook of treatment programs for sexual offenders* (pp. 163–189). New York: Plenum Press.

Johansen, R. K. (2002). *Listening in silence, seeing in the dark: Reconstructing life after brain injury.* Berkeley: University of California Press.

Kazdin, A., Mazurick, J., & Bass, D. (1993). Risk for attrition in treatment of antisocial children and families. *Journal of Clinical Child Psychology, 22,* 2–16.

Kecskemeti, M., & Epston, D. (1995). A proposal for an interview format and practices of appreciation that value teachers' and students' knowledges in schools. Retrieved August 18, 2006, from http://www.narrativeapproaches.com/narrative%20papers%20folder/teacher.htm

Kelley, P. (1995). Integrating narrative approaches into clinical curricula: Addressing diversity through understanding. *Journal of Social Work Education, 31,* 347–357.

Kelley, P. (2002). Narrative therapy. In A. R. Roberts & G. J. Greene (Eds.), *Social workers' desk reference* (pp. 121–124). New York: Oxford University Press.

Kelly, G. A. (1955). *The psychology of personal constructs.* New York: Norton.

Kierans, C. M., & Maynooth, N. U. I. (2001). Sensory and narrative identity: The narration of illness process among chronic renal sufferers in Ireland. *Anthropology & Medicine, 8*(2/3), 237–253.

Kimmel, A. J. (1988). Ethics and values in applied social research. Beverly Hills, CA: Sage.

Kleinman, A. (1988). *The illness narratives: Suffering, healing, and the human condition.* New York: Basic Books.

Kristhardt, W. E. (2002). The strengths perspective in interpersonal helping: Purposes, principles, and functions. In D. Saleebey (Ed.), *The strengths perspective in social work practice* (3rd ed., pp. 163–185). Boston: Allyn & Bacon.

Kutchins, H., & Kirk, S. A. (1997). *Making us crazy. DSM: The psychiatric bible and the creation of mental disorders.* New York: Free Press.

Laird, J. (1995). Family-centered practice in the postmodern era. *Families in Society, 76,* 150–162.

Lamott, A. (1994). *Bird by bird: Some instructions on writing and life.* New York: Anchor.

Law, I. (1997). Attention deficit disorder: Therapy with a shoddily built construct. In C. Smith & D. Nylund (Eds.), *Narrative therapies with children and adolescents* (pp. 282–306). New York: Guilford Press.

Lawrence, C. R. (1987). The id, the ego, and equal protection: Reckoning with unconscious racism. *Stanford Law Review 39,* 317–388.

Lax, W. D. (1995). Offering reflections: Some theoretical and practical considerations. In S. Friedman (Ed.), *The reflecting team in action: Collaborative practice in family therapy* (pp. 145–166). New York: Guilford Press.

Lee, J. A. B. (2001). *The empowerment approach to social work practice: Building the beloved community* (2nd ed.). New York: Columbia University Press.

Lettvin, J. Y., Maturana, H. R., McCulloch, W. S., & Pitts, W. H. (1959). What the frog's eye tells the frog's brain. *Proceedings of the Institute of Radio Engineers, 47,* 1940–1051.

Lieberman, J. A., Stroup, T. S., McEnvoy, J. P., Swartz, M. S., Rosenheck, R. A., Perkins, D. O., et al. (2005). Effectiveness of antipsychotic drugs in patients with chronic schizophrenia. *New England Journal of Medicine, 353,* 1209–1223.

Lobovits, D. H., & Freeman, J. C. (1997). Destination grump station— getting off the grump bus. In C. Smith & D. Nylund (Eds.), *Narrative therapies with children and adolescents* (pp. 174–194). New York: Guilford Press.

Lobovits, D., Maisel, R. L., & Freeman, J. C. (1995). Public practices: An ethic of circulation. In S. Friedman (Ed.), *The reflecting team in action: Collaborative practice in family therapy* (pp. 223–256). New York: Guilford Press.

Lyle, R. R., & Gehart, D. R. (2000). The narrative of ethics and the ethics of narrative: The implications of Ricoeur's narrative model of family therapy. *Journal of Systemic Therapies, 19*(4), 73–89.

Madigan, S. (1993). Questions about questions: Situating the therapist's curiosity in front of the family. In S. Gilligan & R. Price (Eds.), *Therapeutic conversations* (pp. 219–230). New York: Norton.

Madigan, S. (with commentary by Grieves, L.). (1997). Re-considering memory: Re-remembering lost identities back toward re-membered selves. In C. Smith & D. Nylund (Eds.), *Narrative therapies with children and adolescents* (pp. 338–355). New York: Guilford Press.

Madigan, S. (1998a). Destabilizing chronic identities of depression and retirement: Inscription, description and deciphering. In S. Madigan & I. Law (Eds.), *Praxis: Situating discourse, feminism & politics in narrative therapies* (pp. 207–230). Vancouver, Canada: Yaletown Family Therapy.

Madigan, S. (1998b). Practice interpretations of Michel Foucault: Situating problem externalising discourse. In S. Madigan & I. Law (Eds.), *Praxis: Situating discourse, feminism & politics in narrative therapies* (pp. 15–34). Vancouver, Canada: Yaletown Family Therapy.

Madigan, S. (2003, May). *Counterviewing injurious speech acts: Destabilizing eight conversational habits of highly effective problems*. Workshop handout, Louisville, KY.

Madigan, S., & Epston, D. (1995). From "spy-chiatric gaze" to communities of concern: From professional monologue to dialogue. In S. Friedman (Ed.), *The reflecting team in action: Collaborative practice in family therapy* (pp. 257–276). New York: Guilford Press.

Madsen, W. C. (2004). Sustaining a collaborative clinical practice in the "real" world. In S. Madigan (Ed.), *Therapeutic conversations 5: Therapy from the outside in* (pp. 133–146). Vancouver, Canada: Yaletown Family Therapy.

Madsen, W. C. (2007). *Collaborative therapy with multi-stressed families* (2nd ed.). New York: Guilford Press.

Mahoney, M. J. (2003). *Constructive psychotherapy: A practical guide*. New York: Guilford Press.

Maisel, R., Epston, D., & Borden, A. (2004). *Biting the hand that starves you: Inspiring resistance to anorexia/bulimia*. New York: Norton.

Man-kwong, H. (2004). *Overcoming craving: The use of narrative practices in breaking drug habits*. Retrieved November 4, 2004, from http://www.dulwichcentre.com.au/OvercomingCraving.htm

Markus, H., & Nurius, P. (1986). Possible selves. *American Psychologist, 41,* 954–969.

McCarthy, J. (2003). Principlism or narrative ethics: Must we choose between them? *Medical Humanities, 29*(2), 65–71.

McKenzie, W., & Monk, G. (1997). Learning and teaching narrative ideas. In G. Monk, J. Winslade, K. Crocket, & D. Epston (Eds.), *Narrative therapy in practice: The archaeology of hope* (pp. 82–119). San Francisco: Jossey-Bass.

McMillen, J. C. (2004). Posttraumatic growth: What's it about? *Psychological Inquiry, 15,* 48–52.

McMillen, J. C., Morris, L., & Sherraden, M. (2004). Ending social work's grudge match: Problems versus strengths. *Families in Society, 85,* 317–325.

Miller, A. (1984). *Thou shalt not be aware: Society's betrayal of the child* (H. Hannum & H. Hannum, Trans.). New York: Farrar, Straus and Giroux.

Miller, W. R., & Rollnick, S. (2002). *Motivational interviewing: Preparing people for change*. New York: Guilford Press.

Minnow, M. (1993). Surviving victim talk. *UCLA Law Review, 40,* 1411–1445.

Minuchin, S. (1974). *Families and family therapy*. Cambridge, MA: Harvard University Press.

Mitchell, J. B. (1999). Narrative and client-centered representation: What is a true believer to do when his two favorite theories collide? *Clinical Law Review, 6,* 85–126.

Monk, G. (1997). How narrative therapy works. In G. Monk, J. Winslade, K. Crocket, & D. Epston (Eds.), *Narrative therapy in practice: The archaeology of hope* (pp. 3–31). San Francisco: Jossey-Bass.

Monk, G., & Gehart, D. R. (2003). Sociopolitical activist or conversational partner? Distinguishing the position of the therapist in narrative and collaborative therapies. *Family Process, 42,* 19–29.

Morgan, A. (2000). *What is narrative therapy?* Adelaide, Australia: Dulwich Centre Publications.

Morkel, E. (2002). *When narratives create community: Standing with children against stealing.* Unpublished master's thesis, University of South Africa, Pretoria.

Morris, D. B. (2002). Narrative, ethics, and pain: Thinking with stories. In R. Charon & M. Montello (Eds.), *Stories matter: The role of narrative in medical ethics* (pp. 196–218). New York: Routledge.

Moules, N. J. (2003). Therapy on paper: Therapeutic letters and the tone of relationship. *Journal of Systemic Therapies, 22*(1), 33–49.

Mueller, C., & Kirkpatrick, L. (2007). *Federal evidence* (3rd ed., Vol. 5). St. Paul, MN: Thomson/West.

Murphy, K. E. (1997). Rejoinder to Professor Kopels: Is the NASW *Code of Ethics* an effective guide for practitioners? In E. Gambrill & R. Pruger (Eds.), *Controversial issues in social work ethics, values, and obligations* (pp. 124–125). Boston: Allyn & Bacon.

Myerhoff, B. (1982). Life history among the elderly: Performance, visibility and remembering. In J. Ruby (Ed.), *A crack in the mirror: Reflexive perspectives in anthropology* (pp. 99–117). Philadelphia: University of Pennsylvania Press.

Myerhoff, B. (1986). "Life not death in Venice": Its second life. In V. W. Turner & E. M. Bruner (Eds.), *The anthropology of experience* (pp. 261–286). Urbana: University of Illinois Press.

National Association of Social Workers (NASW). (1999). *Code of ethics.* Retrieved August 15, 2007, from http://www.socialworkers.org/pubs/code/code.asp

Neal, J. H., Zimmerman, J. L., & Dickerson, V. C. (1999). Couples, culture and discourse: A narrative approach. In J. M. Donovan (Ed.), *Short-term couple therapy* (pp. 360–400). New York: Guilford Press.

Neimeyer, R. A. (2000). Narrative disruptions in the construction of the self. In R. A. Neimeyer & J. D. Raskin (Eds.), *Constructions of disorder: Meaning-making frameworks for psychotherapy* (pp. 207–242). Washington, DC: American Psychological Association.

Neimeyer, R. A. (2004). Fostering posttraumatic growth: A narrative elaboration. *Psychological Inquiry, 15,* 53–59.

Neimeyer, R. A., & Stewart, A. E. (1998). Trauma, healing, and the narrative emplotment of loss. In C. Franklin & P. S. Nurius (Eds.), *Constructivism in practice: Methods and challenges* (pp. 165–183). Milwaukee, WI: Families International.

Nelson, H. L. (2002). Context: Backward, sideways, and forward. In R. Charon & M. Montello (Eds.), *Stories matter: The role of narrative in medical ethics* (pp. 39–47). New York: Routledge.

Newton, A. Z. (1995). *Narrative ethics.* Cambridge, MA: Harvard University Press.

Nichols, M. P. (with Schwartz, R. C.). (2006). *Family therapy: Concepts and methods* (7th ed.). Boston: Allyn & Bacon.

Nochi, M. (1988). "Loss of self" in the narratives of people with traumatic brain injuries: A qualitative analysis. *Social Science and Medicine, 46,* 869–878.

Nylund, D. (2002). *Treating Huckleberry Finn: A narrative approach to working with kids diagnosed ADD/ADHD.* San Francisco: Jossey-Bass.

Nylund, D. (2004). The mass media and masculinity: Working with men who have been violent. In S. Madigan (Ed.), *Therapeutic conversations 5: Therapy from the outside in* (pp. 177–189). Vancouver, Canada: Yaletown Family Therapy.

Nylund, D., & Ceske, K. (1997). Voices of political resistance: Young women's co-research on anti-depression. In C. Smith & D. Nylund (Eds.), *Narrative therapies with children and adolescents* (pp. 356–381). New York: Guilford Press.

Nylund, D., & Corsigilia, V. (1996). From deficits to special abilities: Working narratively with children labeled "ADHD." In M. F. Hoyt (Ed.), *Constructive therapies 2* (pp. 163–183). New York: Guilford Press.

Nylund, D., & Thomas, J. (1994). The economics of narrative. *Family Therapy Networker, 18*(6), 38–39.

O'Hanlon, B. (1994). The third wave. *Family Therapy Networker, 18*(6), 18–29.

O'Neill, T. (1987). *Man of the House: The life and political memoirs of Speaker Tip O'Neill.* New York: Random House.

Orlinsky, D. E., Ronnestad, M. H., & Willutzki, U. (2004). Fifty years of psychotherapy process-outcome research: Continuity and change. In M. J. Lambert (Ed.), *Bergin and Garfield's handbook of psychotherapy and behavior change* (5th ed., pp. 307–389). New York: John Wiley & Sons.

Pals, J. L., & McAdams, D. P. (2004). The transformed self: A narrative understanding of posttraumatic growth. *Psychological Inquiry, 15*, 65–69.

Paquin, G. (2006). Including narrative concepts in social work practice classes: Teaching to client strengths. *Journal of Teaching in Social Work, 26*(1/2), 127–145.

Paquin, G., & Harvey, L. (1998). A model of marital resolution. *Journal of Couples Therapy, 7*(2/3), 87–101.

Paquin, G., & Harvey, L. (2002). Therapeutic jurisprudence, transformative mediation and narrative mediation: A natural connection. *Florida Coastal Law Review, 3*, 167–188.

Parton, N. (2003). Rethinking professional practice: The contributions of social constructionism and the feminist "ethics of care." *British Journal of Social Work, 33*, 1–16.

Parton, N., & O'Byrne, P. (2000). *Constructive social work: Towards a new practice.* New York: St. Martin's.

Penn, P. (1982). Circular questioning. *Family Process, 21*, 267–280.

Pennebaker, J. W. (1993). Putting stress into words: Health, linguistic, and therapeutic implications. *Behaviour Research and Therapy, 31*, 539–548.

Perlman, H. H. (1957). *Social casework: A problem-solving process.* Chicago: University of Chicago Press.

Petersen, S., Bull, C., Propst, C., Dettinger, S., & Detwiler, L. (2005). Narrative therapy to prevent illness-related stress disorder. *Journal of Counseling and Development, 83,* 41–47.

Pincus, A., & Minahan, A. (1973). *Social work practice: Model and method.* Itasca, IL: F. E. Peacock.

Pipher, M. (1994). *Reviving Ophelia: Saving the selves of adolescent girls.* New York: Putnam.

Poirier, S. (2002). Voice in medical narrative. In R. Charon & M. Montello (Eds.), *Stories matter: The role of narrative in medical ethics* (pp. 48–58). New York: Routledge.

Pozatek, E. (1994). The problem of certainty: Clinical social work in the post modern era. *Social Work, 39,* 396–403.

Prinz, R. J., & Miller, G. E. (1994). Family-based treatment for childhood antisocial behavior: Experimental influences on drop-out and engagement. *Journal of Consulting and Clinical Psychology, 62,* 645–650.

Prochaska, J. O., DiClemente, C. C., & Norcross, J. C. (1992). In search of how people change. *American Psychologist, 47,* 1102–1114.

Rapp, C. A. (1998). *The strengths model: Case management with people suffering from persistent and severe mental illness.* New York: Oxford University Press.

Raskin, J. D., & Lewandowski, A. M. (2000). The construction of disorder as human enterprise. In R. A. Neimeyer & J. D. Raskin (Eds.), *Constructions of disorder: Meaning-making frameworks for psychotherapy* (pp. 15–40). Washington, DC: American Psychological Association.

Raven, M. (1997). *The politics of drug use.* Retrieved July 28, 2007, from http://www.dulwichcentre.com.au/politics_of_drug_use_by_melissa.htm

Reamer, F. G. (1999). *Social work values and ethics* (2nd ed.). New York: Columbia University Press.

Reid, W. J. (2002). Knowledge for direct social work practice: An analysis of trends. *Social Service Review, 76,* 6–33.

Richert, A. (2003). Living stories, telling stories, changing stories: Experiential use of the relationship in narrative therapy. *Journal of Psychotherapy Integration, 13*, 188–210.

Rombach, M. A. M. (2003). An invitation to therapeutic letter writing. *Journal of Systemic Therapies, 22*(1), 15–32.

Romme, M. (1998). Listening to the voice hearers. *Journal of Psychosocial Nursing and Mental Health Services, 36*(9), 40–44.

Roth, S., & Epston, D. (1996). Developing externalizing conversations: An exercise. *Journal of Systemic Therapies, 15*(1), 5–12.

Sacks, O. W. (1983). *Awakenings*. New York: E. P. Dutton.

Sacks, O. W. (1985). *The man who mistook his wife for a hat and other clinical tales*. New York: Summit Books.

Saleebey, D. (1993). Theory and the generation and subversion of knowledge. *Journal of Sociology & Social Welfare, 20*(1), 5–25.

Saleebey, D. (1994). Culture, theory, and narrative: The intersection of meanings in practice. *Social Work, 39*, 351–359.

Saleebey, D. (2001). The diagnostic strengths manual? *Social Work, 46*, 183–187.

Saleebey, D. (2002a). Introduction: Power in the people. In D. Saleebey (Ed.), *The strengths perspective in social work practice* (3rd ed., pp. 1–22). Boston: Allyn & Bacon.

Saleebey, D. (2002b). The strengths approach to practice. In D. Saleebey (Ed.), *The strengths perspective in social work practice* (3rd ed., pp. 80–94). Boston: Allyn & Bacon.

Sanders, C. (1997). Re-authoring problem identities: Small victories with young persons captured by substance misuse. In C. Smith & D. Nylund (Eds.), *Narrative therapies with children and adolescents* (pp. 400–422). New York: Guilford Press.

Sanders, C. (1998). Substance misuse dilemmas: A postmodern inquiry. In S. Madigan & I. Law (Eds.), *Praxis: Situating discourse, feminism & politics in narrative therapies* (pp. 141–162). Vancouver, Canada: Yaletown Family Therapy.

Santisteban, D., Szapocnik, J., Perez-Vidal, A., Kurtines, W., Murray, E., & LaPerriere, D. (1996). Efficacy of interventions for engaging youth/families into treatment and some variables that may contribute to differential effectiveness. *Journal of Family Psychology, 10,* 35–44.

Scheppele, K. L. (1989). Foreword: Telling stories. *Michigan Law Review, 87,* 2073–2093.

Segal, M. (2004). Rebuilding trust in fractured relationships. In S. Madigan (Ed.), *Therapeutic conversations 5: Therapy from the outside in* (pp. 99–110). Vancouver, Canada: Yaletown Family Therapy.

Sells, S. P., Smith, T. E., Coe, M. J., Yoshioka, M., & Robbins, J. (1994). An ethnography of couple and therapist experiences in reflecting team practice. *Journal of Marital and Family Therapy, 20,* 247–266.

Seymour, F. W., & Epston, D. (1989). An approach to childhood stealing with evaluation of 45 cases. *Australian and New Zealand Journal of Family Therapy, 10,* 137–143.

Shulman, L. (1999). *The skills of helping individuals, families, groups, and communities* (4th ed.). Itasca, IL: F. E. Peacock.

Silver, M. A. (2002). Emotional competence, multicultural lawyering and race. *Florida Coastal Law Review, 3,* 219–244.

Simblett, G. J. (1997). Leila and the tiger: Narrative approaches to psychiatry. In G. Monk, J. Winslade, K. Crocket, & D. Epston (Eds.), *Narrative therapy in practice: The archaeology of hope* (pp. 121–157). San Francisco: Jossey-Bass.

Simon, B. L. (1994). *The empowerment tradition in American social work: A history.* New York: Columbia University Press.

Smith, C. (1997). Introduction: Comparing traditional therapies with narrative approaches. In C. Smith & D. Nylund (Eds.), *Narrative therapies with children and adolescents* (pp. 1–52). New York: Guilford Press.

Smith, L., & Winslade, J. (1997). *Consultations with young men migrating from alcohol's regime.* Retrieved October 22, 2005, from http://www.dulwichcentre.com.au/consultations_with_young_men_mig.htm

Snyder, M. (1996). Our "other history": Poetry as a meta-metaphor for narrative therapy. *Journal of Family Therapy, 18,* 337–359.

Solomon, B. B. (1976). *Black empowerment: Social work in oppressed communities.* New York: Columbia University Press.

Specht, H. (1990). Social work and the popular psychotherapies. *Social Service Review, 64,* 345–357.

Steinberg, D. (2000). *Letters from the clinic: Letter writing in clinical practice for mental health professionals.* London: Routledge.

Stockell, G., & O'Neill M. (2001). *Towards collaboration: Raymond's story.* Retrieved August 16, 2006, from http://www.narrativeapproaches.com/narrative%20papers%20folder/toward.htm

Sue, D. W. (2005). *Multicultural social work practice.* Hoboken, NJ: John Wiley & Sons.

Sue, Mem, & Veronica (1999). *Documents and treasures: Power to our journeys.* Retrieved August 17, 2006, from http://www.narrativetherapylibrary.com/catalog_details.asp?ID=100

Talmon, M. (1990). *Single session therapy: Maximizing the effect of the first (and often only) therapeutic encounter.* San Francisco: Jossey-Bass.

Tamasese, K., & Waldgrave, C. (1993). Cultural and gender accountability in the "just therapy" approach. *Journal of Feminist Family Therapy, 5*(2), 29–45.

*Tarasoff v. Regents of the University of California,* 511 P.2d 334 (1976).

Tatum, B. (1997). *"Why are all the black kids sitting together in the cafeteria?" and other conversations about race.* New York: Basic Books.

Taylor, S., & Stein, M. B. (2006). The future of selective serotonin reuptake inhibitors (SSRIs) in psychiatric treatment. *Medical Hypothesis, 66*(1), 14–21.

Tedeschi, R. G., & Calhoun, L. G. (2004). Posttraumatic growth: Conceptual foundations and empirical evidence. *Psychological Inquiry, 15*(1), 1–18.

Tong, R., & Williams, N. (2003, Winter). "Feminist Ethics." In E. N. Zalta (Ed.), *The Stanford encyclopedia of philosophy.* Retrieved June 5, 2006, from http://plato.stanford.edu/archives/win2003/entries/feminism-ethics/

Turner, V. (1969). *The ritual process: Structure and anti-structure.* Chicago: Aldine.

Ungar, M. T. (2001). Constructing narratives of resilience with high-risk youth. *Journal of Systemic Therapies, 20*(2), 58–73.

Ungar, M. T., & Teram, E. (2000). Drifting towards mental health: High-risk adolescents and the process of empowerment. *Youth and Society, 32,* 228–252.

van Gennep, A. (1960). *The rites of passage* (M. B. Vizedon & G. L. Caffee, Trans.). Chicago: University of Chicago Press.

van Wormer, K., & Davis, D. R. (2003). *Addiction treatment: A strengths perspective.* Pacific Grove, CA: Brooks/Cole.

Vassallo, T. (2002). *Narrative group therapy with the seriously mentally ill: A case study.* Retrieved August 17, 2006, from http://www.narrativeapproaches.com/narrative%20papers%20folder/mentalill.htm

Vaughan, S., & Fowler, D. (2004). The distress experienced by voice hearers is associated with the perceived relationship between the voice hearer and the voice. *British Journal of Clinical Psychology, 43,* 143–153.

Waldgrave, C. (1990). Social justice and family therapy. *Dulwich Centre Newsletter, 1*(1), 6–46.

Walter, J. L., & Peller, J. E. (1992). *Becoming solution-focused in brief therapy.* New York: Brunner/Mazel.

Watzlawick, P. (1976). *How real is real? Confusion, disinformation, communication.* New York: Random House.

Weick, A., & Chamberlain, E. (2002). Putting problems in their place: Further explorations in the strengths perspective. In D. Saleebey (Ed.), *The strengths perspective in social work practice* (3rd ed., pp. 95–105). Boston: Allyn & Bacon.

Weingarten, K. (2005). *Making sense of illness narratives: Braiding theory, practice and the embodied life.* Retrieved April 28, 2005, from http://www.dulwichcentre.com.au/kaethearticle.html

Wetchler, J. L. (1999). Narrative treatment of a woman with panic disorder. *Journal of Family Psychotherapy, 10*(2), 17–30.

White, M. (1989). *Selected papers.* Adelaide, Australia: Dulwich Centre Publications.

White, M. (1993a). Commentary: Systems of understanding, practices of relationship, and practice of self. In S. Gilligan & R. Price (Eds.), *Therapeutic conversations* (pp. 190–196). New York: Norton.

White, M. (1993b). Commentary: The histories of the present. In S. Gilligan & R. Price (Eds.), *Therapeutic conversations* (pp. 121–135). New York: Norton.

White, M. (1993c). Deconstruction and therapy. In S. Gilligan & R. Price (Eds.), *Therapeutic conversations* (pp. 22–61). New York: Norton.

White, M. (1995). *Re-authoring lives: Interviews and essays.* Adelaide, Australia: Dulwich Centre Publications.

White, M. (1997). *Narratives of therapists' lives.* Adelaide, Australia: Dulwich Centre Publications.

White M. (2004). *Challenging the culture of consumption: Rites of passage and communities of acknowledgement.* Retrieved November 5, 2006, from http://www.dulwichcenter.com/challenging_the_culture_of_consu.htm

White, M. (2005). *Workshop notes.* Retrieved November 5, 2006, from http://www.dulwichcentre.com.au/Michael%20White%20Workshop%20Notes.pdf

White, M. (2006a). Children, trauma and subordinate storyline development. In D. Denborough (Ed.), *Trauma: Narrative responses to traumatic experience* (pp. 143–165). Adelaide, Australia: Dulwich Centre Publications.

White, M. (2006b). Narrative practice with families with children: Externalising conversations revisited. In M. White & A. Morgan (Eds.), *Narrative therapy with children and their families* (pp. 1–56). Adelaide, Australia: Dulwich Centre Publications.

White, M. (2006c). Working with people who are suffering the consequences of multiple trauma: A narrative perspective. In D. Denborough (Ed.), *Trauma: Narrative responses to traumatic experience* (pp. 25–85). Adelaide, Australia: Dulwich Centre Publications.

White, M., & Epston, D. (1990). *Narrative means to therapeutic ends*. New York: Norton.

Winslade, J., & Cotter, A. (1997). Moving from problem solving to narrative approaches in mediation. In G. Monk, J. Winslade, K. Crocket, & D. Epston (Eds.), *Narrative therapy in practice: The archaeology of hope* (pp. 252–274). San Francisco: Jossey-Bass.

Winslade, J., & Monk, G. (2000). *Narrative mediation: A new approach to conflict resolution*. San Francisco: Jossey-Bass.

Winslade, J., Monk, G., & Drewery, W. (1997). Sharpening the critical edge: A social constructivist approach in counselor education. In T. L. Sexton & B. L. Griffin (Eds.), *Constructivist thinking in counseling practice, research, and training* (pp. 228–248). New York: Teachers College Press.

Witkin, S. L. (1991). The implications of social constructionism for social work education. *Journal of Teaching in Social Work, 4*(2), 37–47.

Witty, C. J. (2002). The therapeutic potential of narrative therapy for conflict transformation. *Journal of Systemic Therapies, 21*(3), 48–59.

Wixson, J. G. (2004). *Letters in the street: A narrative based outreach approach*. Retrieved December 30, 2005, from http://www.dulwichcentre.com.au/lettersinthestreet.htm

Zimmerman, J., & Dickerson, V. (1994). Using a narrative metaphor: Implications for theory and clinical practice. *Family Process, 33*, 233–245.

Zimmerman, J., & Dickerson, V. (1996). *If problems talked: Narrative therapy in action*. New York: Guilford Press.

Zimmerman, M. A. (1990). Taking aim on empowerment research: On the distinction between individual and psychological conceptions. *American Journal of Community Psychology, 18*, 169–177.

# About the Author

This book is about the therapeutic uses of stories: those we create, those we live, and those we leave behind. Its writing is itself a story, a tale of heroism, integrity, commitment, and compassion. Just as stories can keep someone's voice alive for members of his or her club of life, so, too, does this book.

Dr. Gary W. Paquin wrote in this book about being a cancer resister. Gary's stance against his cancer is a story of valor and optimism. Yet it is just one story among the many that defined Gary's personhood. Gary was also a husband and father, a son and brother, a clinical social worker and social work educator and scholar, a mediator and attorney, a person of deep faith and intense spirituality, and a generous and wickedly funny friend. Gary lived his belief in social justice; his life exemplified the slogan "practice random acts of kindness," which he did every day, sometimes without even conscious awareness, so deeply were empathy and generosity part of the fabric of his being.

Gary died just before the book's proof copy came back from the editor. The finishing touches to the manuscript were done by Dr. Charlotte Paquin, Gary's wife and best friend, and Dr. Sandra Wexler, a longtime friend, with encouragement and advice from Dr. Harvy Frankel, Dr. Ann Hartman, David Epston, and Dr. Sophia Dziegielewski. The truths in the book are Gary's; any errors are Sandra's and Charlotte's.

Even before Sandra and Charlotte became involved in completing this work, many others had contributed to it and helped to shape its final form. On Gary's behalf, we thank the many clients and colleagues with whom he practiced over the years. We also acknowledge the students, academic colleagues, and field instructors from whom he learned so much about being a social worker. There are, as well, the many individuals who worked with Gary in professional trainings and workshops, both those he gave and those he attended. Not only have many people shared their lives and thoughts with Gary, but some also have generously shared their unpublished work for use in this book. In particular, we thank Dr. Stephen Madigan, Jill Freedman, Dr. Gene Combs, Trina Crowe, and Lorraine Hedtke. Finally, we acknowledge the contributions to this work, and to the field of narrative practice more generally, made by Michael White. The voices of all of these individuals, and so many others whose names we do not know, echo through these pages and make this book a much richer story as a result.

Gary is sorely missed. It is not often that one is privileged to encounter a spirit as sincere and joyous as his. But Gary's story lives on among all those who knew him. And with the publication of this book, Gary's story is now available to inspire others in the field of social work.

# Index

A
abuse or neglect. *See also* domestic violence
 children and adolescents, 61, 110, 260–62
 clubs and expelling members from, 207
 different abilities and disabilities, individuals with, 61, 110
 historicizing, 130–31
 narrative approach to, 77
 older people, 61, 110
 reporting of, 61, 65, 70, 110
 therapeutic letter about, 182–85
 of women, 37
addiction-based identity, 330
adolescents. *See* children and adolescents
advocacy
 approval of client in, 237
 client's responsibility for, 236
 exercise to develop argument, 251–53
 legal arguments, 237–40
 power issues, 237
 social worker's role in, xiv, 27–28, 235–37, 240–42
 transparency in, 237
agency, 22, 53, 158, 286, 313, 326
aging. *See* gerontology and aging
AIDS crisis, 311
AIDS project, 318
alcohol abuse. *See* substance abuse
Alcoholics Anonymous (AA), 330, 333
alternative stories
 audience of supporters, 170, 204–5
 for children and adolescents, 264
 clubs, 206–8, 211, 229
 coconstruction of (exercise), 171–72
 communities of concern, 211–14, 231–32
 confirmation and support for, 203
 definitional ceremonies, 222
 definition of, 16
 development of, 141, 167, 235
 environment and, 203
 exploration of, 17, 166–67
 externalization and, 93
 for families, 283
 fictional goal, 163
 historicizing, 166–71
 importance of, 157
 internalized other questions, 208–11
 letter-writing campaigns, 212–14
 mediation and construction of, 250–51
 moving too fast toward, 129

 naming, 167
 optimism and, 166
 readiness to explore, 144–45
 relationship to problem story, 144–45, 157, 167, 235
 re-membering, 50, 205–6, 213
American Psychiatric Association, *Diagnostic and Statistical Manual of Mental Disorders*, 2, 52–54, 110, 199, 319–21
anger, 93–97, 135
anorexia and bulimia
 archive, 80, 325
 communities of concern, 325
 conception of self and, 324
 cultural discourse and, 42, 323–24
 externalization, 95–97, 324
 leagues, 215–16, 325
 letter-writing campaigns, 325
 relationships and, 324
anthropology, 1
appreciative ally stance, 48
archive, 79–80, 215, 229–31, 325
assertive behavior, 16
assessment
 narrative treatment and, xiv, 129, 193
 process for, 111–12
 questions to assess problems, 117–19
 social worker–client relationships and, 113
 suicide risk, 113–16
 violence risk, 116–17
Association of Social Work Boards, 2
attention-deficit disorder (ADD/ADHD), 90, 100, 258, 262–64
audience, 17
audiotaped stories, 266–67
auditory hallucinations, 5, 322

B
back-up questions, 145
badness vs. madness, 88
Bakhtin, Mikhail, 16
bed-wetting problems, 146, 158–60, 165–66, 167–70, 259–60, 264, 265–67
beliefs. *See also* culture and cultural, societal discourses
 about death, loss, and pain, 305–6
 deconstructing common beliefs (exercise), 54–56
 stories compared to, 19
best practices models, x

367

better judgment, 51–52
betwixt and between stage, 333
bickering, internalized, 103
bipolar mood disorder, 15–16
borderline personality disorder, 88, 328–29
boundary issues
    reflecting teams and, 219, 220
    written correspondence and, 186, 187–88, 190
Bourdieu, Pierre, 9
bowel-function-control problems, 264–65
brain injury, 304
bravery and courage, 16, 108–10, 146
Bruner, Jerome, 13, 21–22
bulimia. *See* anorexia and bulimia
burn patient story, x–xi

## C

cancer
    authority on, 301
    resisters' lives, 92
capacity building, 6
carnival of possible futures, 16
case conference, 222–24
case files
    client's access to, 193
    definition of people through, 42, 193
    dictation, 192–93
    helping clients through, 193
    intake summary, 192, 193–99
    power of, 42, 193
certificates and awards, 227–28
chaos story, 299–300, 301
characterization, 160–61
cheerleading, 145
children and adolescents
    abuse or neglect of, 61, 110, 260–62
    alternative stories for, 264
    attention-deficit disorder (ADD/ADHD), 90, 100, 258, 262–64
    audiotaped stories, 266–67
    bed-wetting problems, 146, 158–60, 165–66, 167–70, 259–60, 264, 265–67
    bowel-function-control problems, 264–65
    certificates and awards, 228, 229
    communities of concern, 262, 275–77
    as consultants, 260
    creative and expressive arts, 261–62
    cultural discourses about, 257–58, 270–71
    curfew violations, 161–62
    custody of, 238–39
    depression in adolescent girls, 270–71
    empowerment, 37, 271
    externalization, 100, 258, 263, 272
    guilt, 261
    letter-writing campaign example, 212–13
    lists, use of, 258–59
    lying by, 229, 273–77, 294–96
    methods of working with, 258–60
    play, 258
    relabeling, 263, 264
    relationships with, 236
    reporting responsibility and child welfare system, 65, 70
    reputation, interviewing around, 294–96
    resilience-based identity, 271–73
    school as problem, 37, 135–38, 267–70
    sexual pressures, 271
    stealing and lying problems, 229, 273–77, 294–96
    strengths and special talents of, 263, 264, 265–67
    stuffed animal colleagues, 265, 294
    termination, celebration of, 229
    unique outcomes, 259
    violence and, 260–62
    written correspondence to, 264
circulation practices, 78
clean community, development of, 273, 333
clients. *See also* social worker–client relationships
    access to records by, 193
    advocacy responsibility, 236
    appointments, keeping and missing, 41–42, 62–63
    assessment process, 111–12
    better judgment of, 51–52
    consulting your consultants, 79–80, 215, 229–31
    co-research, 16–17
    diagnosis and, 52–54
    discussions of, 81
    engagement of, 106–7
    expert status of, xi, xiv, 1, 19, 38, 215, 229–31, 235, 339
    feedback from, 51
    getting ahead of, 98, 129
    impact of problem on, 131–34, 141, 144
    influence on problem, 141, 145–46
    informed consent, 78–80
    lying by, 27, 229, 273–77, 294–96
    meaning of stories for, 125–27, 164–66
    personal responsibility of, 53
    power of, xii, 41–42
    as privileged author of experience, 17
    referrals to specialists, 65–66, 83
    resources for, 27–28
    respect for, 124, 129–30
    starting where the client is, 129
    use of term, xiii
    values of, 51–52
clinical social work
    examinations for, 2
    focus and goals of, 1–2
    licensing requirements, 2
    practice theory, 2
    values-based approach to, 69
clubs, 206–8, 211, 229, 307, 310–11
*Code of Ethics* (NASW), 66
codes of ethics

*Code of Ethics* (NASW), 59–60, 66, 70, 71, 81, 193
   development of, 60
   ethical decision making, 60
   limitations of and ethical dilemmas, 69–73
   litigation, protection of liability in, 72
   purpose of, 60–61
   reporting responsibility of, 61
   state ethical codes, 61
   violation of, 61
cognitive behavioral strategies, x, 11–12, 19, 65, 101, 322
Coleridge, Samuel, 75
colleagues, stuffed animal, 265, 294
Combs, Gene, 230–31
communications approach, 12
communities of concern
   anorexia and bulimia, 325
   children and adolescents, 262, 275–77
   concept of, 211
   exercise, 231–32
   illness, 300
   leagues, 37, 67, 215–16, 235, 325
   letter-writing campaigns, 212–14, 307, 325
   reflecting teams, 67, 68, 203, 216–22, 232–34, 288
   substance abuse, 333–34
community and human relationships, 68, 204
competence
   compassion and competence, 7
   narrative competence of physicians, 303
   quiet competence, 3, 19
   of social worker, 65–66, 68–69
computer virus analogy, 91–92
conception of self, 23–27, 137–38, 307–10, 323, 325–29
confidentiality
   basis for idea of, 55
   benefits and limitations of, 55
   codes of ethics and, 61, 72, 110
   concept of, 54
   exceptions to, 54–55, 61, 110
   exercise about, 54–56
   leagues and, 216
   written correspondence and, 80–82, 177, 186–87
conflict and mediation. *See* mediation
confronting stage, 272
connection, 48
conscientization, 37, 235
constitutionalism, 22–23
constructivism, 11–12
consulting your consultants, 79–80, 215, 229–31
context, 160–61
co-research, 16–17
counter documents, 173, 178, 235
couple counseling
   blame for problems, 286
   difficulty of, 283
   ethical dilemma exercise, 84–86
   exceptions to problem, 285, 286
   forgiveness, 284–85
   gender practices, influence of, 285
   individuality, 286–87
   internalized other questions, 287–88
   letter-writing campaigns, 213
   multistoried people, 17
   optimistic view, 144
   practice exercise, 288–94
   preferred experiences, 285
   preferred identities and relationships, 285–86, 287
   reauthoring practices, 286
   reevaluation by social worker, 51–52
   reflecting teams, 219, 288
   transparency, 283–84
   unique outcomes, 144
   view of self, effect of problems on, 284–85
courage and bravery, 16, 108–10, 146
COX (cyclooxygenase), 9–10
creative and expressive arts, 261–62
critical legal theorists, 239
Crowe, Trina, 336–37
culture and cultural, societal discourses
   about aging, 297, 304–5
   about children and families, 257–58, 270–71
   about illness, 297, 302
   about women, 38, 43, 76, 98, 130–31, 138, 244
   acceptance of stories of subordinate groups, 238–39
   anorexia and bulimia and, 42, 323–24
   attention-deficit disorder (ADD/ADHD), 262
   benefits of, x
   changing, 138
   conception of self and, 23–26, 137–38, 323
   constitutionalism and, 22–23
   contribution to and impact on problems, 42–43, 134–38
   control of members, 41
   influence of, 7
   internalized discourses, 90, 243
   mediation and, 243, 244, 249–50
   mental health, 319, 323
   negative attributes of subordinate groups, 38
   normal, definition of, 25
   normalization, 40
   ordering of members, 38, 39
   power issues and, 38–40, 76–77
   reality and, 13
   relationships and, 43–47
   schools and education, 267–69
   standards set by, 23, 38–39
   substance abuse, 329–39

values embedded in, 39
curfew violations, 161–62
curiosity, respectful, 48
curious listening, 123–28
curious questioning, 15, 31–33, 272
cyclooxygenase (COX), 9–10

**D**
Davis, Peggy, 46
death
    dying process, 310–13
    exercises, 315–18
    funerals, 314–15
    remembrance of dead, 313–15
Declaration of Independence, 228
deconstructing common beliefs (exercise), 54–56
deconstruction, 27, 235, 243, 331
deconstructive listening, 128–29
deconstructive questions, 134–35
deficit labels, 3–4, 15–16, 138
defining stage, 272–73
definitional ceremonies, 222
deontological analysis, 60
depression
    in adolescent girls, 270–71
    impact on the person, 133–34
    legacy, 313
    naming, 108, 321
    objectification and, 53
    oppression and, 42–43
    referrals for medical care, 66
    resistance to power and, 40–41
    of strengths and resources, 108–10
    taking stand against, 15
    unique outcomes, 147–48, 149–54
diagnoses
    benefits and difficulties of, 52–54, 319–21
    ethical issues and, 83–84
    explanations to client, 112, 113, 199
    importance of, 112
    medication and, xiv, 112
    narrative treatment and, xiv, 199
    personal responsibility and, 53
    process for, 112–13
    reliability and validity of, 199
    stigma of, 320–21
    treatment, financial considerations, and, ix–x, xiv, 62–63, 199
*Diagnostic and Statistical Manual of Mental Disorders* (American Psychiatric Association), 2, 52–54, 110, 199, 319–21
dictation, 175, 192–93
different abilities and disabilities
    abuse or neglect of individuals, reporting of, 61, 110
    cultural discourses about, 297
    modernist thought and, 10–11
    posttraumatic growth, 304
    socially constructed meanings of, 13–14

discourses. *See* culture and cultural, societal discourses
discrimination. *See* oppression and discrimination
diversity
    relationships and cultural discourses, 43–47
    sensitivity to, 69
divorce, 311
domestic violence
    advocacy argument exercise, 251–53
    cultural discourses and, 277–78
    dominant stories, 278–79
    intervention principles, 279
    narrative approach to, 77
    power issues and, 278–79
    prior abuse or oppression and, 278–79, 280
    reporting of, 61
    stories of abusers, 279–81
dominant stories, 16
double-listening, 326–27
drug companies, 83
drug use. *See* substance abuse
DSM. *See Diagnostic and Statistical Manual of Mental Disorders* (American Psychiatric Association)
Dubus, Andre, 17
dying process, 310–13

**E**
eating disorders. *See* anorexia and bulimia
ecological understandings, 5, 14
elderly people. *See* gerontology and aging
elimination problems. *See* bed-wetting problems; bowel-function-control problems
empowerment, 35–37, 69, 271
encropesis, 264–65
engagement, 106–7
enuresis, 146, 158–60, 165–66, 167–70, 259–60, 264, 265–67
environment. *See also* person–environment relationships
    alternative stories and, 203
    critical awareness of, 37
Epston, Ann, 95–97
Epston, David
    ADHD client, work with, 264
    audiotaped stories, 265–67
    internalized other questions, 208–11, 287–88
    narrative approach of, 13
    stealing and lying problems, 273–75
    therapeutic letter, 182–85
ethics
    of caring, 74–77
    *Code of Ethics* (NASW), 59–60, 66, 70, 71, 81, 193
    codes of ethics (*see* codes of ethics)
    confidentiality, letter writing, and, 80–82

diagnoses and, 83–84
ethical analysis, 70–71
ethical decision making, 60
ethical dilemmas and principles, 62–66, 84–86
ethical reasoning, 69–70
feminist ethics, 74
limitations of codes of ethics and ethical dilemmas, 69–73
narrative approach to, 73–74
social worker–client relationships and, 80–82
eulogies, 213
exercises, xiv
advocacy argument, 251–53
alternative story, coconstruction of, 171–72
communities of concern, 231–32
couple counseling, 288–94
curious questioning, 31–33
deconstructing common beliefs, 54–56
ending ceremony, 234
ethical dilemma, 84–86
interviewing a problem, 119–21, 338
marginalization, discussion of, 56–58
mediation initiation, 254–55
memory box, 317–18
professional identity, development of, 28–31
reflecting teams, 232–34
reputation, interviewing around, 294–96
resistance against problems, 149–55
slowing down interview, 138–39
stories to pass on, 316–17
strengths, recognizing, 33
stuffed animal colleagues, 294
substance abuse, 334–38
talking about those we've lost, 315–16
unique outcome, expansion of, 171
written correspondence, 199–201
experience
ambiguity of, 238
authenticating, 45–47
clients as privileged author of, 17
negative experience of identity, 25–26
preferred experiences, 285
as reality, 11
expressive and creative arts, 261–62
externalization
advantages of, 92–97
anorexia and bulimia, 324
authentic belief in, xii
cautions in, 97–98
children and adolescents, 100, 258, 263, 272
concept of, 91–92
engagement, 106–7
ethics of caring and, 75
gerontology and aging, 306–7
how to externalize, 98–100

interviewing a problem (exercise), 119–21
mediation and, 243, 247–48
naming problem, 107–8, 159–60, 321
narrative treatment and, 105–10
of stealing, 277
slowing down interview (exercise), 138–39
social worker responsibilities, 110–13
substance abuse, 330–31

F
families
alternative stories for, 283
externalization and, 92–93
relationship patterns, 281–83
fear, escalating, 102
felonies, reporting of, 61, 63
feminist ethics, 74
fictional goal, 163
fighting, 281–83
financial reimbursement, ix–x, xiv, 62–63, 199
Flexner, Abraham, ix
forgiveness, 284–85
Foucault, Michael
power and narrative treatment, 38
strategies to extend influence of problems, 101
truths and divisions between people, 39–40, 76–77
Freedman, Jill, 230–31, 301
Freire, Paulo, 37, 235
Freudian theory, 7, 20, 24, 205
frogs, 12
funerals, 314–15

G
gender issues
gender roles, 285
mediation and, 243, 244
modernist thought and, 10–11
narrative approach to, 77
questioning dominant reality, 37
socially constructed meanings of, 13–14
Gergen, Kenneth, 8, 13
gerontology and aging
abuse or neglect of older adults, reporting of, 61, 110
beliefs of social workers and, 305–6
challenges of working with, 305–6
clubs, 307, 310–11
conception of self, 307–10
cultural discourses about, 297, 304–5
dying process, 310–13
exercises, 315–18
external constraints on, 309
externalization, 306–7
legacy, 311–13
letter-writing campaigns, 307
medicalization of problems, 305

modernist thought and, 10–11
narrative treatment, 306–10
re-membering, 307, 310
remembrance of dead, 313–15
responsibility for aging, 298
socially constructed meanings of, 13–14
stories to pass on, 310–13, 316–17
grief, redefinition of, 89
grief theory, 313–15
guilt, 104–5, 261, 312

## H

Health Insurance Portability and Accountability Act, 65, 186
Hedtke, Lorraine, 315–16
Helms, Janet E., 46
hero stories, 301
historical truth, 310
historicizing alternative stories, 166–71
historicizing problems, 130–31
historicizing self-description, 25
historicizing unique outcomes, 166–71
honest reputation, 229, 273–77
  honesty meetings, 275–77
  honesty parties, 229, 275, 277
  honesty tests, 274–75, 276, 277
honor before helping, 106
hopefulness, 48
hopelessness, 103–4, 132, 181–82

## I

identity. *See* self
illness
  authority on, 301
  brain injury, 304
  chaos story, 299–300, 301
  communities of concern, 300
  concept of, 11
  cultural discourses about, 297, 302
  journey story, 300–301, 304
  listening to narratives, 298–99
  modernist thought and, 9–10
  narrative approach to medicine, 303–4
  narratives about, 298–301
  postmodern philosophy and, 11
  posttraumatic growth, 302, 304
  quest story, 300–301, 304
  resisters' lives, 92
  responsibility for, 297
  restitution story, 299, 301
*The Illness Narratives* (Kleinman), x–xi, 75
immigrants, undocumented, 69–70
inclusion, 49
individualism, 94, 302
individuality, 286–87
individuation discourse, 270–71
informed consent, 78–80
inherent dignity and worth of a person, 67–68
instances of direct change, 167

intake summary
  diagnosis, 199
  family history, 192, 196
  formulation (assessment), 192, 198–99
  history of presenting complaint, 192, 195–96
  identifying information, 192, 193–94
  medical condition, 192, 196–97
  narrative approach to, 193–99
  presenting complaint, 192, 194–95
  substance abuse, 192, 197
  treatment contract, 192
integrity and trustworthiness of social worker, 64–65, 68
internalized bickering, 103
internalized dialogues, 101
internalized discourses, 90, 243
internalized other questions, 208–11, 287–88
interviews
  back-up questions, 145
  curious questioning, 15, 31–33, 272
  deconstructive questions, 134–35
  internalized other questions, 208–11, 287–88
  meaning of stories, questions to explore, 164–66
  motivational interviewing, 132
  narrative perspective, 127–29
  problem, interviewing a (exercise), 119–21
  relative influence questions, 146
  resistance against problems (exercises), 149–55
  slowing down interview (exercise), 138–39
  smalling questions, 146
invitation, letters of, 177–78
isolation, therapies of, 228

## J

Japanese culture, 38–39, 323
jargon, professional, 189–90
Jenkins, Alan, 279–80
journey story, 300–301, 304
Julie's story, 230–31
just therapy, 46–47

## K

Kant, Immanuel, 74
Kelly, George, 12
Kleinman, Arthur, x–xi, 75
knowledges, 10

## L

landscapes
  landscape of action, 157–62
  landscape of consciousness, 158, 162–64
language
  impersonal, 135
  professional jargon, 189–90
  reality and, 7–8, 11

Law, Ian, 262
laziness, externalization of, 99–100
leagues, 37, 67, 215–16, 235, 325
legal arguments, 237–40
legitimacy, 101
letter writing. *See* written correspondence
letter-writing campaigns, 212–14, 307, 325
life model framework, 2
liminality, 229
listening
  apprehension of professional, xi
  curious listening, 123–28
  deconstructive listening, 128–29
  development of richer stories, 19
  double-listening, 326–27
  effects of, xi
  illness narratives, 298–99
  information gathering through, xi
  not-knowing stance, 26–27, 124–25
  to story as a story, 15
lists, 190–92, 201, 258–59
local knowledge, 215
lying, 27, 229, 273–77, 294–96

M

madness vs. badness, 88
magic and wizardry, 259
marginalization, discussion of (exercise), 56–58
marriage, experience of, 87–88
mediation
  alternative stories, construction of, 250–51
  content of, 244
  cultural discourses and, 243, 244, 249–50
  definition of, 242
  exercise to initiate, 254–55
  externalization and, 243, 247–48
  language and, 249
  mental health and, 321
  narrative mediation and role of social worker, xiv, 242–43
  neutrality of mediator, 243–44
  problem-focused mediators, 244
  problem stories, disputes as, 244–45
  process of, 242, 244, 245–51
  rule-setting, 250
  side effects, 321
  written correspondence and, 251
medicalization of problems, 305
medical model
  definition and redefinition of conditions and, 89
  diagnoses, treatment, and financial considerations, ix–x, xiv, 62–63, 199
  medical bioethics, 62, 75–76
  mental health system based on, 41–42, 62–63
  narrative approach to, 303–4
  research-based best practices, x
medication

attention-deficit disorder (ADD/ADHD), 90, 263
  choices about, 112–13
  definition and redefinition of conditions and, 89
  diagnosis and, xiv, 112
  effectiveness of, 112–13
  narrative treatment and, xiv, 83
  noncompliance and discontinuation of, 112–13
  value of, xiv
mental health
  auditory hallucinations, 5, 322
  categories of behaviors, 319
  conception of self, 323
  cultural discourses about, 319
  cultural discourses and, 323
  diagnoses and labels, 319–21
  interviewing exercise, 338
  mediation and, 321
  resilience-based identity, 271–73
  stigma of, 320–21
mental health system, 41–42, 62–63
mental karate, 259
Mental Research Institute, 12
merit-based hiring and promotion, 76
metaphors, 124
micro-aggression, 46
migration of identity metaphor, 332–33
modernist thought, 8–11
motivational interviewing, 132
multistoried people, 17, 21
Myerhoff, Barbara, 205

N

Narcotics Anonymous, 330
narrative
  definition of, 18
  landscapes, 157–64
  making sense of world through, 170–71
  scientific/logical thinking compared to, 157–58
narrative ethics, 73–74
narrative psychology, 1
*Narrative Therapy* (Freedman and Combs), 230–31
narrative treatment
  assumptions about social work practice and, xii, 1
  benefits of, 18
  clients as experts, xi, xiv, 1, 19, 38, 215, 229–31, 235, 339
  contradictory expectations, 7
  criticism of, 27–28, 235, 330–31
  dangers of following models, xiii
  documentation of treatment, 187–88
  focus and principles of, x, 14–17, 339
  medication and, xiv, 83
  models for, xii–xiii, 17
  population-specific techniques, xii

power issues and, 35–37
role of social worker in, xi
social work values and, 66–69
strengths-based social work and, x, 1, 18
theoretical foundations of, xi, 1, 13
training opportunities, 339
treatment, use of term, xiii–xiv
National Association of Social Workers (NASW)
   client's access to records, 193
   clinical social work, goals and focus of, 1–2
   *Code of Ethics*, 59–60, 66, 70, 71, 81, 193
negative imagination/negative comparison, 102
neighbor mediation exercise, 254–55
nervousness, 79–80, 93, 145
new associations, 49
New Zealand therapists, 46–47
normalization, 40
note-taking during sessions, 179–80
not-knowing stance, 26–27, 124–25

O
objectification, 53
older people. *See* gerontology and aging
O'Neill, Thomas "Tip," 8
openness, 48
oppression and discrimination
   acceptance of stories of, 239
   authenticating experience of, 45–47
   conscientization, 37, 235
   definition and maintenance of problems through, xi
   depression and, 42–43
   domestic violence and, 278–79, 280
   empowerment, 35–37
   integrity and trustworthiness of social worker and, 64–65
   marginalization, discussion of (exercise), 56–58
   micro-aggression, 46
   modernist thought and, 10–11
   narrative approach to, 77
   objectification and, 53
   relationships and cultural discourses, 43–47
   societal issues and context of problems, 135–38
optimism, 143–44, 166
outcomes
   preferred outcomes, 141, 148
   unique outcomes (*see* unique outcomes)

P
paralyzing guilt, 104–5
people as problems, xii, 3–4, 15–16, 90, 91
people over problems, x, 339
perfection, demand for, 104
personal construct theory and therapy, 12

person–environment relationships
   accommodation of environment, 39–40
   clinical social work and, 2
   exercise to discuss, 54
   as focus for social work, ix, 2, 39–40
   importance of environment, 64
   problem-based assessments and, 5
pharmaceutical companies, 83
physicians and narrative approach to medicine, 303–4
play, 258
plot, 161–62
point of view, 163
political candidates, 320
political forces, xii, 38
postmodern philosophy. *See also* social constructionism
   constructivism, 11–12
   difficulty of understanding, xiii
   language, reality, and, 7–8, 11
   reality and, 10
posttraumatic growth, 302, 304
poverty
   anger and frustration at, 94
   changing approaches to, 89–90
   cultural discourses, 323
   war on poverty, 8
power issues
   advocacy, 237
   culture and, 38–40, 76–77
   empowerment, 35–37, 69, 271
   men and abuse situations, 278–79
   narrative treatment and, 35–37
   power disparity between social worker and client, xii
   privilege and, 44, 189
   reflecting teams and, 216–17
   relationship between social worker and client, 38, 43–47, 63–64, 81
   resistance to, 40–42
   separating practices, 40–42
   social constructionism and, 37–38
   teachers and social worker, 269–70
   truth and the acquisition of power, 39
   truth and the exercise of power, 40–42
   women, 76
prediction, letters of, 178
preferred identities, 24, 285–86, 287
preferred outcomes, 141, 148
preferred stories, 309
premodern thought, 8
principlism, 71, 73, 84–85
privilege
   acceptance of stories of subordinate groups, 238–39
   client as privileged author of experience, 17
   power issues and, 44, 189
   recognition of, 43–47, 67
   status of social worker, 43–47, 49, 217

problem-based approach
  assessment data, 4–5
  capacity building, 6
  ecological understandings, 5
  labeling people as problems, 3–4
  pessimism through deficit labels, 4
  strengths-based social work compared to, 6
problems
  client's words for, 321
  conception of self and, 25–26, 137–38
  constitutionalism and, 22–23
  control over, 158–60
  cultural context of, 14
  definition and redefinition of conditions as, 87–91
  evaluation of by client, 131–34
  exceptions to, 285, 286
  experience of, 11
  externalization (*see* externalization)
  historicizing, 130–31
  impact on the person, 131–34, 141, 144
  influence of, mapping, 263
  influence of client on, 141, 145–46
  inherent dignity and worth of a person, 67–68
  internalized dialogues, 101
  interviewing a problem (exercise), 119–21, 338
  leagues, problem-specific, 37, 67, 215–16, 235, 325
  naming, 107–8, 159–60, 321
  objectification and, 53
  oppression and definition and maintenance of problems, xi
  organizing with others against, xii
  partialization of, 9–10
  people as problems, xii, 3–4, 15–16, 90, 91
  personal responsibility for, 53
  personifying, 159–60
  political forces and, xii
  power issues and, 38–39
  questions to assess, 117–19
  reasons for, 88–89
  relationship of alternative story to, 144–45, 157, 167, 235
  resistance against (exercises), 149–55
  sharing strategies, 79–80, 215, 229–31
  socially constructed meanings of, 13–14
  societal issues and impact of, 134–38
  sociopolitical activist stance, 76–77
  starting where the client is, 129
  strategies to extend influence of, 100–105
  strengths against, harnessing power of, 265–67
  taking stands against, 15, 37, 138, 141, 143–44
procrastination, 154–55
prodigal son mediation example, 246–50

prognosis, 298
progress notes, 192
psychiatric pathologies, 89

## Q

questions. *See also* interviews
  back-up questions, 145
  curious questioning, 15, 31–33, 272
  deconstructive questions, 134–35
  notebook of, xiii
  relative influence questions, 146
  smalling questions, 146
  types of questions asked, xiii
quest story, 300–301, 304
quiet competence, 3, 19

## R

*A Race Is a Nice Thing to Have* (Helms), 46
race issues
  importance of, 45
  micro-aggression, 46
  modernist thought and, 10–11
  questioning dominant reality, 37
  relationships and cultural discourses, 43–47
  separating practices, 43
  socially constructed meanings of, 13–14
  stereotypes, 46
rape, 239–40, 260–62, 278–79
reality
  constructivism and, 12
  cultural stories and, 13
  definition of problems and, 88
  development of through stories, 21–23, 245
  experience as, 11
  language and, 7–8, 11
  modernist thought and, 8–11
  postmodern philosophy and, 7–8, 11
  questioning dominant reality, 37
  selection of, 74
  social constructionism and, 13
re-authored life, 16
reauthoring practices, 286
redundancy, letters of, 178
re-engagement, 49–50
reexperiencing events, 160–61
reference, letters of, 178
reflecting stage, 271–72
reflecting teams, 67, 68, 203, 216–22, 232–34, 288
reframing, 145
*Regents of the University of California, Tarasoff v.*, 72
rehabilitation, 5
reincorporation, 229
relapse, 332
relational identity, 284

relationships. *See also* couple counseling; person–environment relationships; social worker–client relationships
  anorexia and bulimia and, 324
  community and human relationships, 68, 204
  conflict and mediation, 242–45
  individuality in, 286–87
  mediation and construction of, 250–51
  obligations to others in, 74
  reexperiencing, 310
  stuffed animal colleagues, 265, 294
relative influence questions, 146
re-membering, 50, 205–6, 213, 307, 310
remembrance of dead, 313–15
reputation
  honest reputation, 229, 273–77
  interviewing around, 294–96
  suicidal reputation, 27
research-derived models, x, 28
resilience-based identity, 271–73
restitution story, 299, 301
re-voicing therapy, 50
*The Rime of the Ancient Mariner* (Coleridge), 75
rite of passage metaphor, 332, 333
romanticism, 8
rules document, 192, 201

S
Sacks, Oliver, 303
Sanders, Colin, 334–36
schizophrenia, 320, 322
schools, 37, 135–38, 267–70
second guessing, 103
self
  addiction-based identity, 330
  conception of, 23–27, 137–38, 307–10, 323
  historicizing self-description, 25
  individuation discourse, 270–71
  migration of identity metaphor, 332–33
  negative experience of identity, 25–26
  preferred identities, 24, 285–86, 287
  relational identity, 284
  resilience-based identity, 271–73
  true self, 24–25
  view of self, development of through stories, 18, 21–23
  view of self, effect of problems on, 284–85
self-determination, exercise to discuss, 54
self-help groups, 64
self-identity, 284
self-narrative, x
separation, 229
service, 66–67
sexual assault, 239–40, 260–62
sexual orientation issues
  homosexuality diagnostic category, 53–54
  modernist thought and, 10–11
  questioning dominant reality, 37
  socially constructed meanings of, 13–14
sexual pressures, 271
short stories, 17
smalling questions, 146
SMART Approach, 263–64
snake story, 18–19, 20, 22
Sneaky Poo, 264–65
social class issues
  modernist thought and, 10–11
  questioning dominant reality, 37
  socially constructed meanings of, 13–14
social constructionism
  conception of self, 24
  concept of, 13–14
  needs, development of, 244
  perform meaning on stories through, 20–21
  power and, 37–38
  as theoretical foundation of narrative treatment, xi, 1, 13
social justice
  exercise to discuss, 54
  narrative approach to, 35–37, 67, 236
  promotion of, 69
  state policies and social workers role in, 63
social work. *See also* strengths-based social work
  challenges to the profession, ix–x
  deconstructing common beliefs (exercise), 54–56
  encroachment on functions of, ix
  fiscal restraint pressures, ix–x
  imperialistic and patriarchal approaches to, 1
  mission of profession, 59–60, 69, 235
  normalizing goals of, 39–40
  values of profession, 59–60, 61–62, 66–69
social worker. *See also* social worker–client relationships
  accountability of, 16
  advocacy role of, 236–37
  anger and frustration of, 93–97
  competence, 65–66, 68–69
  contradictory expectations, 7
  co-research, 16–17
  examinations for, 2
  externalization and social worker responsibilities, 110–13
  impact of narratives on, 48–52
  integrity and trustworthiness of, 64–65, 68
  learning from clients, 51–52
  licensing of, 2, 61
  power of, xii, 41–42
  professional identity, development of (exercise), 28–31
  reevaluation by, 51–52
  reporting responsibility of, 61, 63, 65, 69–70, 110

role of in narrative treatment, xi, xiv, 1, 27–28, 38
solutions to problems, 124, 125, 134
subspecialties, 66
social worker–client relationships
　appreciative ally stance, 48
　assessment and, 113
　collaborative relationships, 18, 19, 36, 107, 129, 235
　diversity and, 43–47
　ethics and, 80–82
　integrity and trustworthiness of social worker, 64–65
　narrative treatment and, xii, 47–48, 225–26
　power and, 38, 43–47, 63–64, 81
　termination and, 224–26
　two-way approach to therapeutic relationships, 48–52
　written correspondence and, 67, 68, 176–77
societal discourses. *See* culture and cultural, societal discourses
sociopolitical activist stance, 76–77
solution-focused approach, x
solution knowledges, 50–51
South Africa's AIDS project, 318
South Africa's Truth and Reconciliation Commission, 239
sparkling moments, 141
special occasions, letters of, 178–79
starting where the client is, 129
statement of position, 190, 192
stealing and lying problems, 27, 229, 273–77, 294–96
stories. *See also* listening
　about suffering, 130
　acceptance of stories of subordinate groups, 238–39
　alternative stories (*see* alternative stories)
　audiotaped stories, 266–67
　beliefs compared to, 19
　benefits telling, x–xi
　conception of self and, 23–27
　cultural stories, 7
　curious listening, 123–28
　development and origins and, 7
　disputes as, 244–45
　dominant stories, 16
　expansion and exploration of, 18–20, 66–67, 145
　inherent dignity and worth of a person, 67–68
　internalization of, 23
　landscapes created by, 157–64
　legacy, 311–13
　making sense of world through, 170–71
　meaning of for client, 125–27, 164–66
　modernist thought and, 10
　modification of, 124
　as more important than listener's version of, xiii
　multistoried people, 17, 21
　perform meaning on, 20–21
　preference over theory, 14–15
　preferred stories, 309
　reading vs. telling, 303–4
　reality, development of through stories, 21–23, 245
　reflecting teams, 67, 68, 203, 216–22, 232–34
　repetition of, 20, 22
　richer stories, development of, 19, 93
　understanding meaning of events through, 20, 21
　value of, 27
　view of self, development of through, 18, 21–23
　written stories, 20
strengths against problems, harnessing power of, 265–67
strengths-based social work
　benefits of, 3–5
　challenge of, 3
　context-specific nature of strengths, 3
　definition of strengths, 1
　externalizing strengths, 108–10
　focus and goals of, 3
　increase in use of, 2
　model and principles of, 5–6
　narrative as source of strength, 6–7
　narrative treatment and, x, 1, 18
　populations helped by, 2–3
　problem-based approach compared to, 6
　rehabilitation, 5
　strengths, recognizing (exercise), 33
stuffed animal colleagues, 265, 294
substance abuse
　addiction-based identity, 330
　allies, supporting, 331–32
　clean community, development of, 273, 333
　communities of concern, 333–34
　cultural discourses, 329–39
　deconstruction, 331
　denial of influence, 332
　exercises, 334–38
　externalization, 330–31
　intake summary, 192, 197
　letter-writing campaigns, 213–14
　migration of identity metaphor, 332–33
　narrative treatment, criticism of, 330–31
　relapse, 332
　rite of passage metaphor, 332, 333
　12-step recovery programs, 330, 333
　written correspondence, 333–34
suffering, x–xi, 11, 94, 130, 298–99, 301, 302
suicide
　assessment for, 63
　assessment of risk, 113–16

suicidal reputation, 27
supervision, 222–24
supportive teams, 203
systems framework, 2, 92–93

## T

taking-it-back practices, 49, 304
*Tarasoff v. Regents of the University of California*, 72
teachers and social worker, 269–70
teams
    audience of supporters, 107, 204–5
    clubs, 206–8, 211, 229, 307, 310–11
    communities of concern, 211–14, 231–32
    exercises, 231–34
    leagues, 37, 67, 215–16, 235, 325
    reflecting teams, 67, 68, 203, 216–22, 232–34, 288
    supportive teams, 203
teleological analysis, 60
Temporary Assistance to Needy Families (TANF) agency advocacy example, 240–42
termination
    abandonment feelings, 228
    celebration of, 228–29
    certificates and awards, 227–28
    ending ceremony planning (exercise), 234
    narrative approach to, 203, 224–26
    premature, 71, 225
    process for, 228–29
    social worker–client relationships and, 224–26
    unilateral, 102, 225
    when to end, 226–27
thank-yous, 188–89
theme, 162–63
thoughts, power of, 322–23
tough kid story, 21
toys, 265, 294
training opportunities, 339
transference reactions, 48
translation of session, 190
transparency, 68, 218, 237, 283–84
trauma
    alternative stories, 326
    conception of self and, 325–29
    double-listening, 326–27
    precious things taken away by, 327
    restorying incident, 325–26
treatment, use of term, xiii–xiv
treatment contract, 192
triangulation, 93
trouble
    resilience-based identity, 271–73
    societal issues and context of problems, 135–38
    stories behind, 74
Truth and Reconciliation Commission, 239
truths
    acceptance of, 138
    changing, 138
    conditionality of, 10
    deficit labels, 15–16, 138
    divisions between people through, 39, 76–77
    exercise of power and, 40–42
    historical truth, 310
    modernist thought and, 7, 9, 10
    narrative treatment and, 14–15
    past truths compared to current truths, 39
    postmodern philosophy and, xi, 10
    power acquisition and, 39
    repetition of stories and, 22
    social constructionism and, xi
    traditional treatment and, 14–15
Tutu, Desmond, 239
12-step recovery programs, 330, 333
two-way approach to therapeutic relationships, 48–52

## U

Ungar, Michael, 271–73
unique outcomes
    alternative stories, readiness to explore, 144–45
    children and adolescents, working with, 259
    clues to, 144–46
    definition of, 97, 141–42
    evaluation of event as, 142, 147–48
    examples of, 142–43
    exercises, 149–55, 171–72
    exploration of meaning of, 165–66
    focusing on, 144–45
    historicizing, 166–71
    optimistic view and, 143–44
    patience and persistence and, 148

## V

values
    of client, 51–52
    embedded in culture, 39
    neutral, objective values, 239
    of social work profession, 59–60, 61–62, 66–69
violence. *See also* domestic violence
    assessment of risk, 116–17
    children and adolescents and, 260–62
    externalization of, 98
    in family life, 257
    potential of, reporting of, 61, 65, 72, 110
voice, 163–64
voice hearing, 5, 322

## W

war on poverty, 8
Weingarten, Kaethe, 300
welfare recipients, 8
White, Michael, 13, 91, 97, 205, 326–29

who we are
  postmodern theories of, 7
  stories and, 21–23
wisdom, 302
wizardry and magic, 259
women
  abuse of, 37
  cultural discourses and, 27, 38, 43, 76, 98, 130–31, 138, 244
  distress, 38
  eating disorders (*see* anorexia and bulimia)
  feminist ethics, 74
  political factors that affect, 38
  power issues, 76
  relationships and cultural discourses, 43
worldviews, 8–11
worry, 103
written correspondence
  advocacy letter example, 240–42
  anorexia letter example, 95–97
  audiotaped stories instead of, 266–67
  boundaries and, 186, 187–88, 190
  briefer documents, 190–92
  to children and adolescents, 264
  common errors, 188–90
  confidentiality and, 80–82, 177, 186–87

  contract clarification, 174–75
  counter documents, 173, 178, 235
  impact of, 173, 176–77
  letter-writing campaigns, 212–14, 307, 325
  lists, 190–92, 201, 258–59
  mediation and, 251
  narrative-style letters, 175
  note-taking during sessions, 179–80
  to other professionals, 174, 175, 189
  practice exercises, 173–74, 199–201
  practice for, 177
  presenting idea to client, 177
  professional jargon, 189–90
  reasons for, 173, 175–77
  rules document, 192, 201
  signatures, 176
  social worker–client relationship and, 67, 68, 176–77
  statement of position, 190, 192
  thank-yous, 188–89
  therapeutic letters, writing, 179–85
  time to compose, 186, 187
  translation of session, 190
  treatment documentation, 187–88
  types of letters, 177–79
  value of, 175–77, 185, 333–34
written stories, 20